Learning Together

The Agricultural Worker's Participatory Sourcebook

Susan Stewart

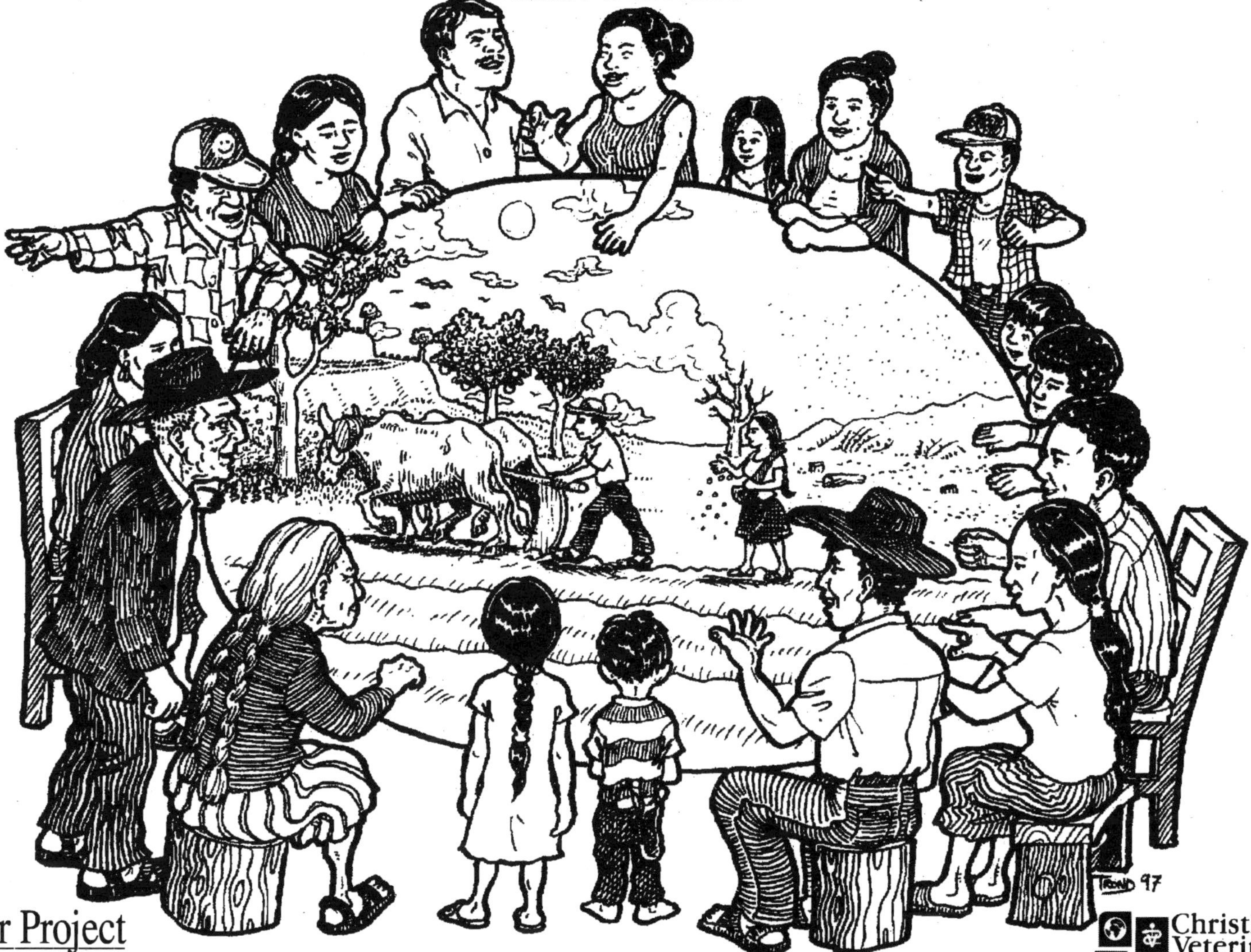

Heifer Project International

Chapters by B.J. Lundquist, Jennifer Shumaker and Karen L. Stoufer
Illustrations by Trond Scheen Korssjøen

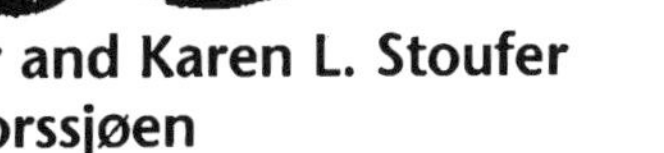

Christian Veterinary Mission

How to use this Sourcebook

This book was designed for any agricultural or livestock worker who is or will be training farmers. It is for people designing training programs or making decisions about training programs, and for farmers and professionals who are trainers. It is written by agricultural people for agricultural people. Agricultural trainers from more than 25 countries on five continents have shared their ideas here about what works for them in training adults.

This book is different from most manuals and texts. Most books describe everything they want you to know, then give you exercises to practice it. In this Sourcebook, many exercises are in the text to stimulate you to think about how you would respond to an exercise as you read through the text. The exercises can also be used later for training workshops.

There are three ways this book can be used:

1. Read it all the way through.
2. Skim it to get the main points. To do this, look at what stands out most to you, generally:
   - The things in boxes
   - The pictures
   - And the things written in bold.

   As you skim the book, you will get an idea of the areas most useful to you. You can then read those in greater depth.
3. Use it as a reference book. It was primarily designed for this purpose. Go to the section or area related to the activity you are planning and study it. Use it to get ideas to get your own creative thoughts going.

These pictures will help you to find:

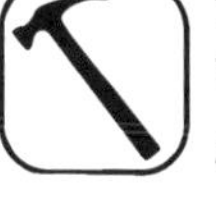

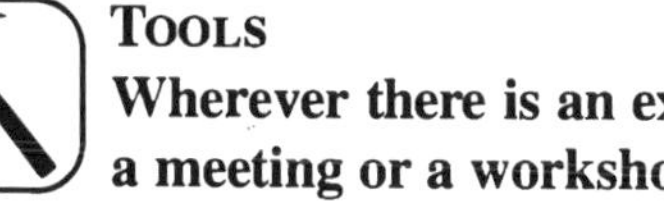

Tools
Wherever there is an exercise you can use in a meeting or a workshop.

Tips
Wherever there is a hint or a tip to make the training go smoothly.

Questions
Wherever a common question is asked.

Steps
Wherever several steps are described to complete a task.

As you can see, this book has tabs on the side to help you to find the chapters quickly.

There are four sections in the book and the tabs for all the chapters in a section are the same color.

This sourcebook is cross-referenced in many places. It will help you to have a greater understanding of a topic if you read the cross-reference.

This manual is organized in terms of issues related to training, rather than in terms of specific technical agricultural topics. It is organized into four sections.

The **first section,** chapters one through three, is about how adults learn and the most effective training methods for adults. It includes who should be trained and who should facilitate the training.

Section two chapters four through eight, discusses the training cycle step by step. It begins with defining the need for training and the content and moves through planning, implementation, and evaluation of a training program.

Section three, chapters nine through eleven, focuses on some important issues in livestock and agricultural training. These topics – gender, traditional knowledge, and good communication and group work – will positively influence agricultural training if they are included in the program.

The fourth section, chapters twelve through fourteen, is a reference section. In this section are tools for participation with examples of how to use them. There are also suggestions for making your own training materials and other relevant reference materials.

Sections one and two present many of the basic concepts behind participatory adult education. **If participatory adult learning is new to you,** section one will give you the background to be able to use it.

If you have been using participatory training and will be training facilitators, section one will give you some ideas. To help train others, each concept of participatory training is illustrated with an example of a drawing, game or role playing exercise which could be used to teach the concept to someone else. As you prepare your training of trainers sessions, please consider including the important concepts in section one and section three.

If you are beginning to plan a new training program, or to revamp an existing one, section two will take you through a program step by step.

Sections one through three describe many training tools such as small groups, brainstorming, etc. Section four outlines the use of each of these tools. Each tool has a definition, a description of its use, a discussion of pros and cons and other uses, and an example from a real situation. As you read through sections one through three, refer to the reference section to discover how to use each tool. Then adapt each tool to your situation as you plan your training workshop.

There is great interest in training community agricultural and livestock workers who will later assist their communities. Many examples in this book were taken from Community Livestock Worker training programs. The same concepts apply to agricultural or forestry workers or to individual community members, only the subject matter will change. The examples are given to illustrate the tools and techniques and are not intended to limit the application of the participatory training approach to any relevant content.

ISBN 978-1-886532-54-0

IN MEMORIAM

Philip Mark Bounds, DVM

January 22, 1955 – September 7, 1995

A pilgrim who found his "elsewhere" in service.
The service which transformed him, and others with him,
into something better and beyond.

He was our mentor, and anmchara*:
Quick to encourage a new and different idea,
looking, and using all he had to fill someone else's needs,
bursting with creativity.

He gave us laughter,
challenged us to stretch and grow,
modeled a simple yet complex faith,
unafraid to question deeply, and to love deeply.

A part of him stays with our team and a part goes forth in this book.

❧

*anmchara; An Irish word meaning soul-friend. Someone to be trusted over a whole lifetime.

Thanks

Without the effort of many people, this book would not have been born. The PROPECO project team in Bolivia learned and created together, and they were taught and influenced by many people. It is the spirit of that creative and mentoring action that is imbued in these pages. In the Sourcebook, individuals and programs who first suggested an idea for an exercise are mentioned by name. Exceptions are the exercises in common use by many programs and those developed by the PROPECO team.

Thank you to all of the farmers, trainers, and administrators from several programs who gave their time, ideas, and encouragement for this book.

The key people who collaborated in the development of the ideas and tools in this book are:

- In Bolivia: Florentino Llavera, Alijandrina Espinoza, Lucio Hualpa, Monica Mendez, Jose Zanabria, Lourdes Alarcon, Teofilo Belmonte, Teofilo Choque, Bernadina Rojas, Dori Coca, Gregorio Carmona, Zaida Alavrez, Roger Hinojosa, Tomas Duran, Hacinto Menchaca, Margaret Hicks, Victor Alvarez, Lina-Maria Nivea Obando, Tom and Dee Yaccino. The team from the Center for the Training of the Woman Farmer (C-CIMCA) especially Evelyn Barron.
- In Nepal: Narayan Ojha, Goma Shrestha, Bal Krishna Maharjan, Padam Kumari Gurung, Bhola Kumar Shrestha, Yam Kumari Shrestha, Hans Olov Green, Ron Stoufer, Peter and Mary Quesenberry, Helena Vesterinen, Walton McCaslin, Yamuna Ghale, Dr Mahendra Bhattarai, Paul Daughtery, John Collum, Dr. Prakash Raj Shrestha, Shyam Paudel, Irene Christensen, Peter Lowe.
- In The Phillippines: Ding Navarro, Evelyn Mathias-Mundy, Paul Mundy, Eseng Quintos, Ed Sabio, Lito Pastores. Jim Orprecio, Daisy Catchero, Dr Mila Gracia Ejercito, Bing Flores, Father Elias Salomon, Nestor Maghanoy, Elmer Sayre.
- In Thailand: Pramote Eva-Amnuay, Niwatchai Suknaphasawat, the people of Pang Kham Noi.
- In Uganda: A. Beinempaka, Mugamba Women's Cooperative Group, Margaret Makuru, Stan Burkey, Val Sheen, Brad Frye
- In Kenya: Suzanne Kiamba, Gilbert Namuonja, Josephine Wangechi, Susan VanLinden, Jacob Wangnama, Wendall Cantrell

Thank you for the creativity and time of B.J., Jennifer, and Karen as they put their extensive experience into a form we could all learn from and use in the chapters on "Local Knowledge", "Evaluation", and "Follow-up."

Thank you to the dedicated people who reviewed the sourcebook and gave suggestions, especially: Jennifer Shumaker, Kit Flowers, Margaret Stewart, Helen Giardella, Jim Hoey, James DeVries, Alison Meares, Anna Lawrence, Beth Miller, Brad Frye, Nikki Bonilla, Cyndie McLachlan and Karen Stoufer. Thank you for the editorial talents of Conrad Shumaker. Thank you also to the chief midwife of the Sourcebook, Jerry Aaker for his encouraging, correcting and guiding.

And finally, special thanks to International Program Director for Heifer Project, Dr Jim DeVries and Christian Veterinary Mission Executive Director, Dr. Kit Flowers who believed the Sourcebook was possible from start to finish.

This is our book. A starting place for ideas to be shared and to join all of us who work in participatory agriculture. May we continue learning and growing together.

What is in this book?

Section 3: ISSUES IN AGRICULTURAL TRAINING

Section 4: RESOURCES, TOOLS AND REFERENCES

Proceed with caution!

This Sourcebook is a group of ideas, methods, and techniques which have been successful in many agricultural training programs around the world. **This book is not a recipe book for success in an agricultural training program.** Examples of methods and tools are included to encourage your creativity. The purpose is to share new ideas and tools with people who are working with their *communities* for change.

Village and *community:* these two words are often used interchangeably in this book. However sometimes the word *village* is used to define a rural place. Sometimes *community* is used to suggest the idea of a group of people working together.

"No individual knows exactly how to do it. No one has all the answers, and no one is totally ignorant. Each person has different perceptions based on their own experiences."
–Freire, 1973

So this book does not have all of the answers! Every workshop is unique. Every village situation and every region is unique. The workshop should be designed with the participants according to their needs. The key is to work with creativity, initiative and perseverance. The planning process for a workshop is itself a learning opportunity for all those involved. It gives the workshop planners tools to be applied in other areas of their communities.

Participatory: A process where local people and outsiders work together to accomplish their goals. It is based in an attitude of respect, valuing of the other's ideas, and dialogue.

Many people believe a "participatory approach" to training is just a set of methods, tools, or "games" such as role playing, puppet shows, and songs. IT IS MUCH MORE! Methods, tools, and techniques cannot be used in a philosophical or theoretical vacuum. The first chapters of the book cover the philosophy behind the participatory approach. You will also find in the reference section other books and manuals which provide more information in greater depth on the theory behind the practice. The philosophy with which you approach participation in training will affect your attitude toward the participants. **If someone attempts to use the methods without embracing the philosophy, the results will be manipulation, rather than participation.** This then becomes a further way to discourage change, cloaked in the words "participatory."

So please use the materials here: challenge them, shape and mold them to your unique situation, and please share your results with us!

Agriculture is also social

The professional's view of agriculture is often physical and technical.

When I (Susan Stewart) began to work with men and women farmers to improve animal production in the lowland jungle of Bolivia, I did not look beyond the immediate causes of poor production. I thought that skinny, poorly producing animals were caused by lack of proper management, poor breeds, and pastures. The situation was made worse by farming the jungle with its thin topsoil, flooding, wind and water erosion. To me, the poverty of the people was due to poor agricultural production. I thought that training in land and animal management, credit, and improved breeds of animals and pastures would revolutionize the people's production. If only families could improve their management of animals and pastures they would have increased income which would translate into healthy, happy families.

My view of the situation, of people's needs, was largely physical, based on the physical surroundings. I thought that each individual farm family could change with physical inputs and improve their lives. This limited world view on my part was understandable. After all, I was a veterinarian, an expert, trained to provide physical solutions to physical problems. I had little social or political awareness.

Agriculture has a strong social side.

But then I became close to some of the men and women with whom I was working. From working with farmers in veterinary practice, I already had a healthy respect for their knowledge, ingenuity, and patience far beyond my own in dealing with their land and animals. But as friendships developed and deepened, I began to grasp the depth of the farmers' strength in adversity and the breath of their faith in action. They taught me about the human side of their needs. They didn't sit me down and explain the world to me. They opened their lives and their homes. I shared in their problems and dreams as they lived each day. We struggled together to prevent the loss of animals and crops, which could also mean the loss of a child, a home or hope. Sometimes they survived. Sometimes they didn't.

Bit by bit I learned that, **although many of the problems in agricultural production and marketing had some physical causes, they also had social causes at their roots.** They were often caused by the way individuals and groups treated or acted on the lives of other people. Many times I saw the loss of animals, crops and dreams because of the unthinking actions of some or the tremendous greed of others.

Here are some examples of problems in livestock production which have social roots:

- A very poor family in the Philippines has a few animals which are thin and non-productive. They have learned about forage trees and sloping lands pasture systems. But they do not plant them because of their fear of losing the land. Once the pastures are established, the land owner will take away the land without reimbursing the farmer for their labor or trees and pastures.

- Multinational corporations are patenting local knowledge in India in medicinal plants, insecticides, and technologies and selling them back to the villages from which they originated, for profit. Corporations now claim they own the intellectual property rights to the traditional, village-owned technology. The corporations profit from the products and the royalties. The villagers receive nothing. The same farmers who created the technology now have to pay for it, often in emergency situations.

- An influential farmer in the community organizes with a non-government organization to drill a well on his property. He has presented them with a plan for how it will be used by the community. Shortly after the well is completed and paid for, arguments begin. The argument ends with the community prohibited from using the well. The water is now used solely by the family and animals of the influential farmer. The other families have a poor water supply resulting in continued poor production of their animals.

- Farmers have decided to eliminate Brucellosis from their herds. They negotiate with the government agency to help them in a testing campaign. When the test results are finished, the government veterinarian refuses to brand the positive animals. It is election time and he does not want to create bad feelings. The positive cows are sold to unsuspecting people in neighboring villages, creating a greater hazard to families and animals.

Training for change and action

Community Livestock Workers (CLWs) and trainers who are farmers have experienced agricultural problems with social roots in Bolivia. As a result, they decided to become *Agents of change* in their villages.

Agents of change: A person who acts to facilitate change in their community. They can cause people to think about new ideas or reflect on a current situation. (See diagram on pg. 48 "Role of the Facilitator")

Community Livestock Worker (CLW): A person who works in and for their community with livestock care and agricultural extension.

- They worked together with village women to organize the sale of their sheep to get better prices in order to dig a good well close to their houses. The men in the community had refused to build a well for years. Now the community has clean water for their livestock and families, and the milk production has gone up.

- They worked with local livestock producers' organizations to build an effective livestock credit program. Now members have access to a credit system that does not bankrupt them. They pay back the first female offspring of the animal which in turn is passed to another family.

- They insured that expensive, inappropriate, and expired medicines are no longer carried by the local medicine shops.

- They helped their communities make an annual plan and act on it in order to solve many community problems and work toward their common vision.

The CLWs have developed skits and puppet shows to get the people in their villages thinking, talking, and acting in order to deal with some of the root causes of poor animal production and sales. Some of the methods they developed are included in this book.

In some cases, the CLWs and *facilitators* have met with difficulties and problems in working as change agents. They fight everything from apathy to outright hostility on the part of some of the people affected. The men in the community where the women dug the well refused to participate in the process. The government vet destroyed their efforts at organizing a Brucellosis campaign. The corrupt leader of a local livestock organization tried to discredit the CLWs publicly because they were demanding accountability for the organization's expenses. Many have tried to discourage them or render their work ineffective. But the CLWs have seen the positive results of their work, and they continue as agents of change in spite of the pressures to conform to the status quo.

Facilitator: The person who guides the training or change process. They help people to look at a situation, define their vision, seek out new information and plan change. (See "Facilitators of training," pg. 39)

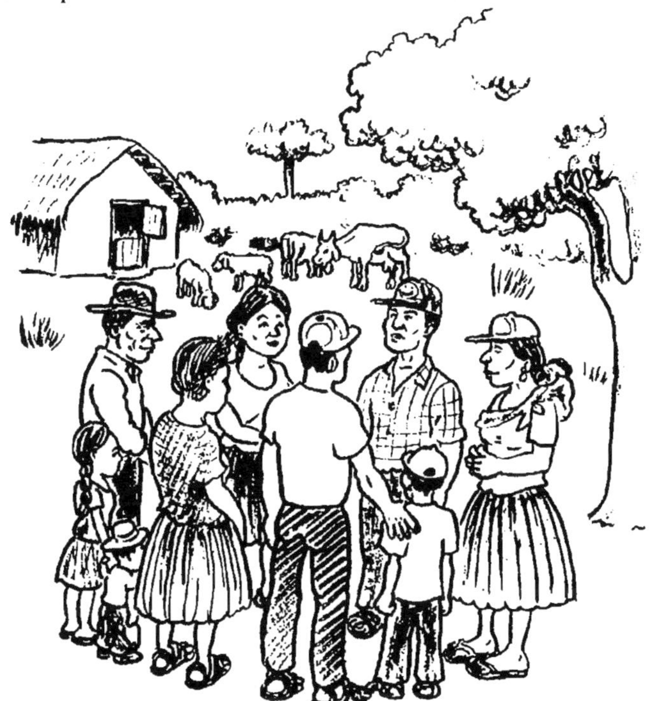

A powerful training program

When we begin a training program we want to encourage people's growth. We want to equip them for the future and for change. Because participatory training can cause change, it can also affect power, authority, and control. **Therefore, training of any kind is not neutral. Every type of training can either maintain the status quo or change it.**

Why?

- Participatory training says at the outset that **the views of the village people are important.** Their views have substance and are often more appropriate than the views of the "experts."

- The participatory approach is designed to help people to look at their present situation, analyze it, and act on it for positive change. It is also designed for personal and group growth. Growth means change. Growth or change will effect any power balance.

- Participatory training brings the knowledge of the few into the hands of poor farmers for their use.

- Participatory training **helps people to respect their own knowledge and understanding.** This can cause a shift in the balance of power.

This book is about training for change and action. Power, control and authority are all part of the participatory process no matter where it is found. **Change is threatening for many,** especially for those who benefit from the status quo. Tensions, fights and conflicts may arise in the process of change. Everyone who participates should be aware of this.

As trainers we should not ignore the consequences of the training. If by sharing local knowledge of natural pest management, village people forfeit their intellectual property rights to a large corporation, should we take appropriate steps in the situation, or be unwitting partners to it? If by producing more, the farmer will only be paid less for their animals because of intermediary control rather than supply and demand, should our training program address marketing? If planting agroforestry pasture systems will cause farmers to lose their land, should that be ignored? **Dealing with the issues of power, conflict, control and authority will always be a part of a participatory training program.**

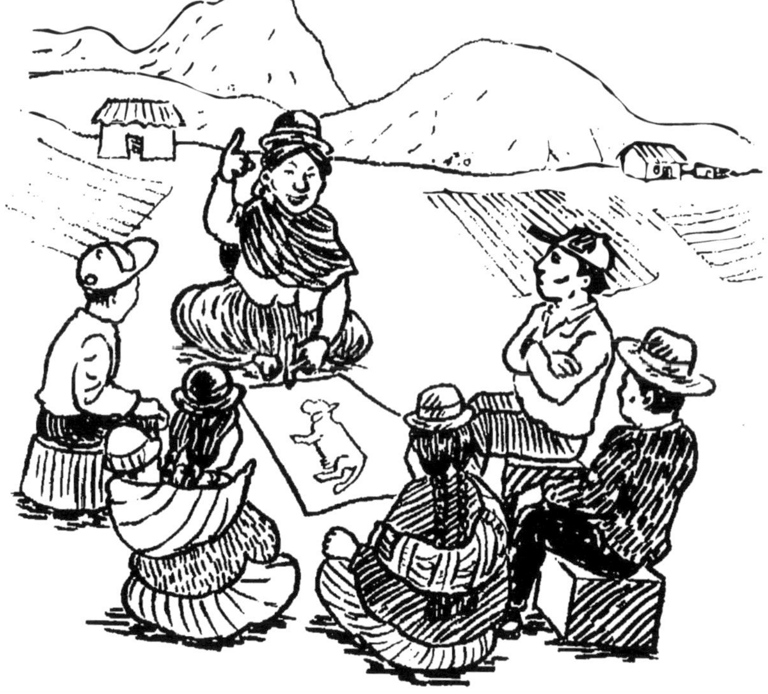

About participatory livestock programs

The lessons shared here were often learned the hard way through the development of many different programs such as the Community Based Livestock Project (PROPECO) in Bolivia. PROPECO is a program which focuses on livestock production and marketing, wise use of soil, water, and land, and strengthening of local organizations. It centers around a training program designed together by farmers and outsiders for men and women farmers.

Nine years ago the PROPECO team set out to develop a training program which might deal with the physical and some of the social causes of livestock production problems. We had attended a two-day workshop about the effectiveness of participatory training in human health programs and were armed with a copy of *Helping Health Workers Learn.* (Werner and Bower 1982) As a team we explored some of the ideas in the book and then developed a participatory workshop for farmers. We based the workshop on what the men had identified as their most important problems with cattle. The workshop centered around common cattle diseases, parasites, nutrition, and pasture and land management. We included some social issues, such as wise buying of medicines from sometimes tricky shops and accurate weights of animals to negotiate with intermediaries. The topics were appropriate because the farmers had chosen them. The topics addressed urgent problems the farmers saw daily.

After two years of giving very popular workshops in several communities, the team did an evaluation to see which of the topics taught were being used on a regular basis. The team discovered that some of the things discussed in the workshop were being applied and had dramatically improved animal production. The simple fact that many farmers were now feeding iodized salt had caused a tremendous decrease in calf deaths and goiter. Many people were now deworming their animals and seeing improvement. But the deworming was sporadic. Only some of the communities were vaccinating their cattle. People were practicing better pasture rotation and control of their animals. But the establishment of improved pastures and forage trees was very slow. Although the farmers left the workshop enthusiastic about providing a clean water supply for their animals during the dry season, they still did not have water available. There was not a wide use of improved management in other animals such as sheep, goats, and pigs.

The farmers had left the workshops excited about management changes. Why did they not implement more change?

- The farmers explained that for worming and vaccinating, the products in the vet pharmacies were too expensive for one farmer alone. That meant they had to organize to vaccinate and deworm together. Unfortunately, the organization was difficult and sporadic. There were always problems with who should go and buy the vaccine, when and how much people would pay, who would organize everyone to bring their animals to be vaccinated.
- Many farmers explained that when they had planted new pastures and trees on their land, the neighbor's animals or fire from the next land plot had destroyed all of their work.
- A government program had offered people loans for shallow ponds which they had dug. These were all dry during the dry season.

- Women were the primary caretakers of the animals. But in some communities, the men had not permitted the women to attend the workshops. We added to the problem by making the workshop about cattle, which are traditionally viewed as the men's property. So the women, who cared for the other animals, did not apply things learned in the workshop to the other animals.

We learned from that first evaluation that our focus in the training program had been wrong. We had approached the whole training as if individuals, armed with new knowledge could make changes, just because they decided to. We did not consider many of the other factors, outside of the individuals' control, which would affect his or her successful change. We did not consider the larger social, political, and spiritual context of the community. We did not deal with the effectiveness of the local organization for vaccination and worming or for controlled burning regulations. We had not discussed the larger connections to other programs and negotiating with them for what was best. When we asked what topics should be included, the men's voices were loudest and were heard. Although women participated in the workshops, they had not participated in the design.

Livestock programs in development have gone in and out of vogue for many years. The problems innate in providing animals, improving production, and developing marketing systems in isolated rural areas have stumped many programs. Vast amounts of money have been spent on very unsuccessful programs where the animals died, did not produce, or destroyed the land.

Yet animals provide the resource base for the vast majority of rural poor around the world. They are the banking system, often providing the buffer between survival and death. When people lose their animals through war, greed, natural disturbances and disease, the family or family members go without schooling, food and health care, and sometimes die.

Characteristics of successful participatory livestock programs:

Programs for livestock production and marketing have been successful where:

1. The village men and women define the priorities of the program from the initial stages.

They determine the needs, analyze the situation, formulate the plan for the solution, look for the necessary resources, implement the plan, and evaluate it when they are finished. These are participatory programs where villagers drive the program. The outsiders participate by sharing tools for community participation, providing resources including some new information, and facilitating productive dialogue.

The basis of this type of cooperation between villagers and outsiders is *dialogue:*

> "It is not our role to speak to the people about our own view of the world, nor to attempt to impose that view on them, but rather to dialogue with the people about their view and ours."
> – Freire 1973)

Dialogue: A free exploration of what others think and mean, while suspending our assmptions and judgements, at least long enough to really listen.
–Aaker and Shumaker, 1996

Dialogue leads to action. Action leads to improved production and marketing and to ways of resolving the social issues of livestock production. The result is improved livelihoods of the people.

2. The program includes livestock production and people in the whole context of the village not only the individual farmers' lives.

Village and personal life have social, political, productive, cultural, and spiritual aspects. Programs which have recognized how animals and animal production link to all aspects of rural village life and have incorporated that into their actions are far more effective. Village people bring this context to their own programs.

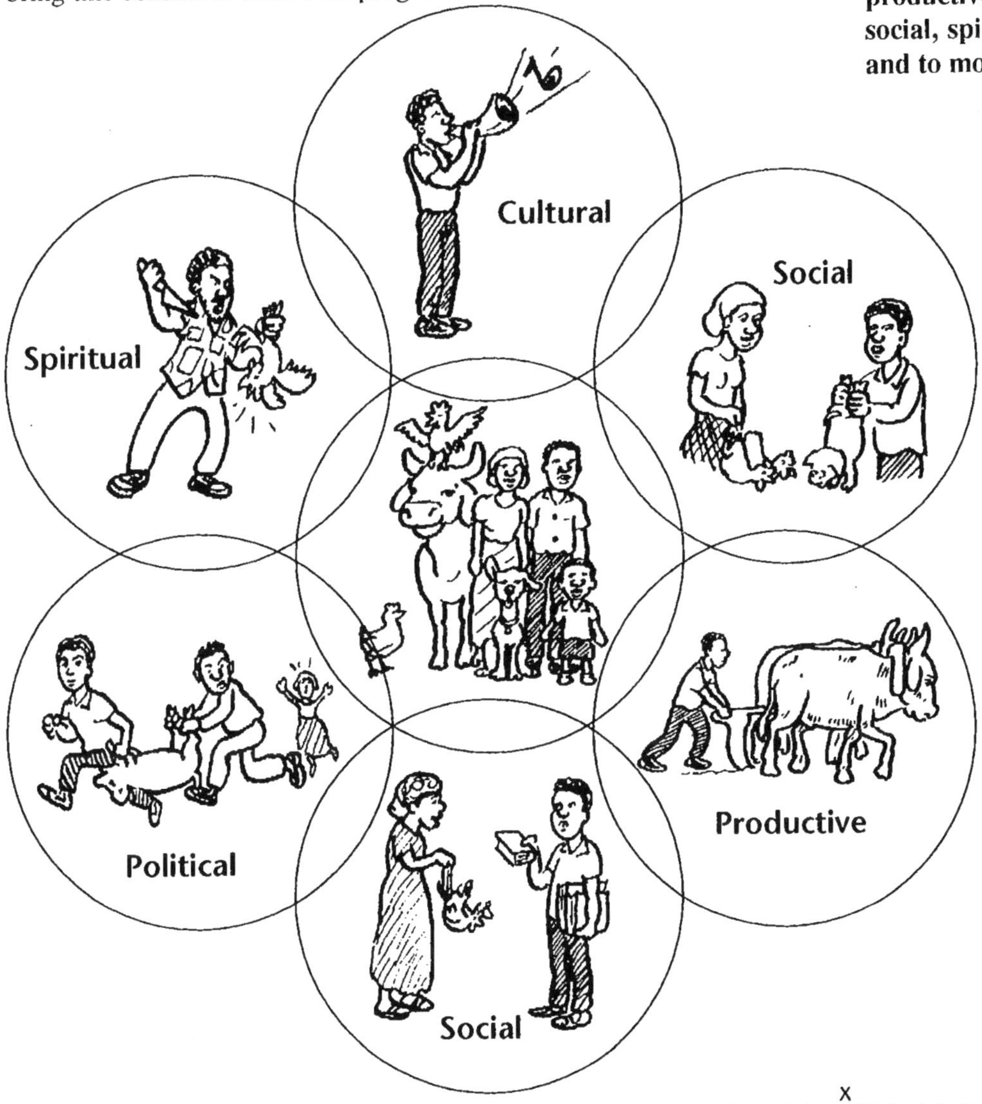

For example:

In PROPECO, many Community Livestock Workers (CLWs) have a Christian commitment to faith and service. They see their role as a CLW as part of that commitment. They have integrated their faith with their personal dealings with village members and their organization, to strengthen their work. Generally, village people make ready connections between the issues in livestock production and marketing and their spiritual values. **Successful programs will not focus solely on economic, productive or technical solutions to problems. They will consider the social, spiritual or political motivation of the community to change and to move toward a vision.**

3. The program emphasizes the role of the local community organizations in dealing with the social issues of livestock production.

The program plans to work with community organizations such as the village governing body, an agricultural cooperative, a church, a livestock association, or others. Through program activities these organizations strengthen their organization, management, communication and accountability skills as they serve their members. These strengthened organizations tackle the tough issues of land tenure, water, marketing, and others. They also help provide the continuity in working toward a vision.

4. Successful programs consider how the local situation fits into the larger context of district and national animal health care programs.

Successful programs help the farmers look at how village organizations and their CLWs will be linked to government and private agricultural production and marketing systems. These programs recognize that the village exists within a larger context. The villagers learn to analyze government and private systems. They also learn to negotiate with people from government and private programs.

The participatory approach is not for villagers alone. Successful programs have helped government and private workers to open a dialogue with the farmers and to look at their systems from the farmers' perspective. In Kenya, government agricultural workers have put into practice a participatory approach in their work which is reflected in more relevant research and more appropriate animal health care systems. In addition, the villagers have access to knowledge about new techniques, medicines, vaccines, and pastures and a way to share their response to new ideas.

This book is a sourcebook on developing and implementing a participatory *training program* in agriculture. It is not the purpose of this book to cover all aspects of the participatory process as it relates to livestock and agricultural programs. There are many good resources available listed in the resources section (pg. 329). These resources are based on experience and understanding of the adult learning process in nonagricultural programs. Although their focus is not agricultural, the information can readily be adapted for the agricultural worker.

Animator: A man or woman farmer who is a facilitator of the participatory process in their own and other communities.

We challenge you to learn from the experiences this book draws on and from the resources listed in the resource section, add your own experiences, and move to a participatory approach in your whole agricultural program, not just in your training program. **A participatory training program will only be truly appropriate and applicable when it is part of a participatory program.** The reverse is also true. A participatory program demands a participatory approach to training.

Many of the ideas and approaches in this book have been developed by the *animators,* Community Livestock Workers, and village people working in the Community-Based Livestock Project (PROPECO) in Bolivia. But other participants, trainers, and advisors from community-based agricultural programs around the world have shared their ideas. The hope is that we all will be encouraged and strengthened in our people-centered, community organization strengthening approach to improving agricultural production and marketing.

The underlying values In a training program

Participatory training opens the world to be explored by learners and educators. It invites people to be *subjects* of their own development rather than *objects* to be moved around like chess pieces. It opens a dialogue and encourages action to change the world into what it might be, for the participants and for their children

Subjects: people who are active decision makers in their own lives. The opposite is to feel like an *object* manipulated or used by others.

> The *popular education* approach to adult learning invites optimal consciousness to do what one is doing in the world as intentionally as possible. Imagine a world of mutual respect, with equitable distribution systems and adequate housing, where it is easier to love. It takes men and women who are subjects of their own lives to design and bring about such a world.
>
> –Jane Vella 1995

Popular education: In Spanish, popular means by and of the people. So popular education is education by and of the people.

People who are *subjects* will base their decisions in their underlying set of values. A training program will help build a vision, as established by the participants. It will also be rooted and grounded in a set of principles and values.

In the PROPECO program in Bolivia we made some decisions about the values we hold. These are the values we use in our team work, with communities and with other organizations.

To help us see our system in visual form we made the following tree for our program:

THE PROPECO VALUE AND VISION TREE

TRAINING PROGRAM
CHRISTIAN CONCEPT OF TRANSFORMATION
GROWTH, ENCOURAGEMENT
PARTICIPATION, EQUITY
GOOD COMMUNICATION
HUMAN RELATIONS
TRUST, WORKING TOGETHER, LOVE
HONESTY, CLARITY, INTEGRITY
SHARING RESOURCES
HOPE IN A DIFFERENT FUTURE
RESPECT FOR LOCAL KNOWLEDGE
SERVICE

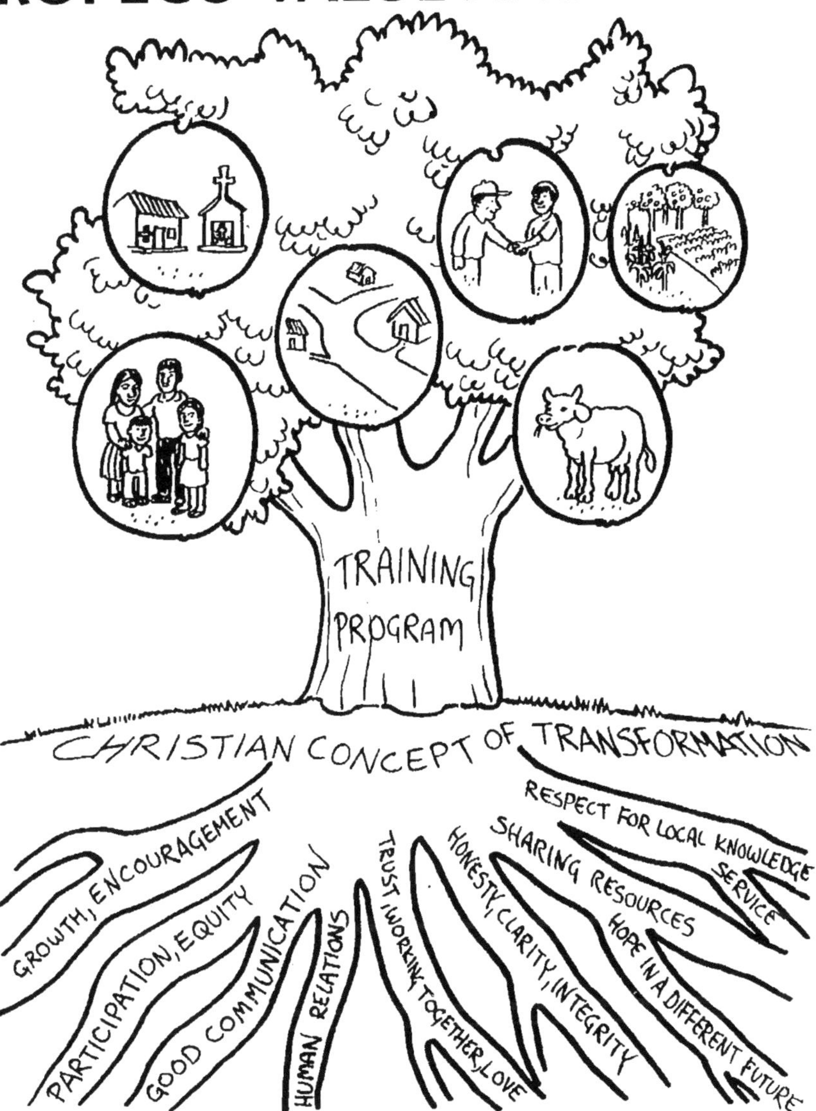

The fruit of the tree of the PROPECO program is the vision we are working toward.
What would your program's value and vision tree look like?

In the Christian Concept of Transformation, which we apply in PROPECO, people's spirituality is at the center of their being. All activities, be they social, economic, or cultural, spring from people's spirituality. Training is about change; change of the whole person or the whole community.

In traditional development, change tends to be linear and strives for more money, more things, more food. *Transformation* means change in a person's or community's situation, values, and attitudes. We can stay where we are and have more of the same, or we can move to a new vision. Transformation is multidimensional and involves the whole person. (DeVries 1992) To move toward the new vision requires putting into practice spiritual values and principles. These values become the guidelines for maintaining the direction toward the vision.

Transformation: The concept of transformation with spirituality at it's center is the conceptual basis of programs of the people of different faiths in different parts of the world.

One of the principles of participation is to allow people to speak. Yet technical training programs often do not encourage people to speak about what is deep inside of them and most important to them. The PROPECO program in Bolivia includes activities to initiate dialogue about specific problems in values or decision-making.

Some examples:

- When participants talk about solutions to the problem of burning one another's pastures by accident, they often talk about working together to solve the problem. They discuss what motivates them to work together in good and bad times.

- When a busy woman decides to accept the responsibility of leadership in a community organization she discusses what motivates her to serve, and to serve well.

In PROPECO, through the discussion of these issues, people share their inner feelings. They will also often reflect on scriptural teachings and the implications for their lives. As a result of this reflection participants and facilitators emerge:

- enthusiastic about their personal vision and direction
- encouraged to continue on toward a common vision
- equipped with tenets to guide them in decision-making.

This aspect of the PROPECO training program is a great encouragement to individual and collective growth. It is good for the people operating and participating in a training program to make decisions about their underlying values and principles. This will provide clarity in the vision and direction of the program. Equally important is the communities' vision of their future based in their values. For *visioning* see "Defining the situation" pg. 73–77.

> As much as human inter-personal relationships must have an ethical foundation, development which touches every facet of life and society should have an ethical, humane foundation in decision making and implementation.
>
> –A. T. Ariyaratne, 1990

Section 1
On learning and teaching

Chapter 3 Facilitators of training

This section will help you to understand the basic concepts behind participatory education in agriculture. What is participatory training? Why is it different from traditional formal education? It will also help you to decide who should receive training and who will make the best facilitators of training.

➜ If you have never used these methods before, begin here.

➜ If you are getting ready to train new trainers, begin here.

Chapter 1

Learning and teaching

This chapter covers the following topics:

How people teach

The most important role of the Community Livestock Worker (CLW)*–the animal health worker, msaidizi, community technician, or extensionist in the community – is to teach. To be successful, the CLW needs to encourage the sharing of experiences, knowledge, and ideas among individuals and organizations. The impact of their teaching will be far greater than that of directly applying their technical skills.

But **how** the CLW teaches and **views their role** as an educator is very important. Agricultural production and marketing training can be presented in a way which builds on people's knowledge, builds self esteem, and helps them to reach out toward their visions. Or, agricultural training can contribute to a lowering of people's self esteem, dependence, and an inability to solve their own problems.

*There are many names for a person who works in their community with livestock care and extension: promoter, village animal health worker, msaidizi, community technician. In this book we will call them Community Livestock Workers. CLW will refer to a person who works in and for their community with livestock care and agricultural extension. If you work with crops or trees, consider this person to be the agricultural promoter trained to work in their community.

Think about the Community Livestock Worker who trains in this traditional way:

OF COURSE your calves are dying!
It is because you do not take care of them.
I will TELL YOU what to do...
So, pay attention!

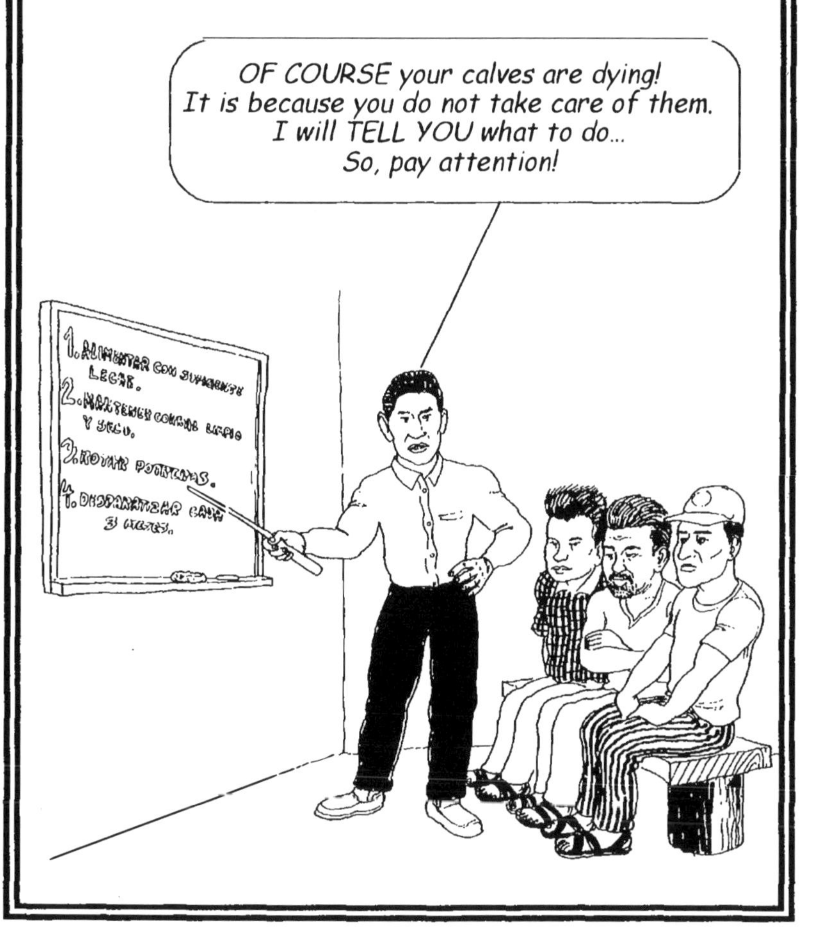

How does this kind of teaching affect the people listening?

If you or the CLWs discuss this question with co-workers, farmers, or leaders you may hear answers such as this or others:

They have heard all of this before, but it doesn't change anything.
The men just sit and listen, they don't share their problems and ideas.
He's talking to the MEN when it's the WOMEN who care for the animals!

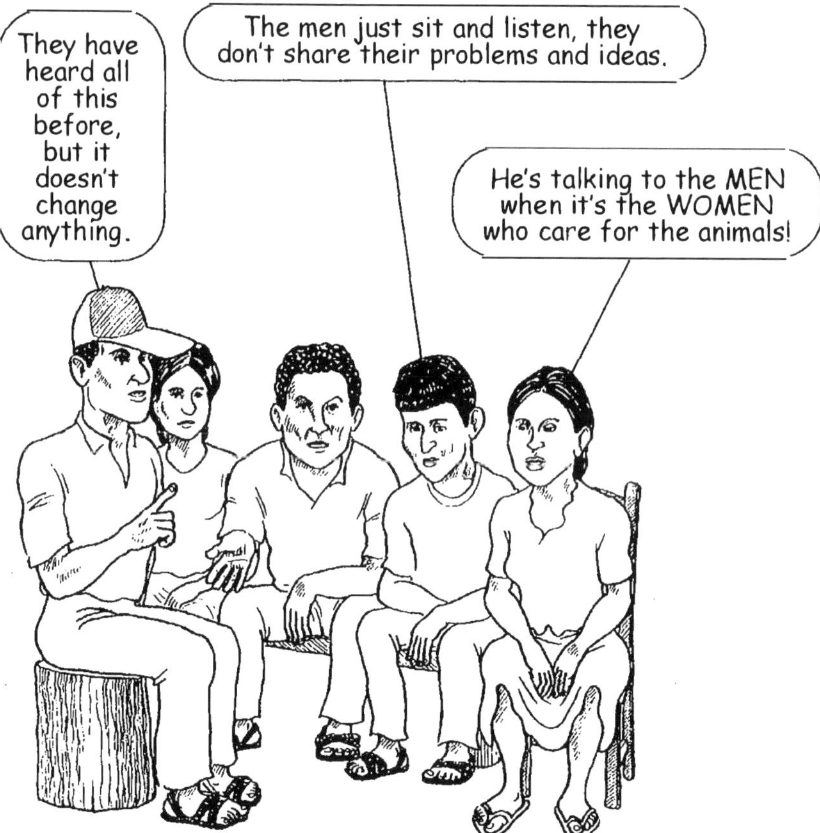

As your group explores this kind of training in depth they can ask:

Why do the men listen to this and not act on it?

Sometimes the men know more than the teacher but they can't share what they know.
Because the teacher makes the men feel worthless.
The Community Livestock Worker acts like they know everything and the men are stupid.
The *women* do the work with the animals but they don't get training.
The message makes no sense for us: if the calf drinks more milk there will be less for the children and they will get sick.
Look at the situation
Reflect on it
Analyze –ask WHY?

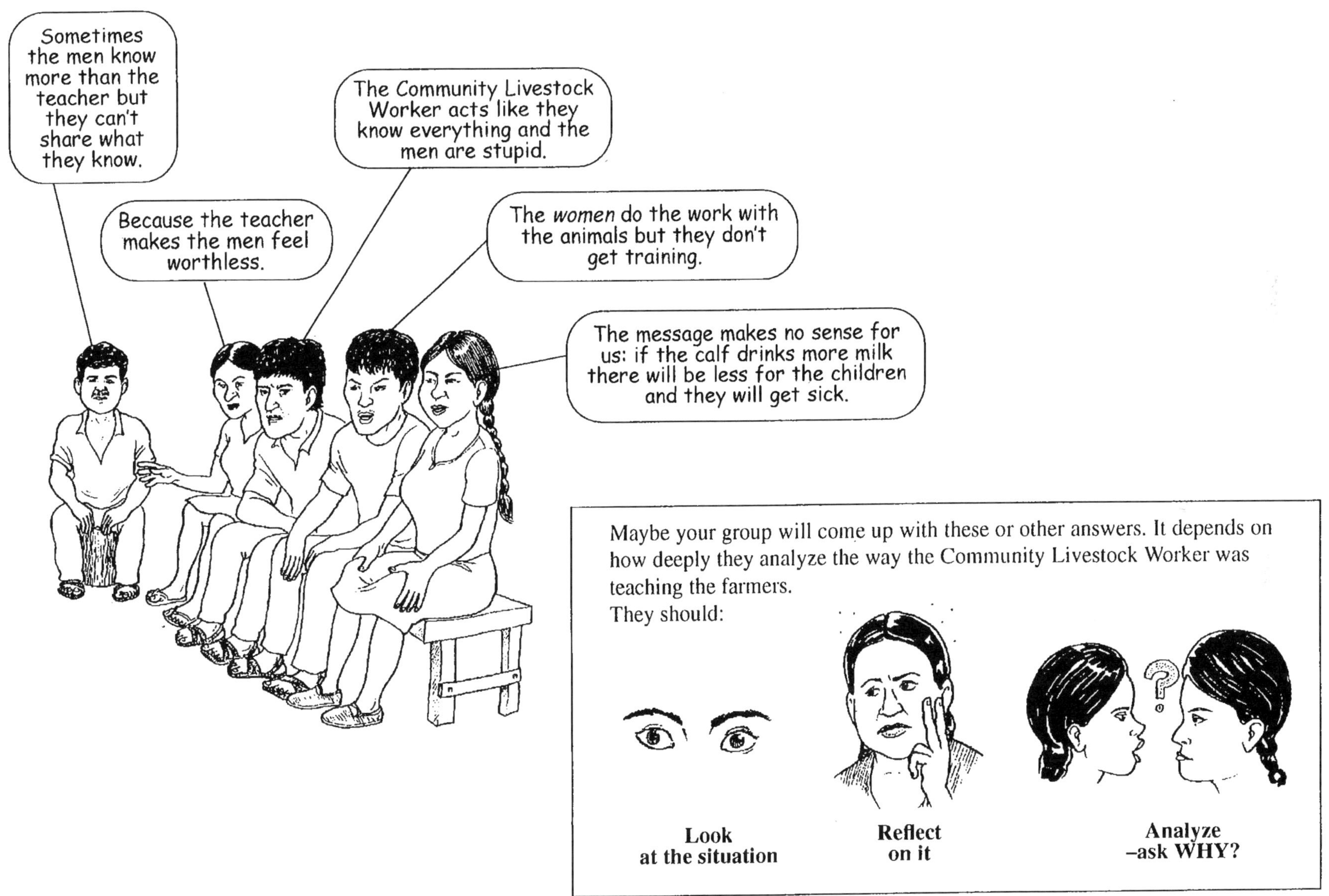

Maybe your group will come up with these or other answers. It depends on how deeply they analyze the way the Community Livestock Worker was teaching the farmers.
They should:

Now think about the way this Community Livestock Worker works in her community at a training session requested by the local organization:

What sicknesses do your calves have most often?
Diarrhea and cough after one month.
Why do they get sick after one month?
They eat pasture and dirt and have less milk.
They have worms.
Ask your group this question
How does this kind of teaching affect the people listening?
You may hear some of these answers:
We all know about these problems and have ideas to share, I think it is good to do it this way.
Everybody is sharing their experience - not just one person.
Why is the livestock worker asking questions? They have the answers-they should tell the people.
Look, the women are there AND they are talking. I bet they will use this right away!
It sure isn't the way we learned in school but maybe it's better because we solve our problems TOGETHER.

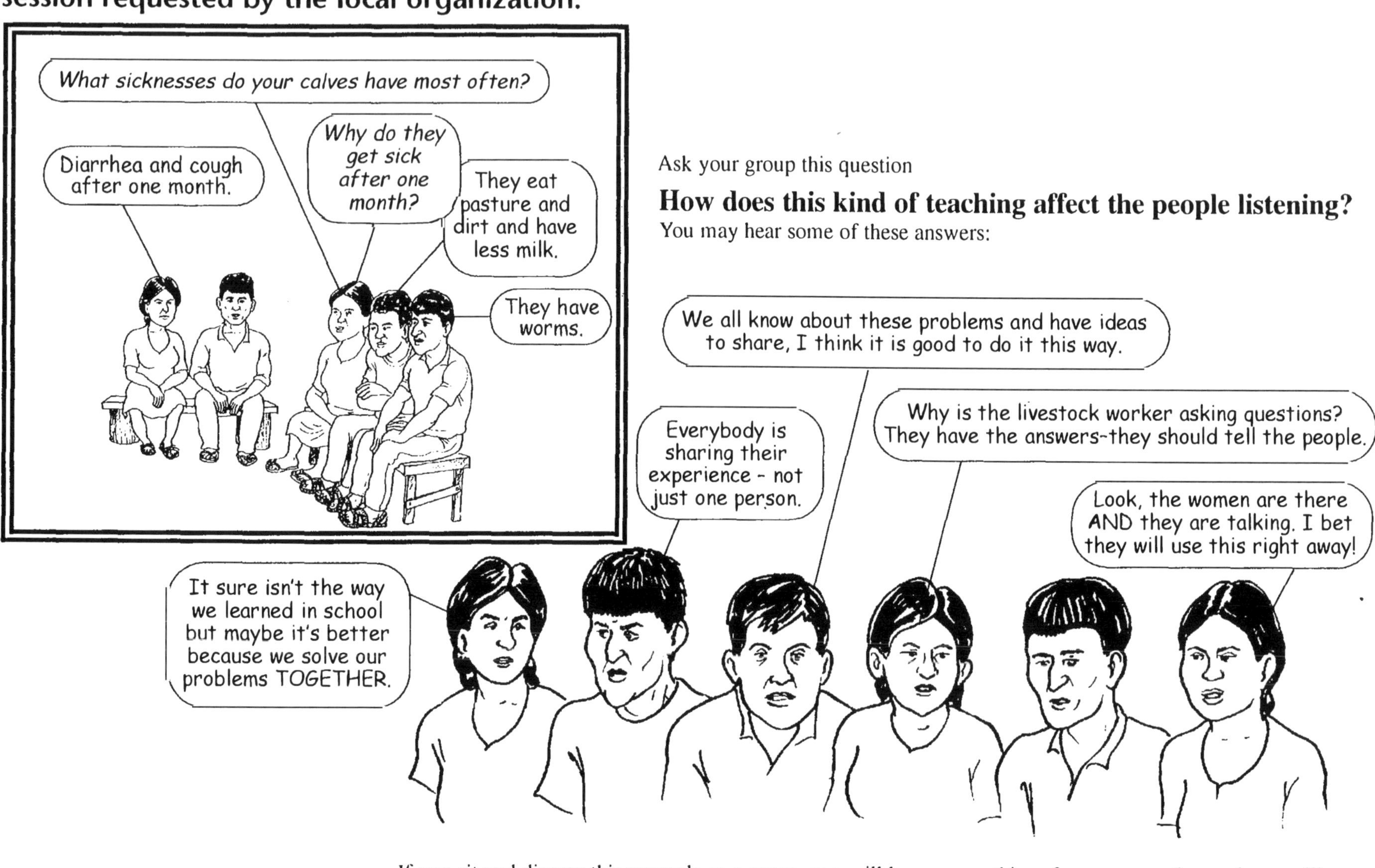

If you sit and discuss this example as a group, you will learn many things from one another and you will be able to consider the difference between two types of education. In this case: **HOW the subject is taught, is as important as WHAT is taught.**

(Adapted from *Helping Health Workers Learn*)

A working partnership between trainers and participants

When we teach are we respecting and valuing one another? Do we have a shared concern in seeing a solution and action result? Are we willing to share our part and encourage others to do so also?

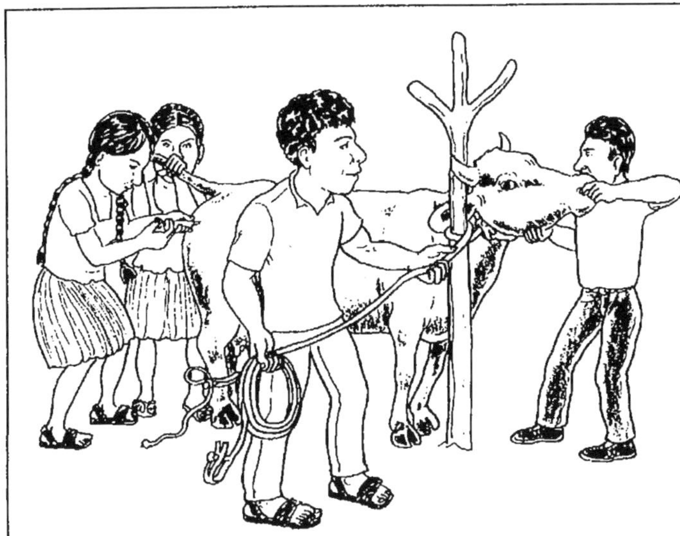

As a facilitator or Community Livestock Worker we are equal partners together with men and women farmers in looking for change. No one has more control. We all recognize that we will contribute something unique and that together we can accomplish something that none of us can do alone.

An exercise about partnership between trainers and the community:

- Ask for two volunteers. They sit at the front of the room with a bunch of bananas (or other food) between them.
- Farther down the room is another volunteer with a blindfold who groans,"I'm dying of hunger." He is the community.

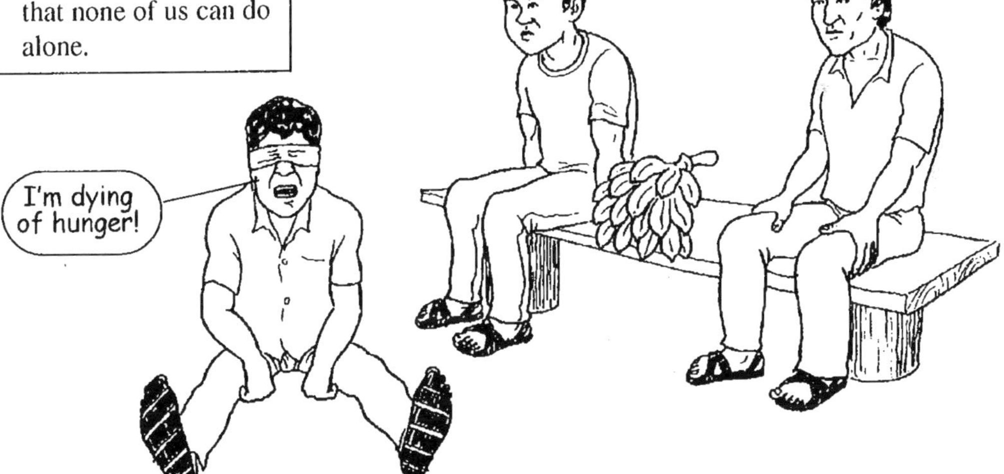

- Say to the two people up front: Help this person.
- Usually, the two up front will talk a bit then go and give the bananas to the groaning person (they may not even remove the blindfold).

• Ask the participants: **What happened here?**

The two men talked and solved the problem of the starving community and gave him a banana.

Why didn't they ask the man what he wanted? Why did they just do it on their own?

They give and he gets used to receiving - then he puts his hand out for more.

It was easy, they didn't think it through.

Because they are paternalistic- they gave him food but they never talked to him about his problems.

• **Does this happen in our community?**

Analyze this question in depth with the participants. How does it happen here?

What is the role of the educator in the community?

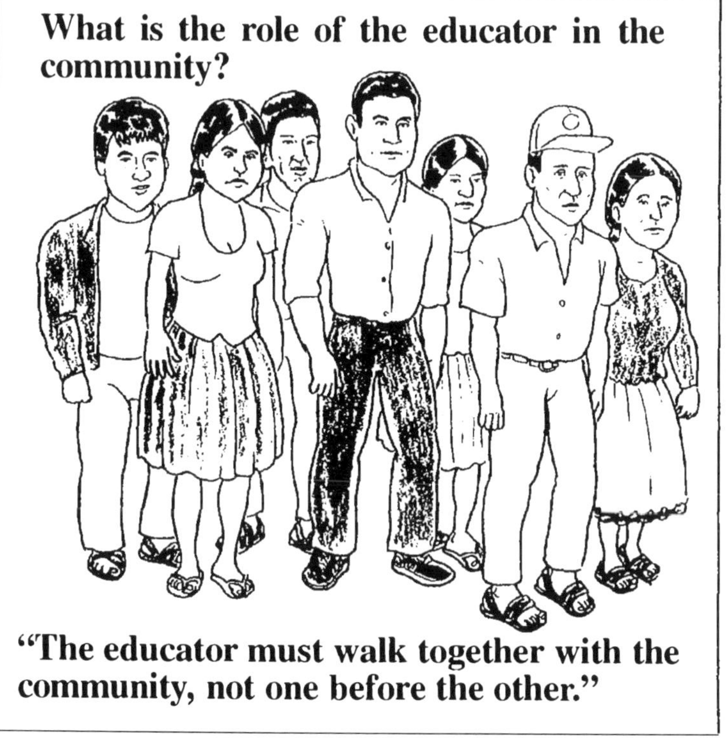

"The educator must walk together with the community, not one before the other."

Source: C-CIMCA Oruro Bolivia

Two types of education

Exercise: Ask participants to discuss two different types of education:

- Divide the participants into four small groups.
- Give each group a set of six pictures (some sample pictures are on the next pages). Each group will also have a different question to answer in their dialogue. The pictures for each group relate to the question the group will answer. (Please note, any pictures used should be appropriate to the cultural context where you are).
- Have each group discuss the pictures and separate them into two distinct types of education. Also have them each answer the specific question for their group.
- They present their results in the plenary session.
- After the results are presented, the whole group should draw conclusions about the two types of education. Write them with big print on large paper in front of the group.

Here are the sample questions given to four groups:

Group 1: What is education for?

Group 2: How does education take place?

Group 3: What does education say to us?

Group 4: What values does the education bring with it?

Tip: Be careful with this type of exercise: it can be leading. The pictures often suggest answers to the questions. Be sure the pictures stimulate an active dialogue between the small group participants.

Here is a sample of how some groups would organize their final conclusions from this exercise on large paper:

TYPES OF EDUCATION

TRADITIONAL	TRANSFORMING
A different reality	From OUR reality
Not Participative	Participative
Doesn't adapt to farmers reality	Broad-based
A "banking" form of teaching	Liberating
Rules	Open
Directed	We solve our own problems
Introduced from outside	Appropriate-practical
Theoretical	In our own language
Discipline	Comes from OUR culture
Humbling	Everyone's ideas are valuable
Academic	Each one is respected and listened to.
Imposed culture from outside	

On the following pages are some sample pictures used in Bolivia:

Source: C-CIMCA Oruro, Bolivia

Group 1: What is education for?

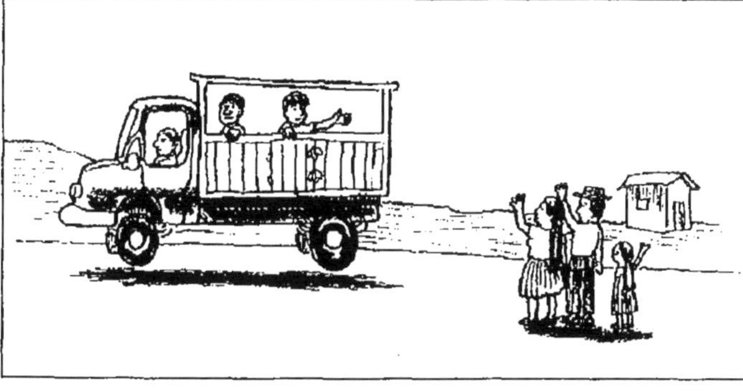

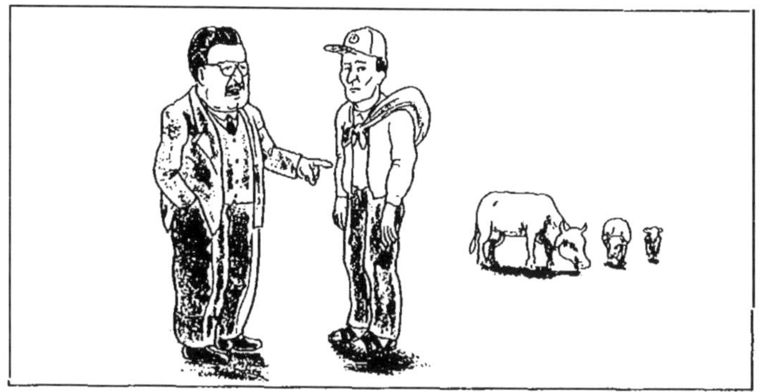

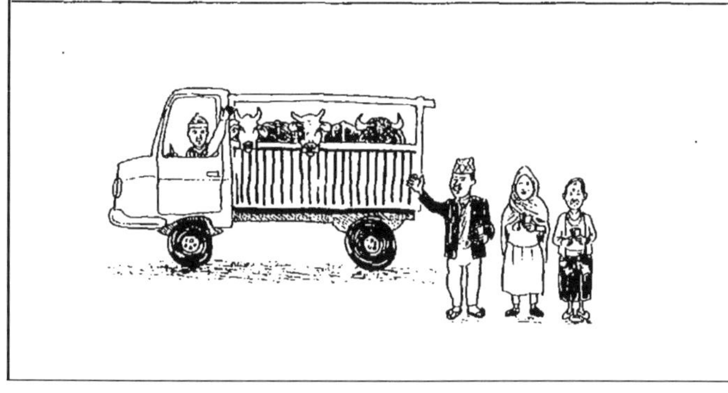

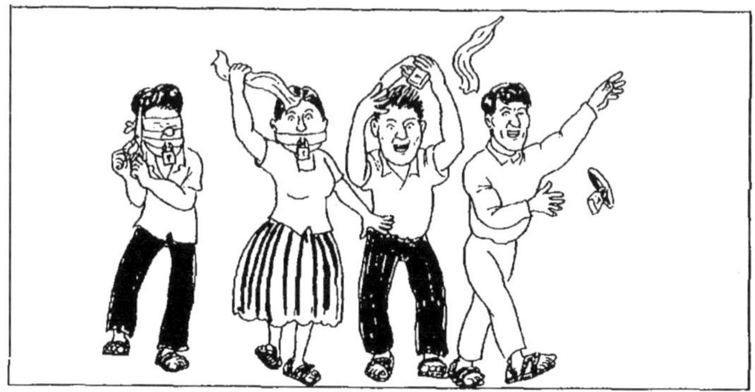

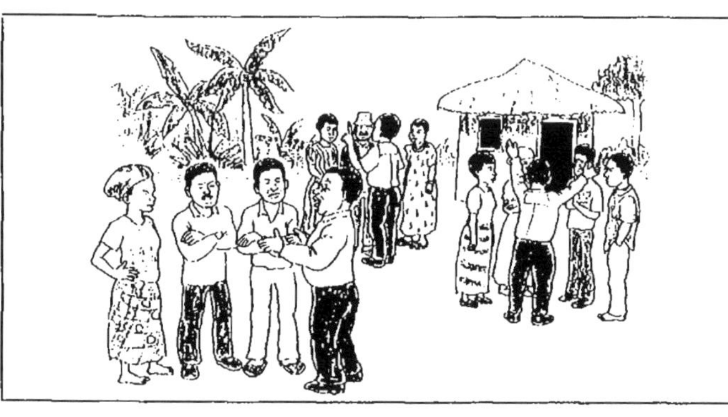

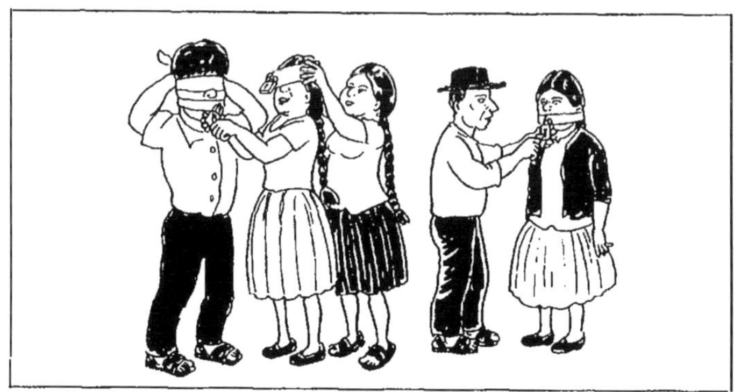

Group 2: How does education take place?

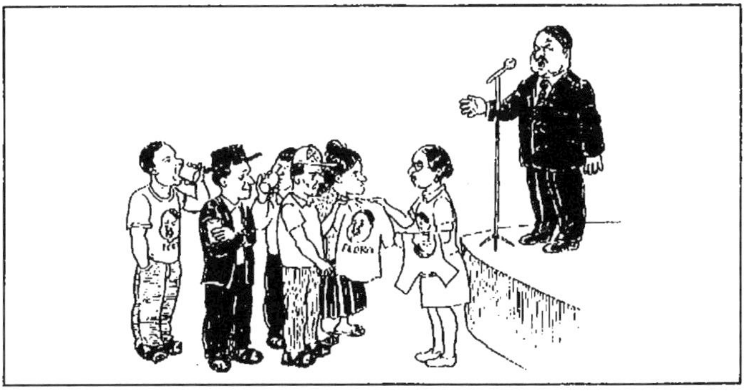

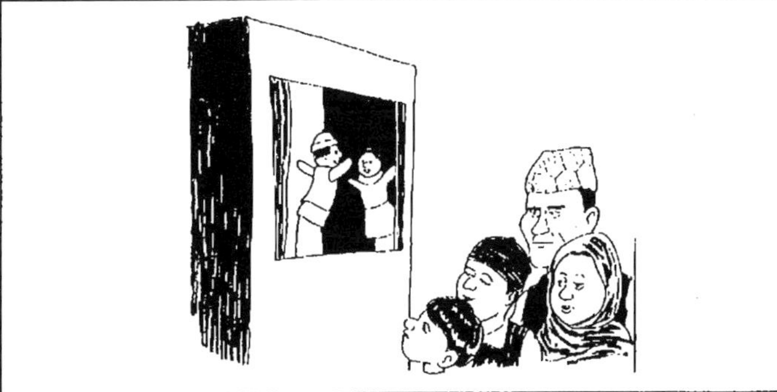

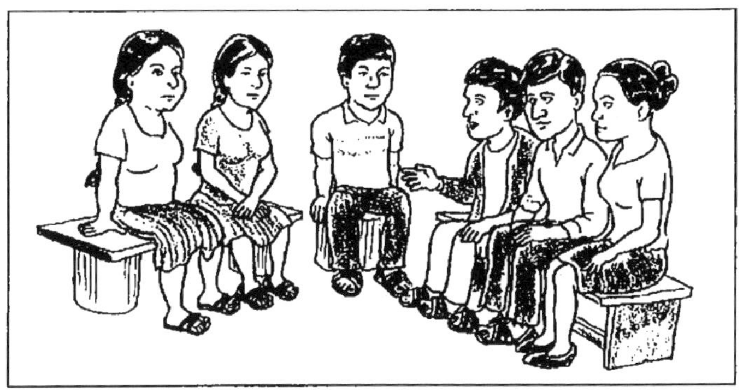

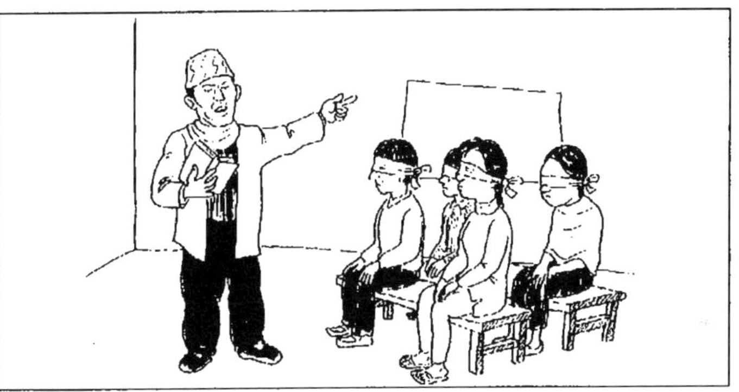

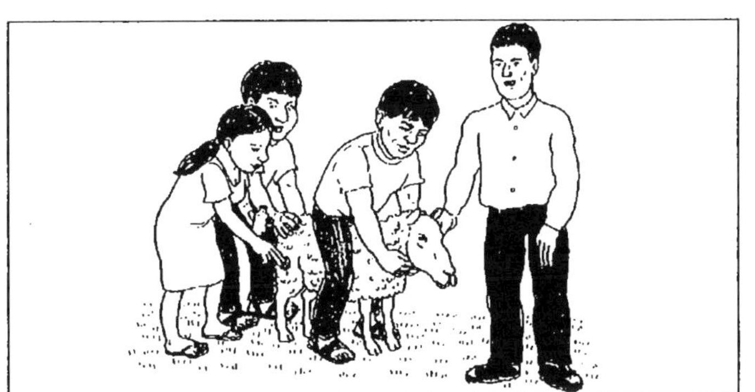

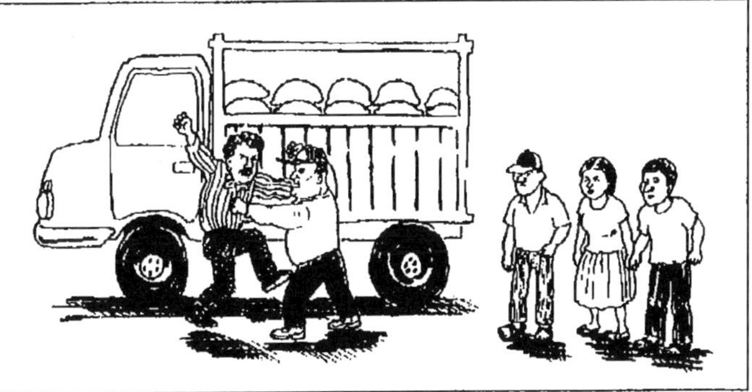

Group 3: What does education talk to us about?

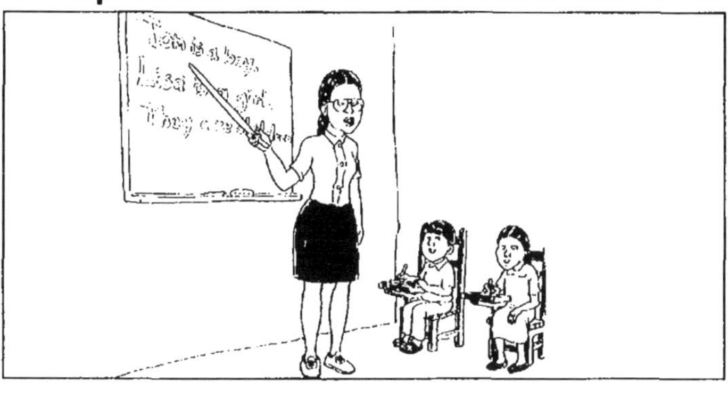

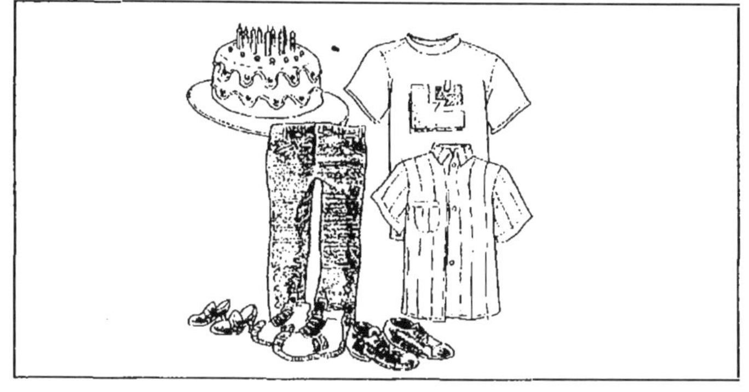

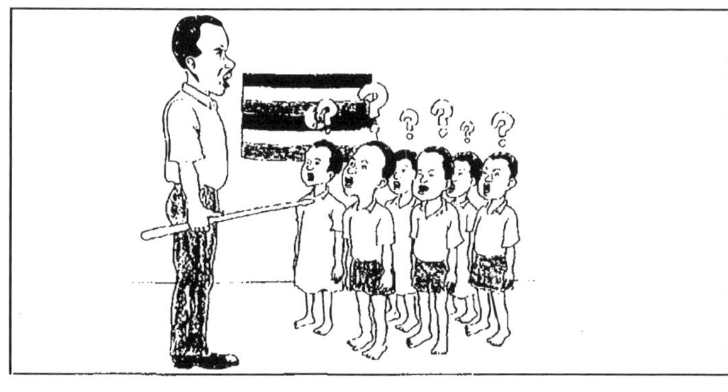

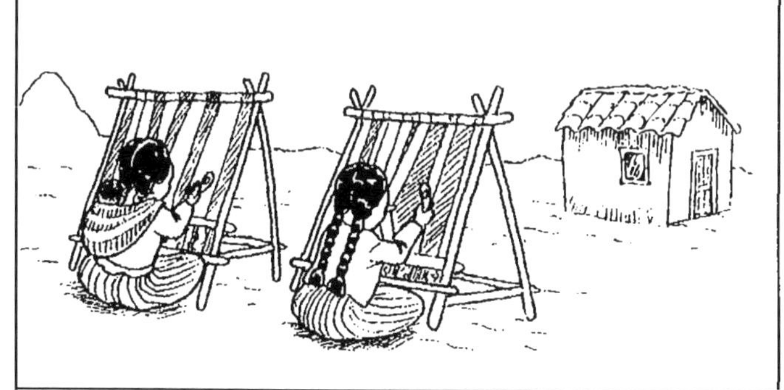

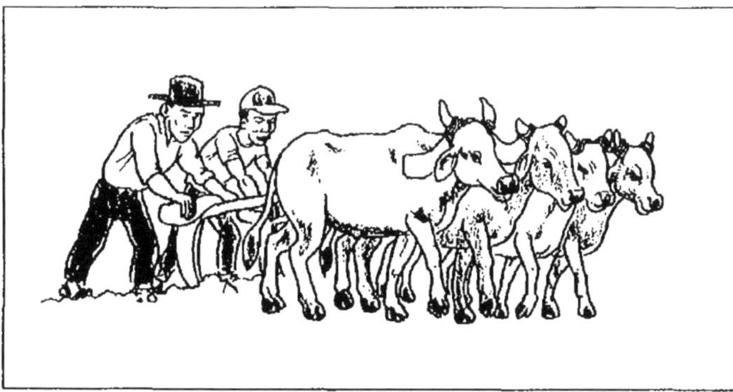

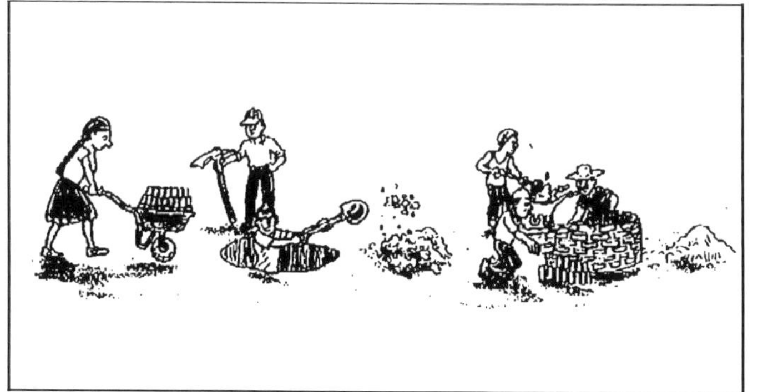

Group 4: What values does education have?

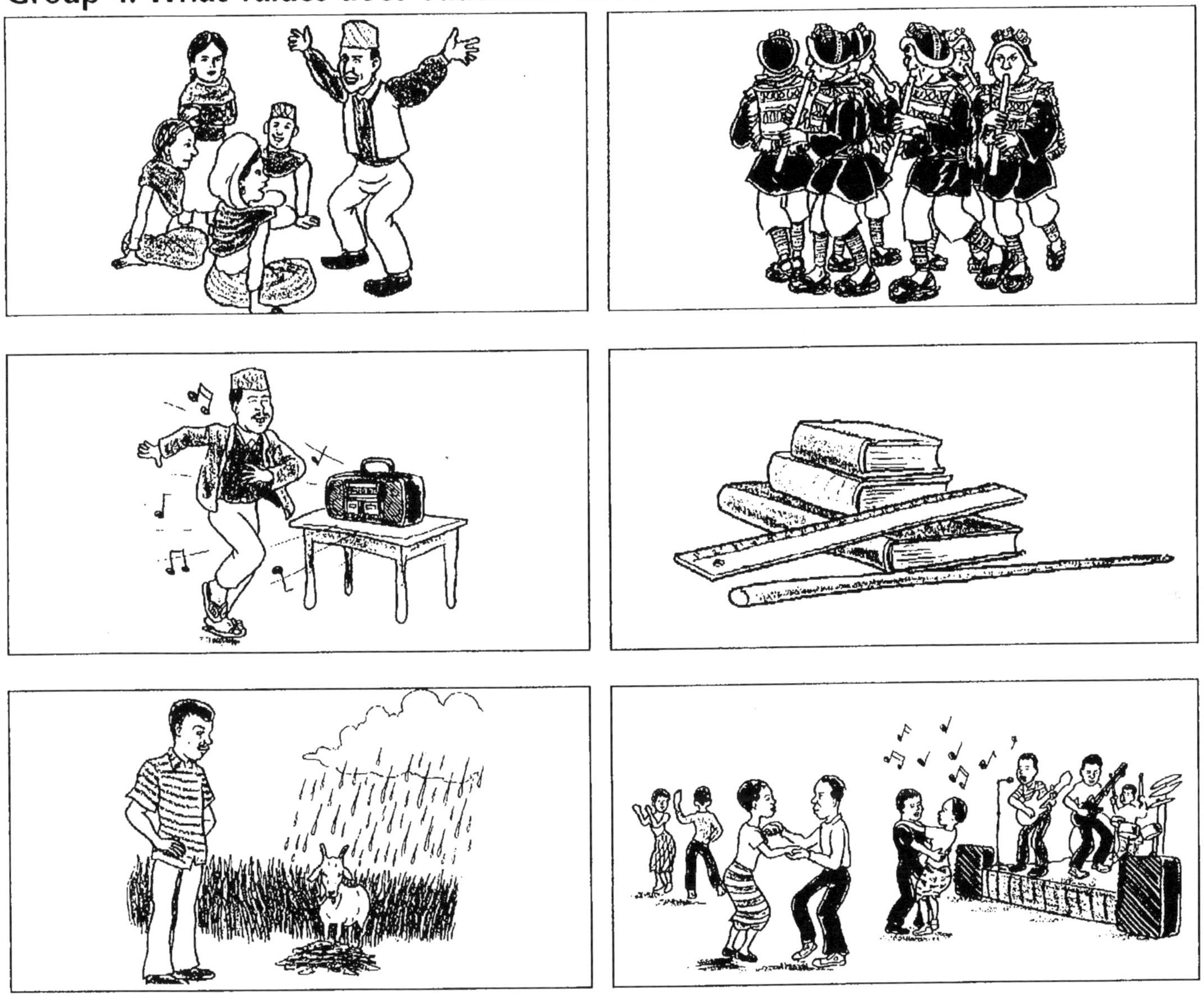

What is typical traditional education like?

• The teacher is in charge.
• Teacher chooses topics.
• Teacher lectures, demonstrates, explains, questions
• Students listen and respond to rote learning
• The answers are already known
• Little discussion
• Teacher knows it all.
• Students are inferior

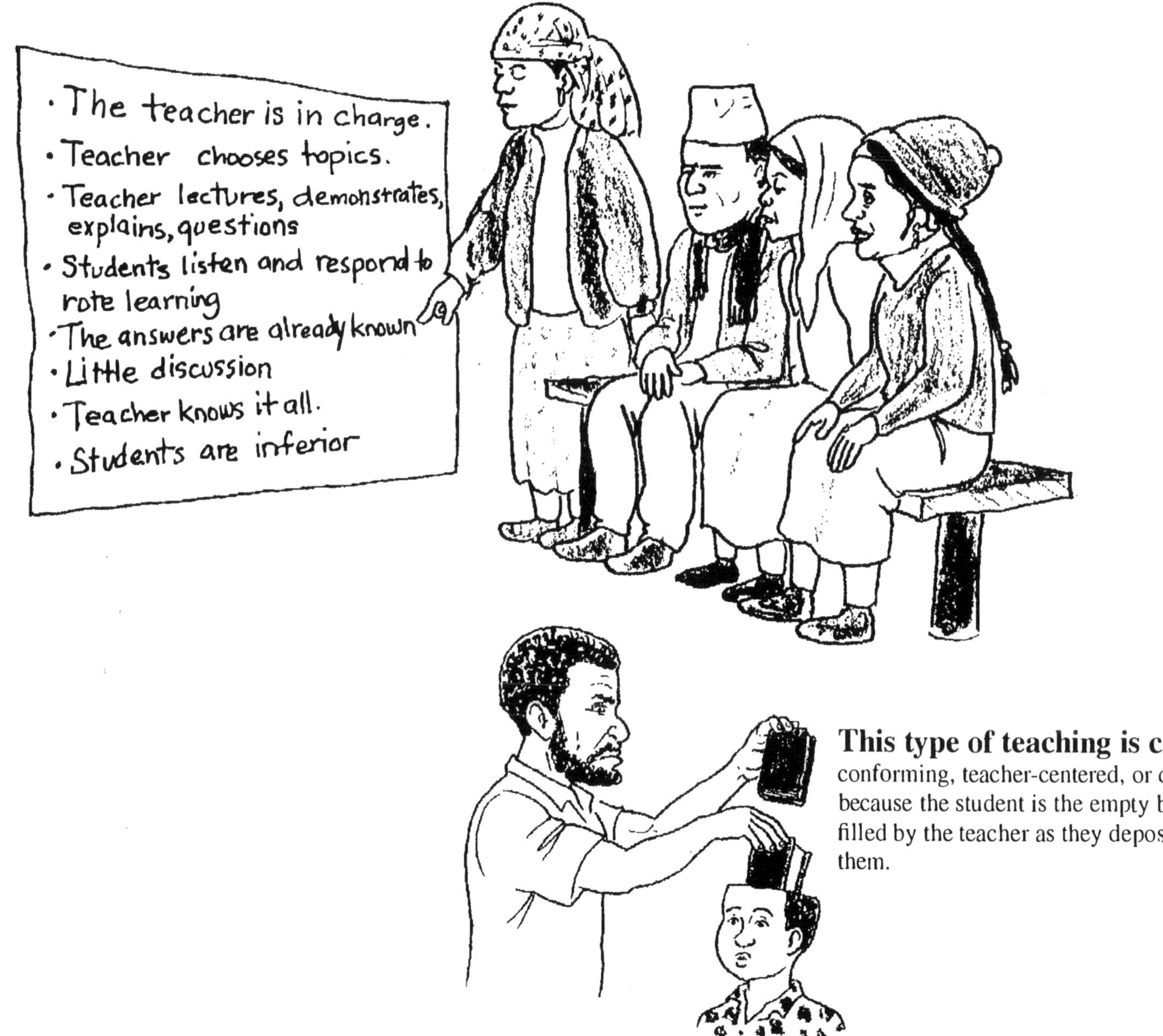

This type of teaching is called banking, conforming, teacher-centered, or dominant education because the student is the empty bank which must be filled by the teacher as they deposit knowledge into them.

What should be the characteristics of good adult education?

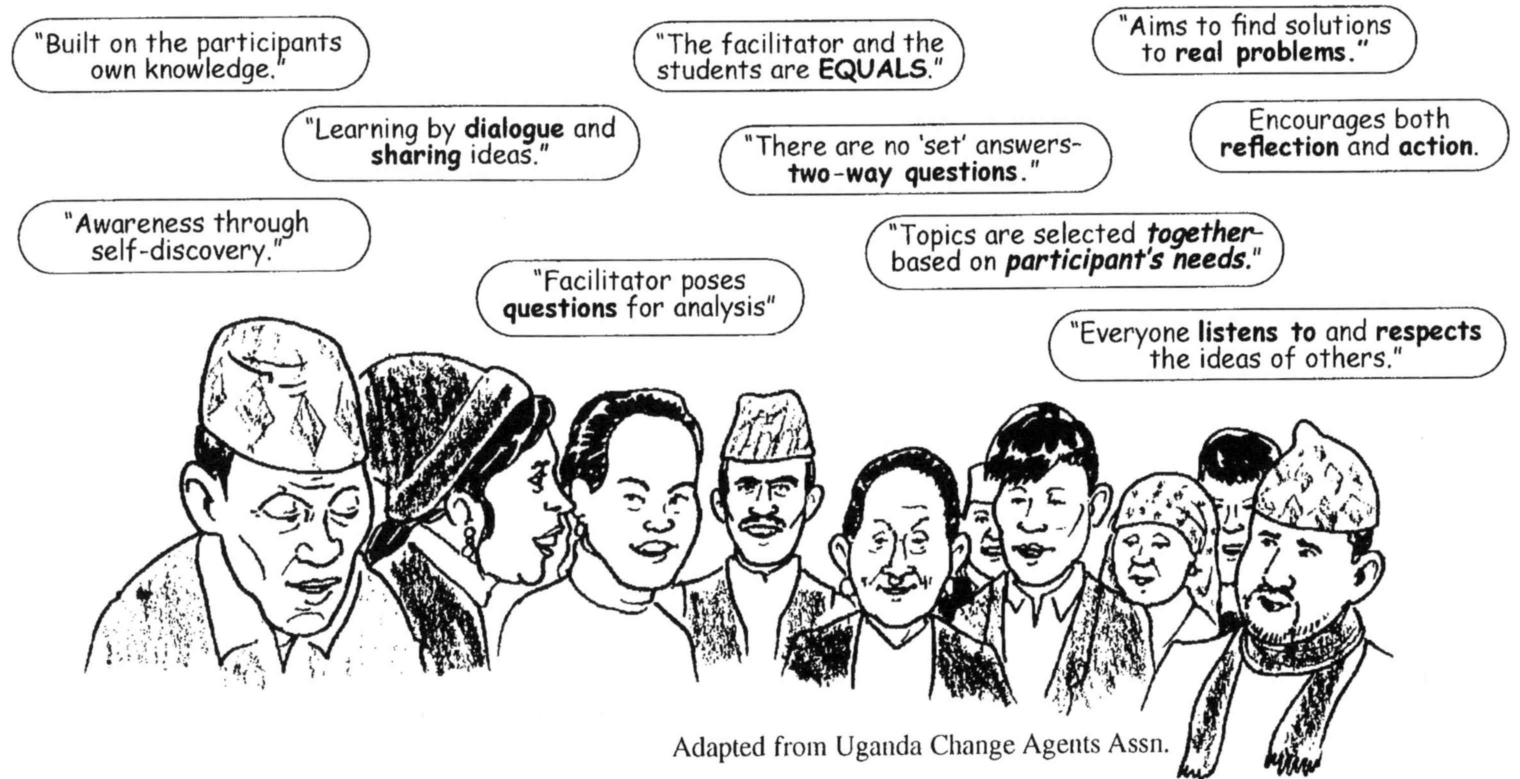

Adapted from Uganda Change Agents Assn.

This type of education is known as liberating or transforming education, the education of the people, or popular education. It is also called problem-solving, learner-centered education for change. The aim of this type of education is to produce critical thinkers who are able to respond flexibly to changing situations, and solve new problems as they arise. The "banking" concept tends to indoctrinate to a social order, producing people who are fixed in their ideas and resistant to change.

We teach the way we have learned.

So unless something happens to make us think differently we will teach the way we learned in school. That is why it is so important to give Community Livestock Workers, extensionists, and farmers the opportunity to analyze in depth their approach to education. They may use the method initially, but unless they have had the opportunity to reflect in depth, they will revert to the banking system when they train.

Your group may have different suggestions about the two types of education but you will all learn a lot from each other.

How adults learn

Two exercises for trainer training about adult learning:

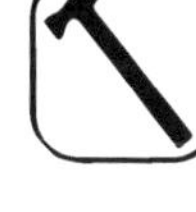

Exercise 1:

Ask your group of new trainers;

How do people learn in the community?

They may respond in many ways, but usually they begin with formal schooling as the only way to learn. As they analyze the question in depth they may identify some of these things:

- apprenticeship
- playing games
- practical experience
- trial and error
- story telling
- helping others work
- solving real problems
- discussions in small groups

Exercise 2:

Adults learn differently than children. Ask your group to **close their eyes and think about the best learning experience they have ever had.**

- Have them define the factors which they feel are the most important to adult learning.
- Each one writes their causes of adult learning on a card.
- Have each person share their causes and paste the cards to the board.
- Put the cards into possible categories, or organize similar cards together.
- Draw a conclusion about the most important factors. (Vella 1995)

Adults learn best when:

✓ They can **share their own experiences.**
✓ The **topic is relevant** to their situation
✓ They need to **know it now;** they can use it right away.
✓ **They discover** a new thing themselves–to know is to do!
✓ They **sense a need to change,** a disequilibrium. Adults need to see that what they now know and use is not adequate for their situation. They must feel a sense of imbalance or discomfort with their current attitude, knowledge or skills.
✓ They have a **good learning environment.**

> **As iron sharpens iron, so one man sharpens another.**
> Proverbs 27:17

These things create a good adult learning environment:

✓ A sense of **respect** for and a valuing of their opinion
✓ **Encouragement** to speak out and participate, to express their ideas
✓ A relaxed, **fun** learning environment.
✓ A **small group** environment. The group itself helps an adult to learn more rapidly, accept and experiment with new ideas, and be encouraged to apply those new ideas in their lives.
✓ Topics and tools which engage the learners mind, feelings, and bodies (they involve what we **think, feel, and do)** very actively.
✓ A **supportive, caring and accepting** environment. This gives an opportunity to experiment and be and think creatively without threat of punishment or ridicule.

For more on the environment for learning see "Implementation" pg. 122–132.

The road to adult learning

The next ten pages will describe each aspect of this chart in depth.

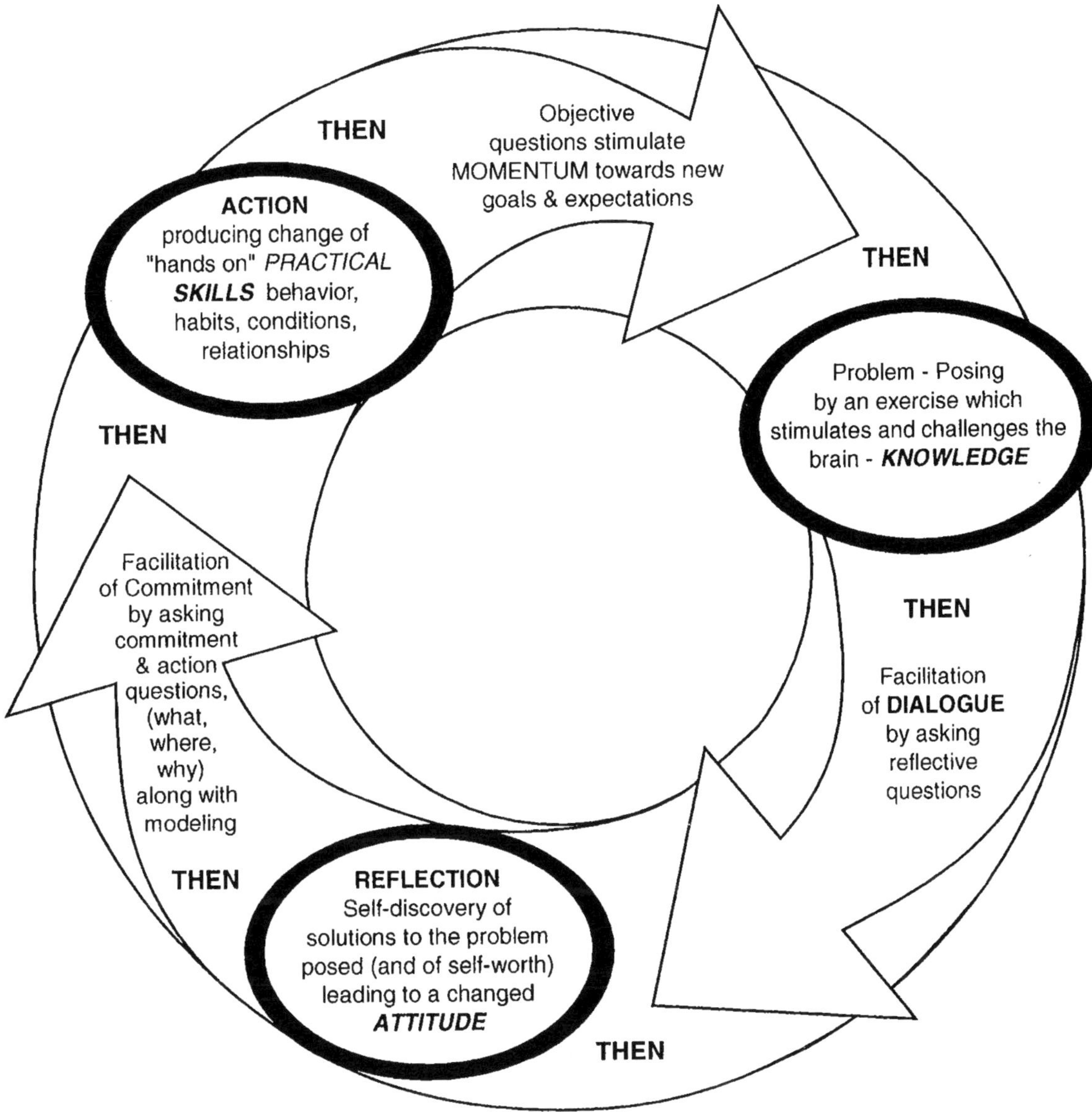

Please notice in this diagram two things:

1. The capitalized words in bold italics–
KNOWLEDGE - ATTITUDE - SKILLS
Every learning experience needs to engage the mind, heart and hands. Information alone does not cause learning.

2. The capitalized words in bold–
DIALOGUE - REFLECTION - ACTION
This is the process by which adults learn. The next pages will walk through this process step by step. This diagram may imply that these are steps to be followed. In fact, the learning process can begin at any point in the process above. It may also skip or combine areas.

Begin the process with a *dynamic* starter

We begin the process with a *dynamic* starter which makes adults aware of their sense of disequilibrium about a situation. This helps them to become engaged in defining the situation.

In the three previous examples a starter was used to begin the discussion on education: The picture, the multiple pictures and the "I'm hungry" game, all used *dynamic* starters. They serve to help people focus on the problem and to get everyone starting from the same spot in a dialogue. This type of activity will be called a *dynamic* in this book because it is a dynamic way to get people involved in a situation. It is an exercise which poses a question to people to stimulate their thinking on a situation. *Dynamics* can include things such as role plays, pictures, games, maps, ranking, or just a well stated open question. For samples of many *dynamics* see "Tools" pg. 235.

See pictures on the following page.

We use *dynamics* with adults because:

1. They help people reach a **sense of disequilibrium.** Adults especially must feel like there is a need to take a closer look at something in order to desire to change. They need to sense that something is not quite right before they want to discuss possible change. The *dynamic* challenges their current knowledge, facts, and awareness. Adults will say to themselves, "Maybe I should take a closer look at this."
2. *Dynamics* get everyone **considering the same situation at the same time.** The differences in experience with a problem create the richness of the dialogue. This is where we all start learning, but we need to start out together.
3. *Dynamics* **pose the problem to be discussed** in a clear way. This is why it is so important that a *dynamic* always ask a question and never present an answer.

   I have seen many role plays in livestock training in which an owner brings a sick animal to a Community Livestock Worker who gives it the appropriate treatment after discussing the symptoms with the owner. The intent is to teach the symptoms and treatment of the disease. Is this a *dynamic?* NO! There is no question asked by the role play. It is just a way of acting out the "correct" information. This is one example of how role plays can be used to disguise the "banking system" of education.

   How could this role play be changed (give an example) so it asks a question?

   Although this type of role play is not appropriate as a *dynamic,* it could be used for participants to report the conclusions of a discussion. It could also be used for CLWs to practice their examination and treatment skills.
4. *Dynamics* set the stage for an atmosphere of active involvement and participation. If the participants develop the dynamic themselves, they are already actively engaged in solving the problem when the discussion begins. Imagine how engaged the people are in the dynamic of the men with the bananas rescuing the starving community!
5. *Dynamics* help people see a direct link from the problem to themselves. They see that the question is directly applicable to their farm, family, or community. Adults need to see this direct link before they want to learn and to change. All dynamics spring from the people's real life situation. With a walk through the village and pastures with the people, looking at a sick animal together, a role play, or a drawing, people begin right away to try to solve the problem.

Some believe that just by playing games, or using role plays and drawings they are doing training with a participatory approach. That couldn't be farther from the truth! Participatory training is a lot more than games, exercises, and *dynamics.* **Although a *dynamic* is an important part of initiating dialogue, a well phrased open question can be just as effective!**

Don't get caught in the trap of thinking that just because you have done a role play your training is participatory. A role play or game can also be used in a banking system of training. The problem-posing approach to education has to do with:

- Using the steps which follow on the next pages: dialogue – reflection – action
- How the dialogue develops among the participants
- The attitude of the facilitators toward the participants and the participants toward each other

Consider these picture *dynamics* – the two on the top ask questions, the two on the bottom give answers:

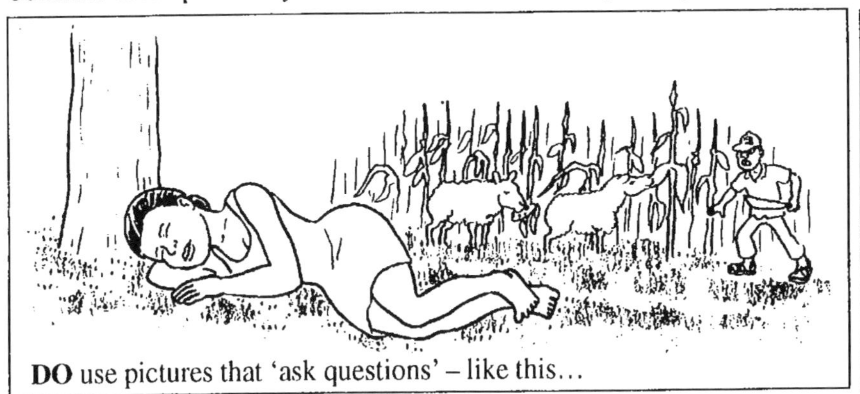

DO use pictures that 'ask questions' – like this…

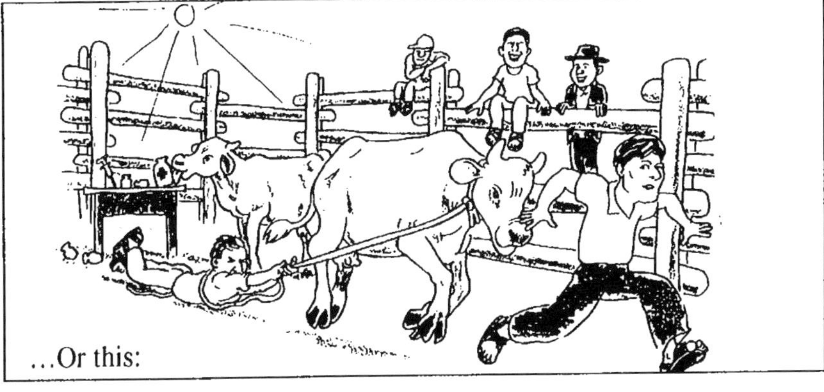

…Or this:

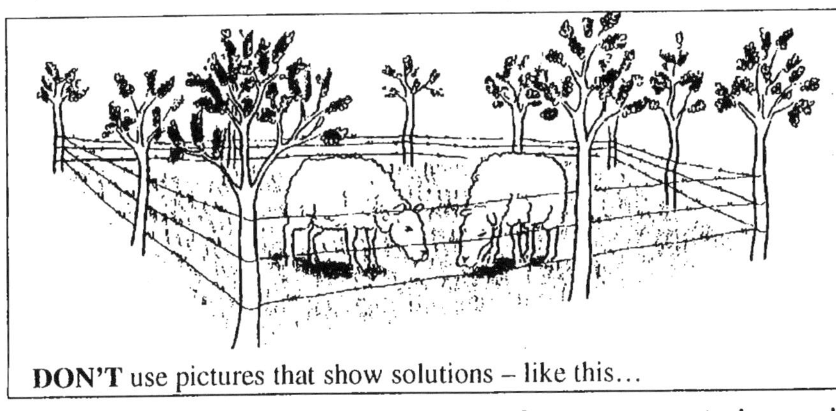

DON'T use pictures that show solutions – like this…

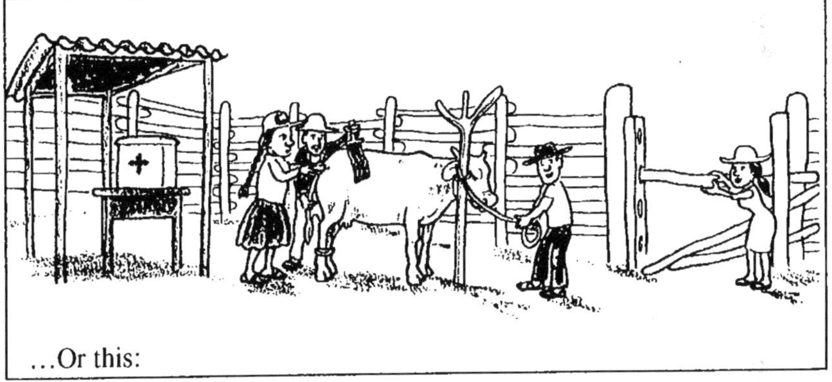

…Or this:

All *dynamics*, be they role plays, puppet shows, games, stories or pictures should pose a question for the participants to ponder. The *dynamic* should not provide the answer!

The *dynamic* 'plants the seed' in the process of growing change. We must still water it and weed it and make sure the climate is right to arrive at change through dialogue and process.

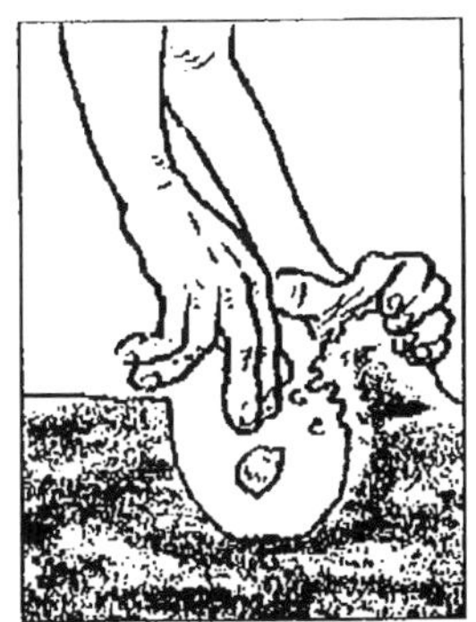

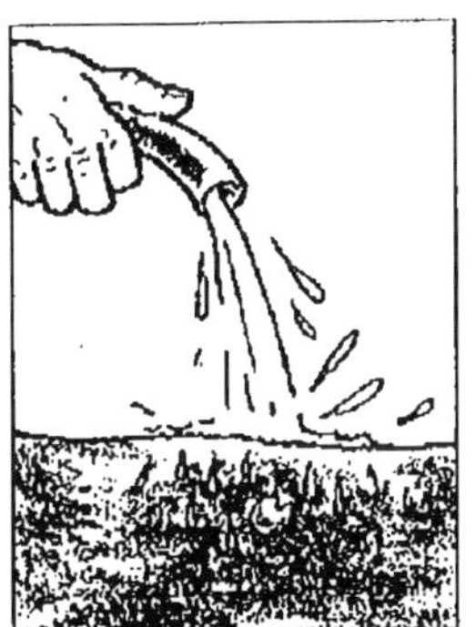

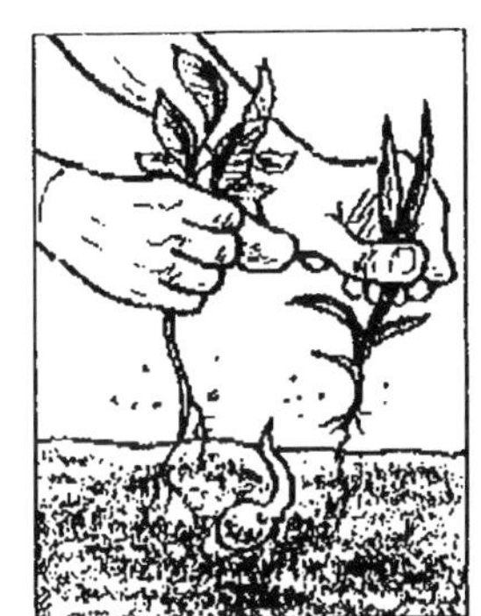

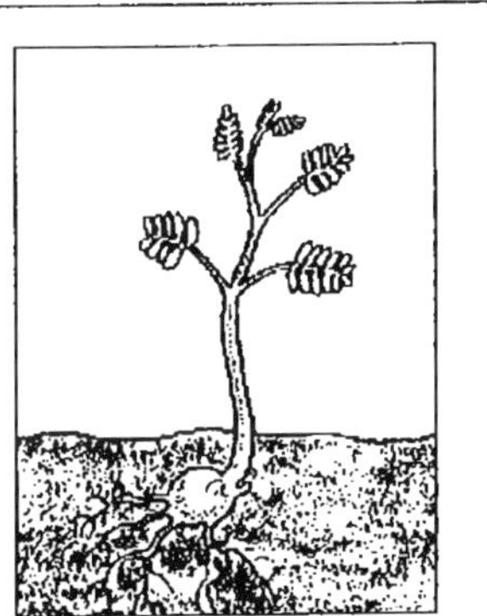

Moving from a *dynamic* to action

Once the *dynamic* has been completed and people are thinking about the posed problem, how do we facilitate movement toward action? This process is virtually the same for group problem solving in a meeting or for facilitating a class session. The class session begins with the presentation of a problem or situation (previously defined by the community in the needs assessment) as does the group problem solving process used in a meeting. Often the session will begin with a *dynamic* which gets everyone thinking about the problem.

Once the *dynamic* has challenged the adults to think about a situation, they move together through Dialogue and Reflection towards Action.

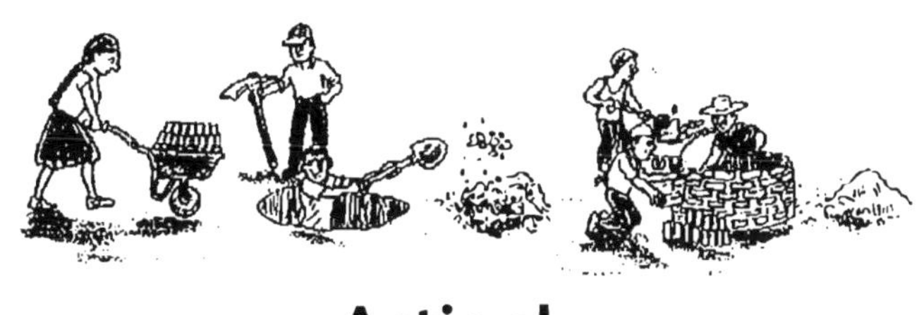

Action!

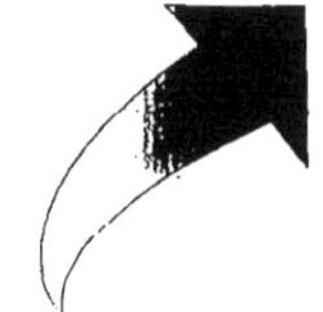

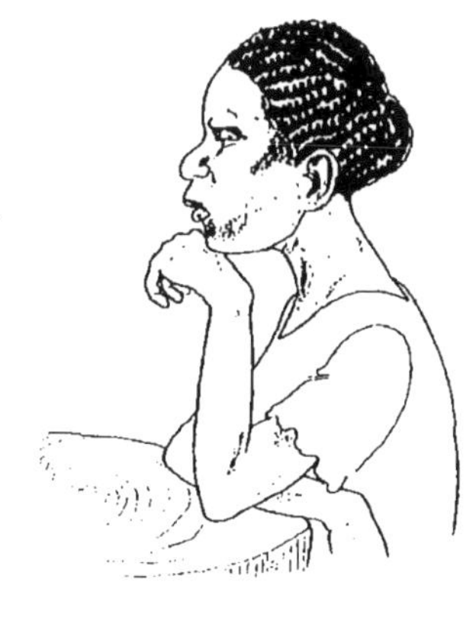

Reflection

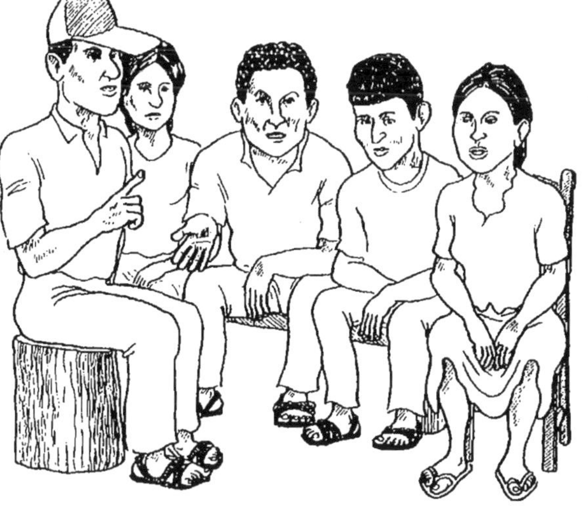

Dialogue

Questions which illustrate the steps in analyzing a *dynamic*

Here is a set of open questions which initially may help you in understanding how to facilitate the dialogue process. These are not the questions you should always use. Appropriate questions will depend on the theme, conditions and cultures.

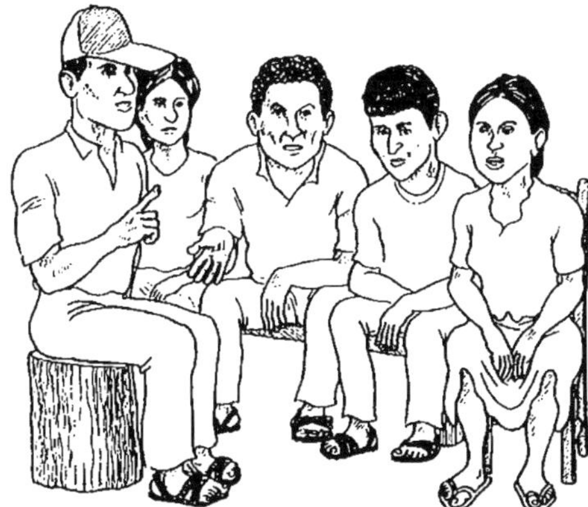

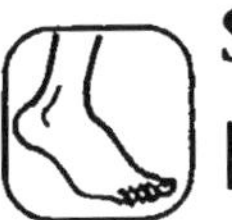

Step one: DIALOGUE

Define the problem or situation:

1. **What did you see happening here?** Arrive at a clear description of the problem. Include feelings but don't suggest blame.

2. **Why do you think it happens?** Help people begin to analyze the problem. If it is a touchy village problem (e.g. the president of the livestock co-op who has run off with the co-op savings) people can begin to analyze it from afar, without it being too personal. The dynamic provides a safer atmosphere to discuss difficult issues.

3. **Does it happen here (in our village, on our farm or in our organization or institution)?** This brings the example home, shows the obvious connection to our reality. Here it is appropriate for people to express their feelings but not to attach blame.

4. **What problems does it cause?** Together make a clear statement of the problem as it relates directly to us.

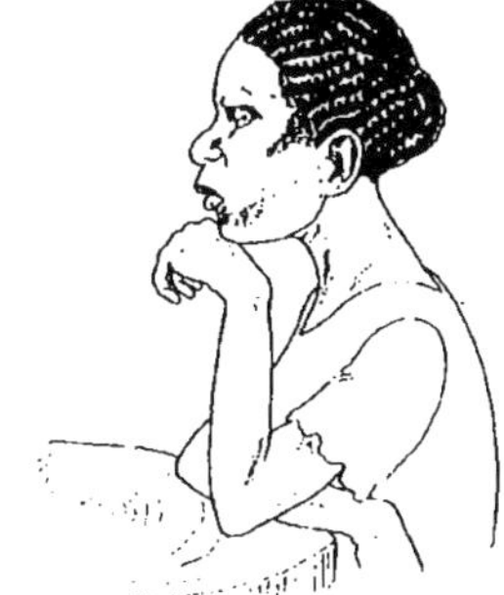

It is indispensable to have a habit of observation and reflection.
–Abraham Lincoln

Step two: REFLECTION

Analyze the problem:

5. **What causes those problems at their roots?** Analyze deeply to get to the root causes of the problems. You can ask "Why is that?" and "But, why is that?" to get deeper. After each answer ask again, "Why?" (See pg. 22–25 "Taking a deeper look at the problem".)

6. **What can we do about it?** This helps us move toward collective or personal action in solving the problems. This is where the possible solutions are proposed

Observe and gather information:

7. **Do we need further information?** This may be a discussion with everyone sharing their experience, including, in some cases, the facilitator. The group may also need to consult an expert or go somewhere to gather the information.

Narrow the alternatives:

The group will have made a list of a number of possible solutions. Now they must critically analyze the options and evaluate alternative solutions. Everyone should offer their solutions without being criticized. It is very important for the facilitator to present the information again at this time. People have shared information in the dialogue and proposed many solutions. The facilitator can help by organizing the information in a way that is easy to understand. This leads to clarity for decision making.

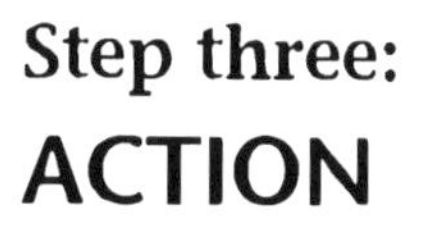

Step three: ACTION

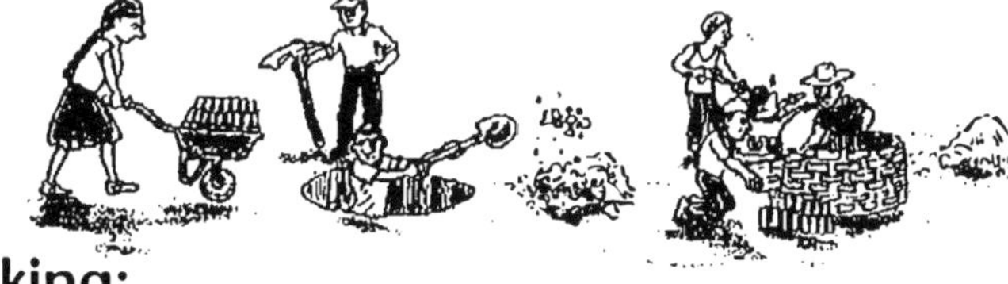

Decision making:

There may be several viable alternative solutions. In the case of a disease treatment there may be local and purchased treatments. What are the advantages and disadvantages of each? Are there reasons why the solution won't work? For group process it is important that there be mutual agreement about the solution or solutions. State the solution so it is clearly understood by all.

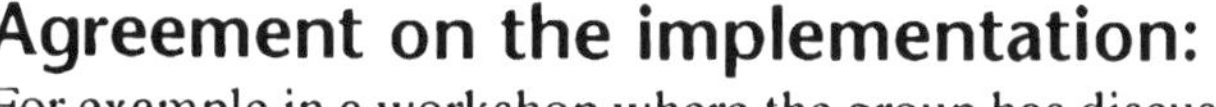

Agreement on the implementation:

For example in a workshop where the group has discussed internal parasites, a plan could be designed for the practicum in the afternoon to deworm the animals. With a community, it may mean a plan for a deworming campaign of all the animals in the community.

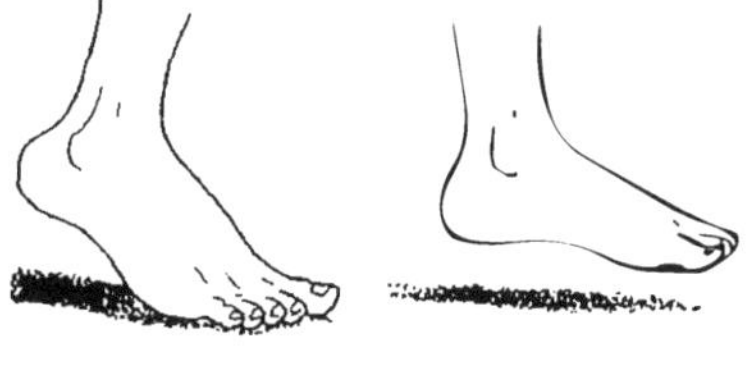

Review the process:

Summarize the process – the problem, the solution, the plan. Group process, planned workshop activities, and community work entail a further step:

Monitoring and evaluation:

Monitor the process on a regular basis. Perhaps the situation has changed or the solution is no longer effective. How did we do? If there was a workshop activity, what were the results of our work? How can we apply this in our community? Even for a solution on an individual level we should reflect on and evaluate our actions.

The key to reflection: taking a deeper look at the problem

This is a series of *dynamics* and information from a workshop for trainers. They are in the order used in the workshop to help a group think through the process of in-depth analysis for action:

Dynamic #1 – Taking a superficial look:

Note: the end of this *dynamic* is on page 25, after the participants think through the reflective process with three other *dynamics*.

- Divide everyone in the workshop into small groups of five or six people. Ask the groups to go outside to look at several things in the community.

Some examples:
- Group 1 - a house
- Group 2 - the health clinic
- Group 3 and 4 - two different families' farms
- Group 5 - a business from a wealthier family (state the business name only)

The significant problems we face cannot be solved at the same level of thinking we were at when we created them.
–Albert Einstein

- When each group comes back, they report on what they have seen. Usually they will report only superficial observations. They might report a house with a dead duck out front and two children, etc. Do not discuss this in great depth. Go on to *Dynamic #2*.
- Note: you can send people out wherever your workshop takes place: in a village or city or on a farm. The idea is to have people begin to look at cause and effect. This initial look gives participants a sense of disequilibrium when they realize they have looked at the things around them quite superficially.

Now enter a time of reflection with the group: Ask, did you look at the house, clinic, farm, or business superficially, with self-interest, or deeply?

Dynamic #2 – How do we look at our situation and analyze it?

These six pictures have been used to create a dialogue about the way we look at a problem:

Look – Analyze – Act

LOOK at the problem:
The CLW and the community look at a cow which is thin and sick.

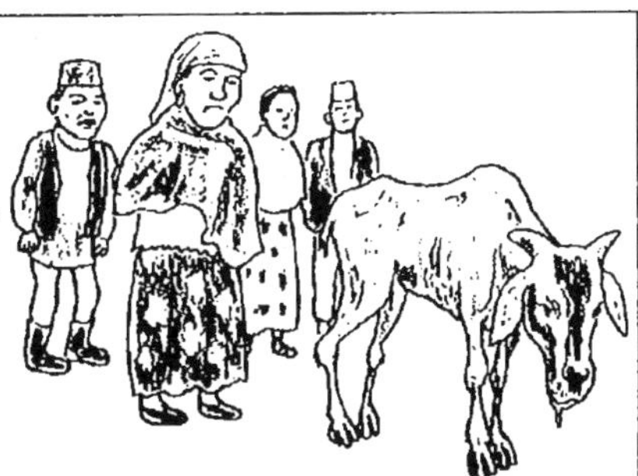

ANALYZE the root causes:
They think through the many causes such as uncontrolled burning, fenceline arguments, expensive medicines…

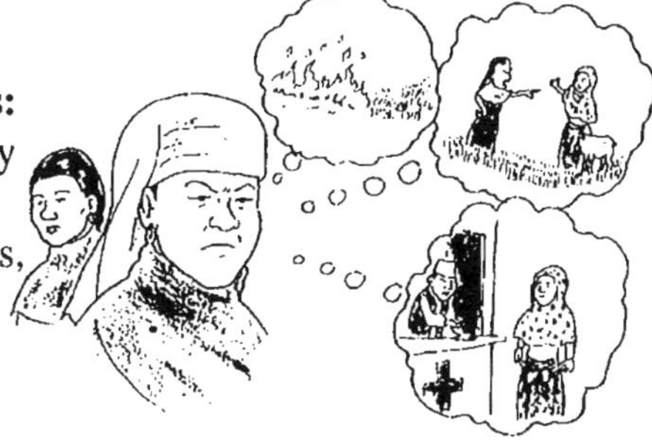

ACT to solve the problem:
They act together to plan their vision for their community with controlled burning, fenced or stabled animals, land which produces well.

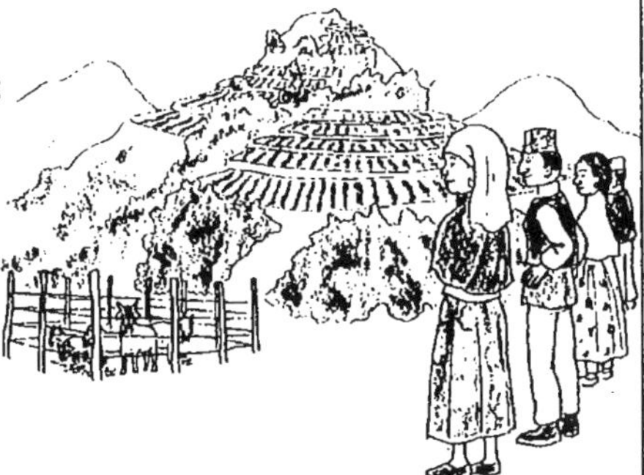

How do we analyze the situation?

We can look at it superficially:
As the woman looks at her pig she sees it has an infected wound. It is sick and could die.

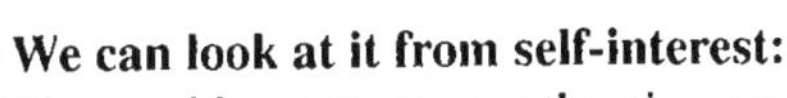

We can look at it from self-interest:
The wealthy woman sees the pig as an economic opportunity. She will buy the pig inexpensively, give it treatment and make money. She does not care that the poor woman will lose and remain poor.

We can look at it in depth, down to the roots:
If the woman examines her pig closely she will find there is a big splinter in the wound. This has been causing the wound and the infection. Now, she can deal with the splinter and the wound and the pig will get well!

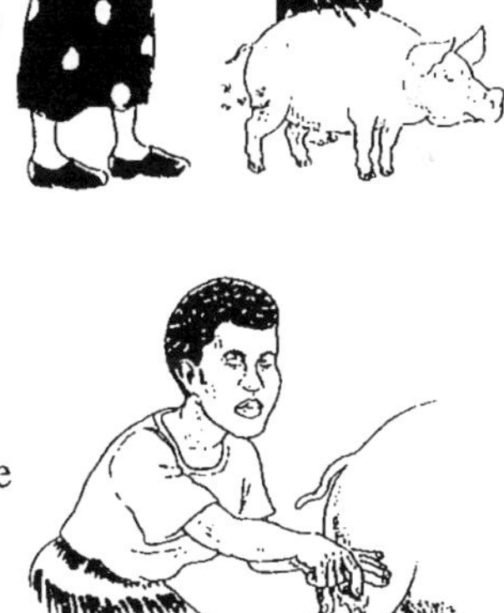

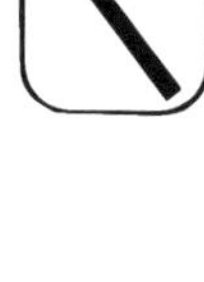

Dynamic #3 – Taking a deeper look.

The six pictures on the previous page have been used to create a dialogue about the way we look at a problem.

Use this simple *dynamic,* together with the pictures to illustrate looking superficially and looking deeply. Use a simple example:

- Take someone's bag and look on the outside. Ask everyone, "What do you see?" This is superficial because you do not know what is inside.
- Take something out of the bag – perhaps a pamphlet. We don't know yet what is inside the pamphlet. Unless we look at what is in the pamphlet we are still examining the bag superficially.
- Take out a wallet. – Inside there is one dollar. Ask everyone, "What is this for?"

They may respond with something like: "To buy bread"

- Then you ask, "But why does she want to buy bread?" They may answer, "To live."
- Then you ask, "But why do you want to live?"

You must keep looking deeper and deeper, keep asking the question, why? why? why? This way you will arrive at the roots of the situation. This way you will have analyzed a situation in depth.

The job of the livestock worker is to analyze deeply and to encourage the community and livestock producers to analyze deeply as well. We can always do a better analysis with many people than we can alone.

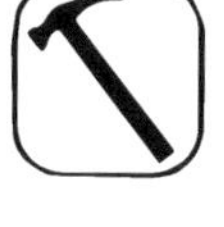

Dynamic #4 – A game to illustrate looking with self-interest:

Use this *dynamic,* together with the picture of the rich woman buying the pig on the previous page to illustrate what looking at something with self interest is all about.

- Divide everyone in the room into four teams by counting off. Ask for a volunteer to represent each team. Put the four people inside a rope which is tied and held in a circle at waist height. Outside the rope at each corner is a pencil, or fruit or something they want to reach.
- Identify the four people inside the rope. Call them: the president of the village organization, the president of the livestock association, the president of the agricultural cooperative, the president of the health committee (or use four other appropriate community leaders).
- Tell the four people, "On the count of three, try to get a pencil." Have the teams root for their president. Generally, all four will struggle with the rope and pull each other until one person gets a pencil. It is good to include both men and women inside the rope.

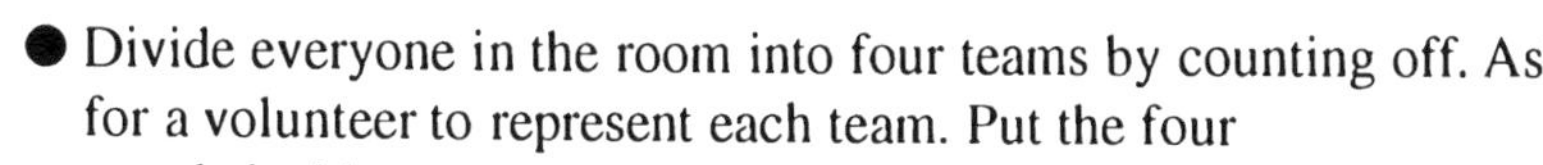

- Ask everyone, "Is this the way the community is?" People may answer many things. They will often comment that many times the community leaders or other people act only out of self interest. They do not think about the others outside of their group who may have other needs. The dialogue can be about looking and acting in self interest. "This is the way they divide us." "They manipulate the community for their ends."
- What could they have done differently? Let the same people play again. This time they will generally talk together and get all the pencils together so each one gets one.

This is the idea of thinking and acting out of self-interest.

Ask everyone to give some examples of how community organizations and outsider institutions also act out of self-interest.

Back to Dynamic #1 – Taking a superficial look, part 2

Now return to the first *dynamic* in this section. It started on page 22.

- What does the group think about how they went out to look at the things in the community (the house, lands, business, health clinic)? Did they look superficially, with self-interest or deeply? The participants should realize by now that they took a very superficial look. Send people out again in their groups to take a deeper look and come back and report.
- Then analyze the results together.

Now you are on the road to looking for the root causes of the problems.

The application of knowledge is where learning occurs:
Telling is not teaching
Listening is not learning.
–John Collum

Finding a solution together

Once we have taken a closer look at the problem and determined the root causes, we can work together toward a solution. But where do the solutions come from?

If the Community Livestock Worker, extensionist, or facilitator comes with a solution to the problem, it is his or her solution, not that of the community. Sometimes the community will choose something different from the Community Livestock Worker's idea. Is that bad?

Consider, for example, this community:

We have talked about the problem that our animals are skinny and don't have milk in the dry season. We decided we want to do something about the pastures. What are your suggestions?
Since we are nearing the rainy season, why don't we plant a bank of dry season pastures and trees for everyone?
Good idea! The co-op has a piece of land we can use.
I don't know which pastures will work the best. I suggest we learn in a workshop about dry season pastures and good organization.
Good idea!
I agree. When can we...

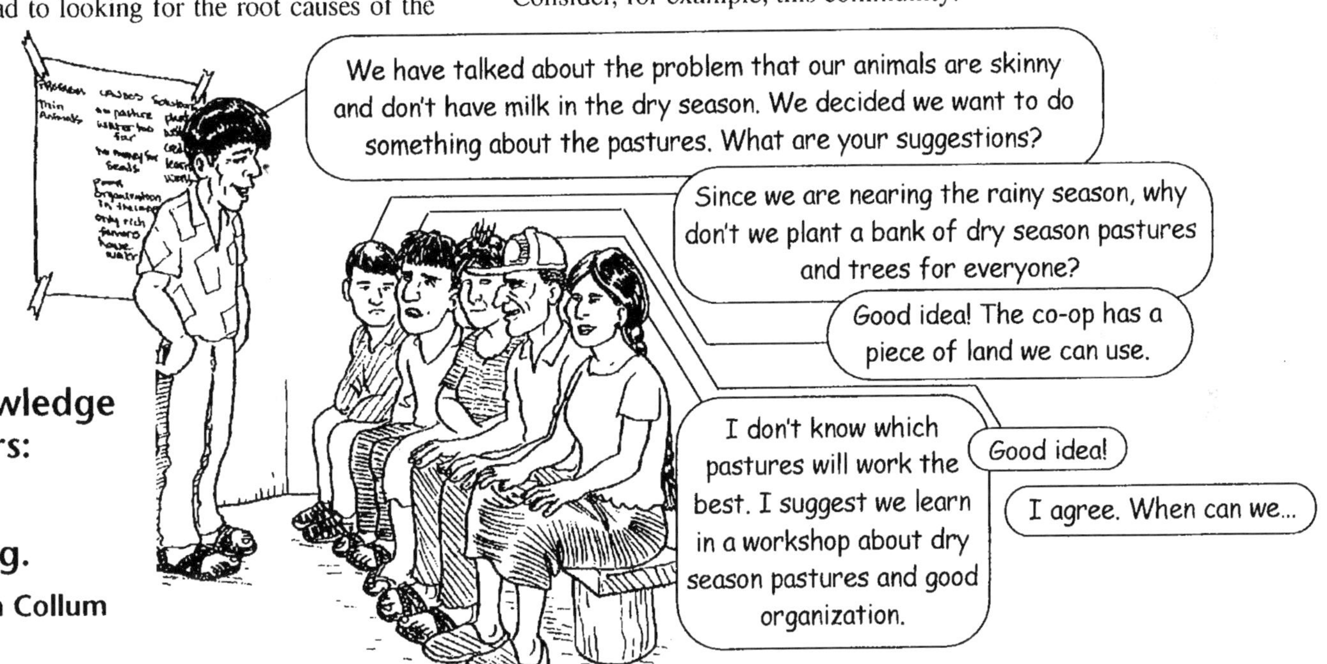

The community here has moved on to collecting information, which follows the process of analysis of a problem and a suggestion of possible solutions. Again, each person will share their thoughts and ideas. The Community Livestock Worker will sometimes need to organize the input of an outsider, or give new information to the community.

Advantages and disadvantages of participatory training

If the learner-centered approach is so successful in helping people to solve their own problems, why haven't more livestock and other agricultural programs adopted it?

Many livestock and agricultural programs with training components are designed with a specific focus in mind:

- That poor farmers have more animals;
- That the small farmer sector produce more rice and corn for the city;
- That the farmers stay on their farms and not move to the city;
- That farmers use methods like zero grazing and terracing to stop soil erosion.

These programs are not focused on the farmers' learning to solve their own problems but on providing solutions to the problems the government and nongovernment institutions see as the most important problems. Also, most professional agriculturalist technicians teach the way they have been taught, which is in a top - down, controlling approach which resists change. Most agriculturalists have not been trained as teachers and have never examined how adults learn best.

As the people who have used the learner-centered approach around the world have shared, there are several advantages and disadvantages to using it.

ADVANTAGES

- It is all-inclusive and everyone can participate without discrimination by sex, age, literacy, etc.
- The people elect the most important topics. It is relevant.
- People can put the information to use immediately.
- Locally available resources are used.
- It builds self-esteem and confidence.
- It encourages villagers to solve their own problems.
- The language is understood by all.
- It creates broad-based support for village initiatives.
- A greater number of new and appropriate technologies are transferred.
- The information is better understood.
- It allows researchers to learn from farmers' experiences.
- It allows the sharing of local knowledge.

DISADVANTAGES

- It takes more time.
- It covers less information in one workshop.
- Smaller groups of people are exposed to new technologies.
- It requires new skills on the part of the trainers.
- Individuals may show resistance because it is an unfamiliar approach.
- It has higher initial cost.
- There are few people in agricultural fields who know how to facilitate this way.
- The facilitator has less control of content and directions.
- It may be politically volatile.

Try discussing advantages and disadvantages with the Community Livestock Workers after they have experienced the problem-posing method. Have them make their own list, and some of the others can be added in. As each is analyzed, it is often seen that many of the perceived disadvantages are really advantages from the standpoint of the participants. The time spent and amount of information given are typical disadvantages listed by agricultural professionals. However, when Community Livestock Workers look at their true purpose, they see it is to assist the community in solving its problems and moving toward it's vision, no matter how long that takes!

As we describe and learn the different tools in this book, we must always remember they are tools for the use of individuals or community organizations. When a community organization understands the difference between the 'banking' approach and the 'problem-posing' approach to education, they can apply the tools to achieve very positive results in their community organization.

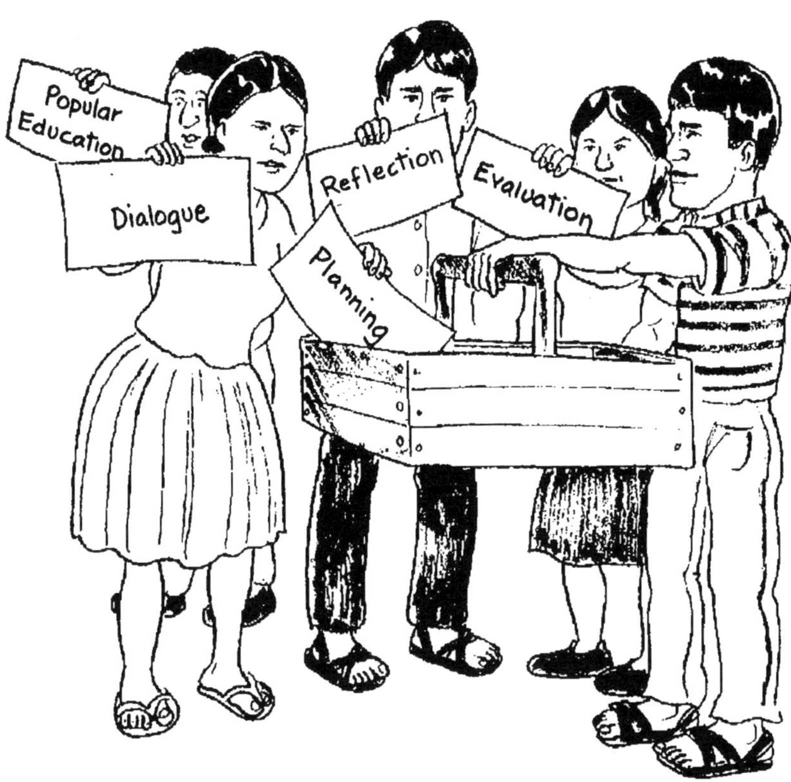

As the CLWs begin to work in their communities, encourage them to share their understanding of the tools in the same ways the tools have been shared with them. Or work with them to help them create new ways of sharing these ideas and discussing them in their village, ways that are appropriate to their village situation.

Chapter 2
Training is for...who?

This chapter covers the following topics:

Training should be available for everyone

There are as many different opinions on who should receive livestock training as there are programs. Should it be herders or owners, young people or older, men or women or children; or should the training be strictly for Community Livestock Workers who will then share their knowledge with their communities?

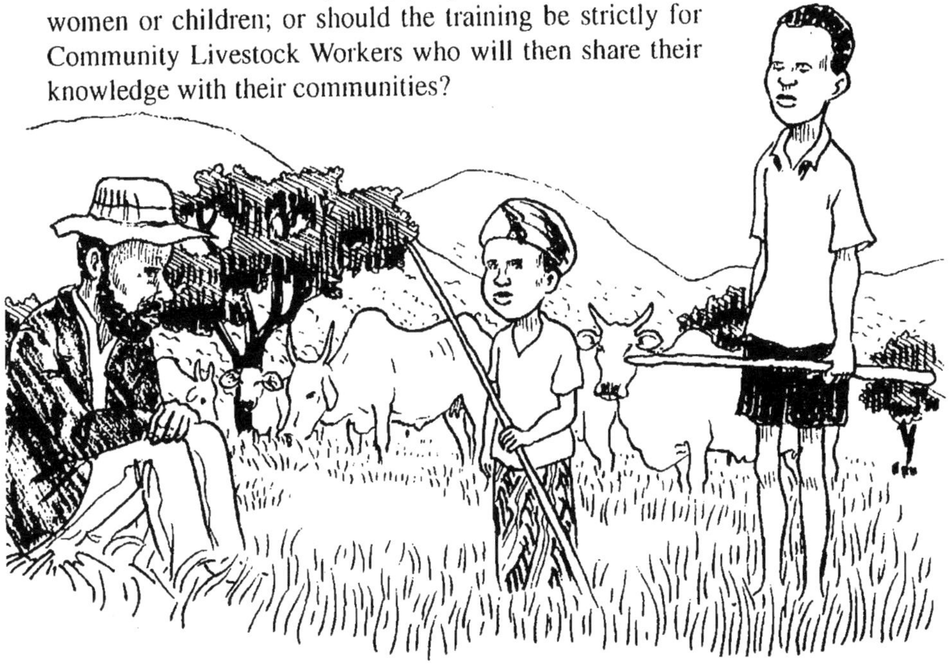

Although some of the information in this book is to help in the training of Community Livestock Workers, our experience leads us to believe that **some training should be available to anyone in the village** who wants it and will put it to use in the husbandry of their animals.

In the PROPECO program in Bolivia we began with training for all farmers' groups who desired it and requested it. Men, women, and young people participated in the workshops. Because the number of people who could participate in the workshops was small (no more than 25 per workshop) the families and villages decided who would be the best participants. This would have been a typical workshop:

My mother sent me because I read and write and herd the cows.
I came because I am the one who feeds and milks the cows.
Me too!
I came because we are sure the women can't learn because they can't read and write.
I came because I just received an animal on credit and I want to care for it the right way.
My mother sent me because she says she is too old to be in a class.

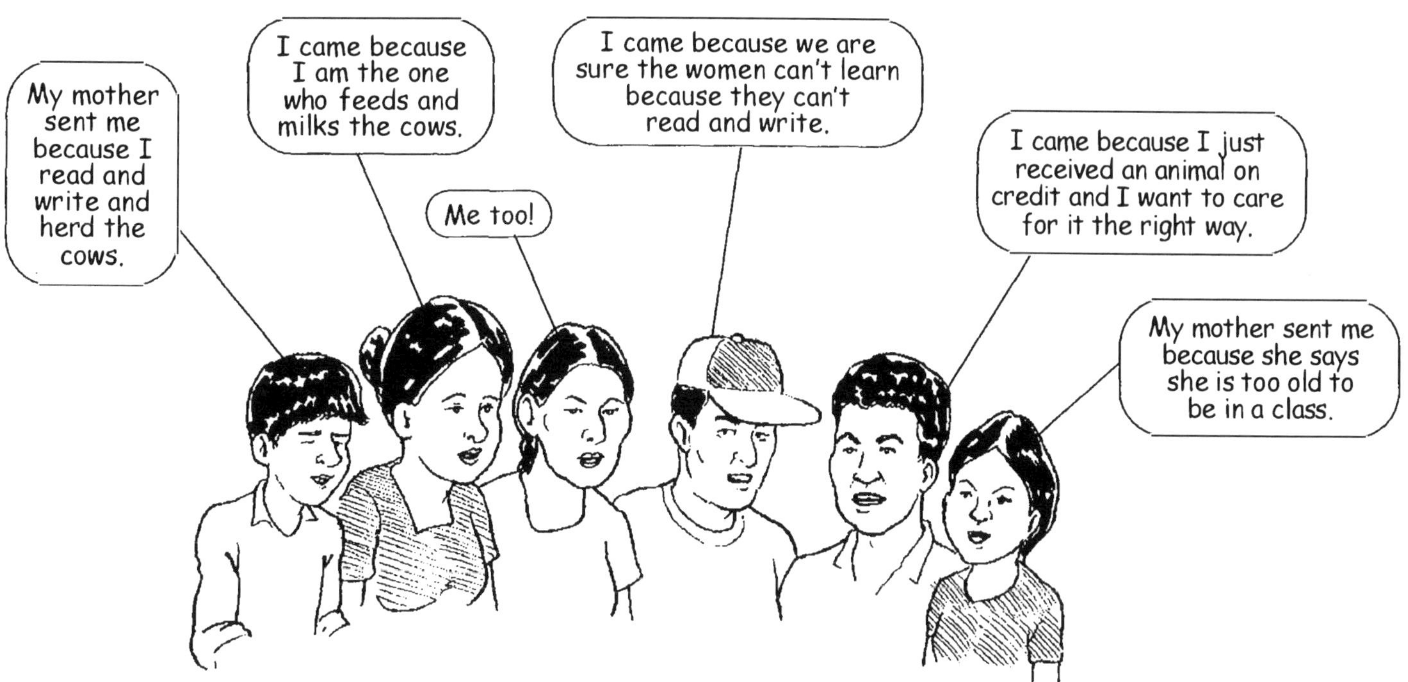

Even though they came for many different reasons, they all learned and were able to apply the information right away to their herds. After they had the workshop, they passed the idea on to other villages that the workshops really were for anyone who wanted them, whether or not they could read and write. Then all the people who came were those who wanted to learn and improve their livestock production.

During an evaluation of the program we asked several women's groups what they thought of the training they had received. This was part of their reply:

The topics we asked for on diseases are the ones we have used least. The ones we use all the time are pasture, vaccinations and deworming.
They presented the topics in a way we could understand.
Our animals are much healthier AND we receive a better price for them.
We vaccinate now and deworm always, and we have better pastures.

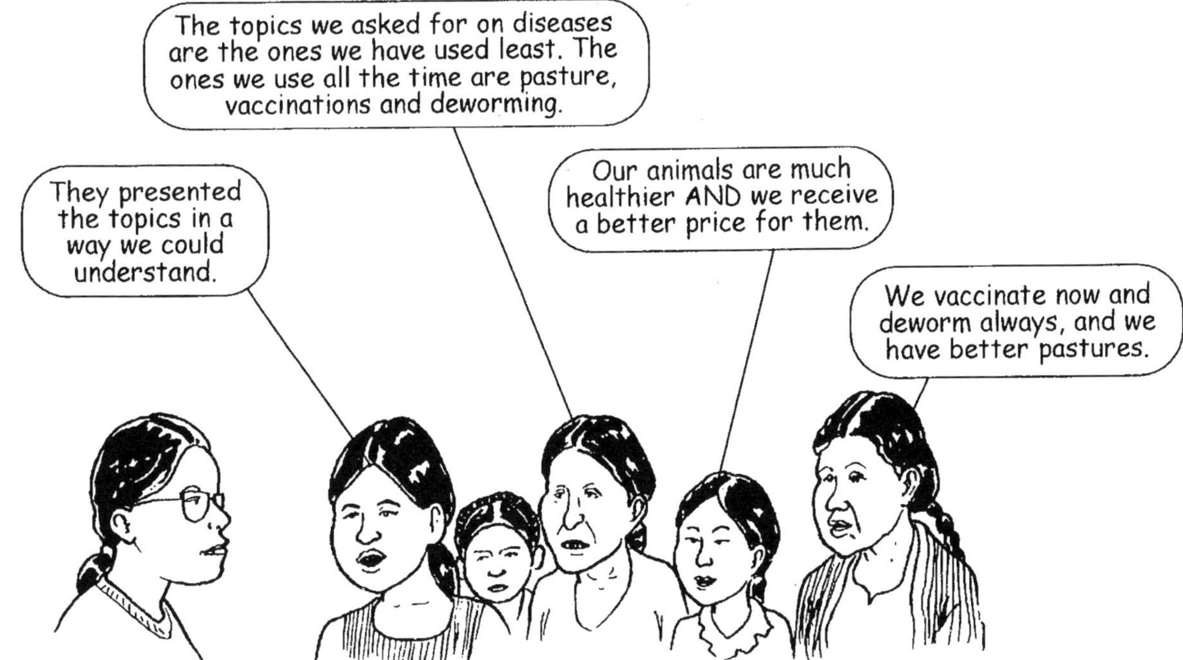

They found they could use the information right away on their farms. In Bolivia the women do the majority of the livestock care, so many changes and improvements occurred in management and production.

In many countries programs give training to Community Livestock Workers or promoters only. In several cases where these programs have been evaluated, the evaluation results say that farmers and herders in general should have received some training for better results. (ITDG 1992)

We have found that farmers with some training in livestock production will:

- Have a greater understanding of the need for and work of a Community Livestock Worker
- Be more supportive of a Community Livestock Worker
- Have a greater desire to implement good animal husbandry practices on their farms
- Be able to derive more benefit from their Community Livestock Worker's training.

Where there is training of CLWs there should also be training for anyone in the community who wants and needs it.

Why train Community Livestock Workers?

CLWs make a difference in their communities!

In a study done in Kenya for ITDG by Sarah Holden (Orito 1995) it was found:

- **CLWs encourage farmers to treat animals** - 62% of farmers in villages with CLWs do something about animal health compared to 44% in villages without CLWs.
- **CLWs heal animals** - When CLWs are used, recovery of animals is 70% while it is only 10% when they are not used.
- 72% of farmers will turn to CLWs as the first course of action when animals are sick.
- There is **lower animal mortality** in areas with CLWs than in those without.
- There are **higher milk yields and earnings** in areas with CLWs in comparison to those without.
- Livestock from areas with CLWs generally bring better prices.

They are effective extensionists

Although it is often easier for an outside expert to gain the respect and attention of community members, experience shows that as Community Livestock Workers gain knowledge, experience, and skills, they work more effectively with community members and have more impressive long-term results. Some of the reasons:

- They **speak the same language** as the community members and in the same way
- They **begin from the same experience base** and can often bring more relevant examples for community members to understand better.
- They have a **support system** within the community.
- They will be **in the community for the long haul,** not leaving when their job is over as an outsider would.
- They apply what they are learning to their own land and herds and **help people see things in action.**
- They help the community see that, yes, we can do it ourselves!

What motivates a CLW?

In Nepal, a group of CLWs shared what motivated them:

✓ They want to apply the training to their own animals. They work to improve their farm production and marketing.

✓ They want to learn more and understand more (personal intellectual growth).

✓ They want to operate a small business with the medicines and/or be able to use the medicine kits some programs provide.

✓ They want to be able to help the community with diagnosis and treatment and to provide a close source of medication and husbandry information.

✓ They want to serve the community.

✓ They want to make the lives of the people better by treating their animals.

Who should be a Community Livestock Worker?

There are various opinions about who should be trained as agricultural workers, Community Livestock Workers and human health workers (See "References" pg. 330). Generally speaking, the person chosen by their community will make a more effective Community Livestock Worker and extensionist than an outsider.

Some criteria for selection in different programs:

The Rural Development Center training program of the United Mission to Nepal has these criteria:

- The CLW must serve an area with at least 500 animals (not counting chickens) within a half-day walk. This enables them to work enough to keep their skills current and to use their medicines before they expire.
- They must be literate so they can buy proper medicines and understand correct dosages and use reference manuals.
- They prefer that they not have graduated from high school, because graduates are not likely to stay in the village to work with their people.
- They must have animals of their own to implement their own advice on.
- They should be settled and respected in the community.
- They should not be very young or very old.

The program makes these suggestions to the community and then the community decides who to send for training.

Training two people in a community:

Other programs suggest to villages that they select two people to be trained, one man and one woman. That way the positive aspects of both can be incorporated into the village livestock care system. They will often work together as a team. Where it has been possible, husbands and wives have made good training teams. This is advantageous because the person in training is growing so much that a couple can sometimes grow apart if the spouse is not also involved in some kind of training.

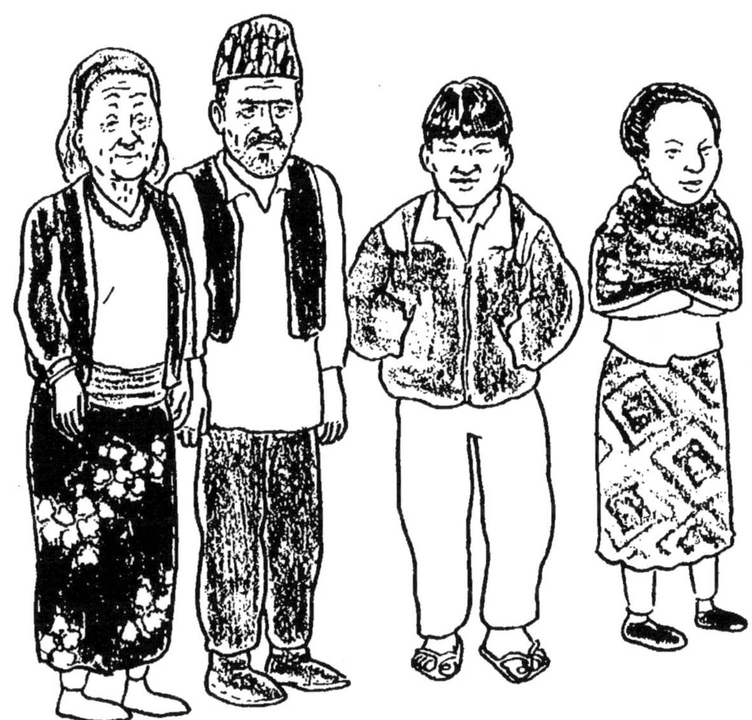

In several programs women are chosen for these and other reasons:

- They are most likely to be in the village when an animal gets sick.
- They are often the caretakers of the animals and are used to seeing their diseases and to treating them with traditional medicine.
- They understand and use the systems of barter with their animals and often are those who make the decisions about sale and price.
- Women Community Livestock Workers will often pass their skills on to their children and to other women and children.
- Women often have strong motivation to initiate social and economic change. They also are responsible for feeding, clothing and sending their children to school, so they want to see their income from their animals increase.
- Often women are more responsible than men. They drink alcohol less and succumb less to the pressure of favoritism. Often women are chosen to handle money.

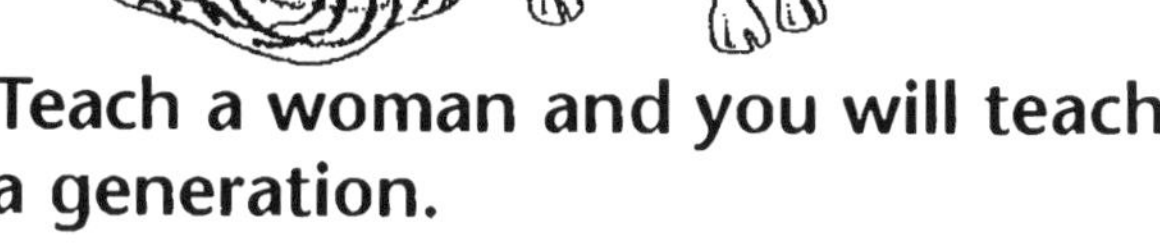

Teach a woman and you will teach a generation.

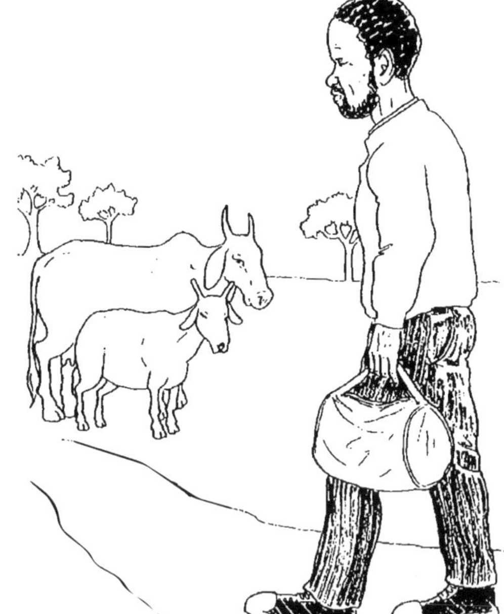

Men are chosen for these and other reasons:

- They are often freer to travel to treat sick animals and to acquire medicines and vaccines and new pastures. They can go alone and at night in emergency situations.
- Many livestock improvement areas are traditionally seen as the domain of the men, such as pasture clearing and planting and tree establishment, well digging, and large livestock marketing.
- Men usually prefer to be led by men, especially where a woman's opinion is not allowed at the village-level organization. Men may be able to have their voice heard for social change sooner than women.

As you can see, there may be some project criteria and some village criteria. This is a partnership so it is good that these criteria are developed and agreed on together.

Community selection of a Community Livestock Worker

Communities can make good choices when selecting their Community Livestock Workers if they are given the chance. However, problems can arise in the process of choosing.

Sometimes, an inappropriate person is chosen to be a Community Livestock Worker as a favor to someone in power.

That boy is lazy and didn't do well in school.
True. But the president can make that decision.
My son likes animal production and has been to high school. I'm sure you'll agree he should be the one to go to training.

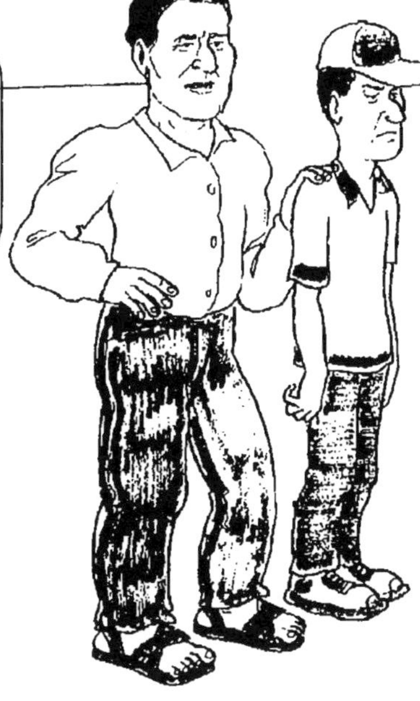

Some institutions offering CLW training send a letter to the community outlining what they feel the abilities and skills and requirements for a Community Livestock Worker are. Then they leave the choice up to the village. In Bolivia, though, the trainers decided to help the villages make decisions in the selection of their Community Livestock Worker. Here we share the process they used with each community:

A Community Livestock Worker selection process

This process is completed with a community over two evening meetings. Often there is a break of up to two weeks between meetings. It is important to review the results of the first meeting before beginning the second meeting.

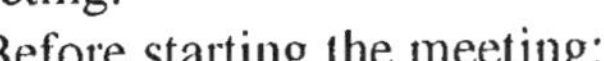

Before starting the meeting:

- **Visit every house** in the community to invite the people to attend the meeting.
- **Prepare two rooms** that are big enough to hold the people and have lighting.
- Cut sheets of paper for use in small groups.
- Prepare large paper and markers for each room.
- Have enough pencils for each small group.

A Community Livestock Worker Selection Process

Objective	Method	Materials
1. The trainers state the reasons for this meeting.	Explain that we are here to discover the needs and desires for a Community Livestock Worker. Also, explain the process to date and the institution or local organization involved.	• A copy of a bulletin explaining the program to be left with the village
2. The village makes a list of the work they would like their CLW to do in their community.	Locate women in one room, men in another. In each room, by numbering off, divide everyone randomly into groups of 5-6 people. Ask each small group to answer the question, "Why do you want to have a CLW?" Give each group a small sheet of paper to write the tasks of a CLW. In separate plenary sessions ask both the men and the women to share their ideas and make a combined list. In a joint plenary session both lists are presented. Make one common list with categories: preventive/curative/organizational.	• Small sheets of paper, one for each small group, • pencils for each group, • large paper for two rooms, • markers
3. The village defines what the Community Livestock Worker needs to do their work.	The men in their group and the women in their's discuss , "What will the CLW need to be able to do this work?" Using the list of work they have made, the leader can ask, "If you were the CLW, what would you need to do a vaccine campaign?" Or, "If you were the CLW, what would you need to cure animals?" They can keep discussing and making the list. The list could be divided into: Materials / Community Support / Other needs. Once each group has their list finished, they share it in the plenary session with everyone present and make one joint list.	• large white paper for each room • markers
4. The village analyses what type of person makes the best Community Livestock Worker and defines their criteria for selection.	Use the example of house building to start the discussion. Ask, "What does the central post of a house need to be like to build a good strong house?" (Show a picture of a house with a weak center post.) Help the people to understand that a good CLW will need specific strengths, just as a central post does. In the divided groups (of men and women) have each group develop a list of the qualities of a good CLW. In plenary the groups can share their thoughts and one final list is made.	• large papers • markers • picture of a house
5. The community defines and begins to solve some of the problems of being a Community Livestock Worker.	Sociodrama: A livestock worker in their house. Several people come with different animal problems and obligate him to treat them. One person wants a vaccination campaign, but there is no money from the first campaign. He blames the worker. A second person wants to send the worker to the city for training but does not want the community to pay the costs. A third person wants the worker to go to the city to buy medicine for his sick cow. The worker leaves his house talking of his frustration and thinking about quitting his work. In plenary, discuss the drama and make a list of the problems of being a Community Livestock Worker.	• Several people to be in the drama • paper • marker
6. The community defines their commitment to the Community Livestock Worker.	Depending on how everyone is working together, divide them into small groups by sex or randomly. Have each small group make one good suggestion about how they would be willing to support the local CLWs and solve some of the potential problems of the worker. Present this list to the village president so the community can make this decision in their regular community meeting when they write the contract with the CLW.	• large papers • markers
7. The community makes their decision about who to select for training.	The president and the village decide if they will select the person now or at their next regular meeting. They discuss the importance of a contract between the village and the CLW .	

When the villages made their lists of criteria for the people selected to be Community Livestock Workers they included:

OUR COMMUNITY LIVESTOCK WORKER IS:

- Honest and makes good decisions
- Doesn't drink or gamble
- Trustworthy • Kind
- Responsible • Listens to other's ideas
- Not Dominating
- Sincere and equal to others
- Owns property in the community (or family)
- Interested in livestock work
- The family agrees
- Can read and write
- A proven good leader
- Takes part willingly in community activities
- No preference to the wealthy or powerful
- Not too young and not too old

A note about gender:
You might ask, **"Why did you divide into groups of men and groups of women?**

In many communities women are not normally invited to community meetings, or if they are, they do not speak in the meeting. Nevertheless, in many poor villages women play important roles in the management and treatment of animals. Often the women are present when the animals get sick, since the men are off working or in the fields.

Recognizing that the women probably would not speak out in a village meeting with men present, but that they had many valuable experiences to share, the trainers decided to create an atmosphere where the women could talk.

When the women began to share their list of ideas, it turned out they had a more profound view of what was needed in a Community Livestock Worker for the village. The men recognized this:

The women have some really good ideas. Maybe they should be the CLW...

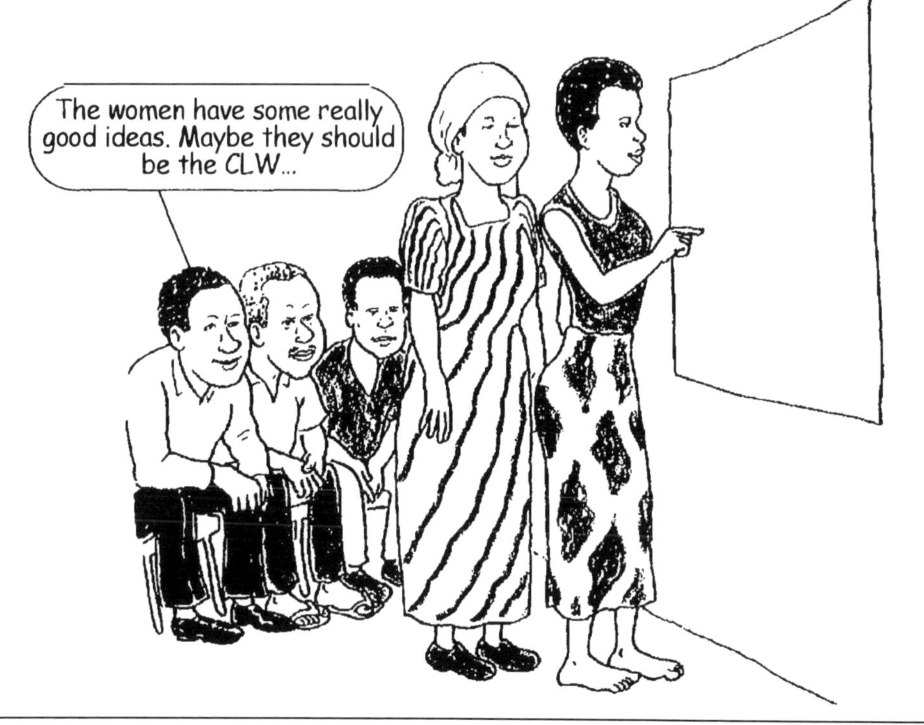

In this way many communities of the San Julian and Berlin regions of Bolivia made their decisions about who should be their Community Livestock Workers. They chose women and men, old and young, traditional healers and modern farmers. These people now serve as effective Community Livestock Workers.

Chapter 3
Facilitators of training

This chapter covers the following topics:

Selecting facilitators

What type of people make the best facilitators of training?

The selection of the facilitators and advisors of training is as important as the selection of participants in the training.

The facilitators model what they know and understand about learning and teaching in their actions toward the participants and others. **It is very important to have facilitators who model an approach to educating that is learner-centered and encourages change.**

If the facilitators show by their actions and manner that they think they are better than the participants, if they boss them around or talk down to them, the CLWs will behave similarly toward the people in their community.

Facilitator: The person who guides the participatory process. Also called a trainer. This guiding can be in workshops, meetings, or individual interactions. See "Role of the Facilitator," chart pg. 48.

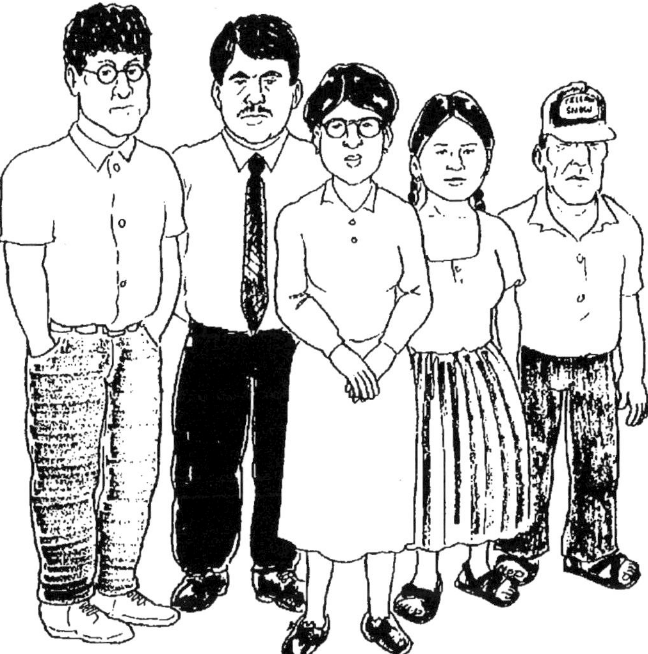

See "Learning and teaching, how we teach," pg. 3.

Professionals as facilitators

Agronomists, veterinarians, soil scientists and other professional experts are often quite eager to share what they have learned and what they "know" to be right with farmers. They feel that all their training has been focused toward this end.

We teach the way we have learned!

But, how did the professional learn in school?

Many professionals have the banking system of learning so deeply impressed upon them that they do not even consider exploring another way of teaching. Many years of the banking system of school were drilled into me as I became a veterinarian. There are times when I slip back into the old system, without thinking, even though I am committed to learner-centered education.

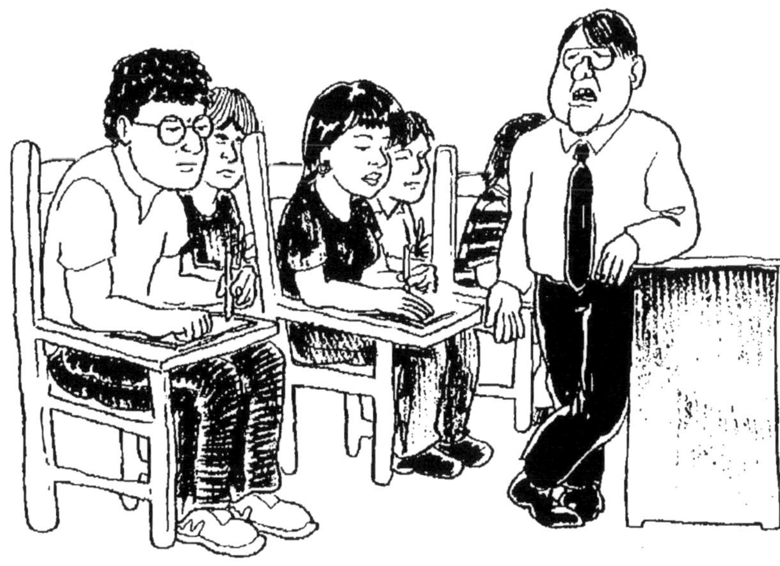

A professional's concept of learning and teaching must be challenged for them to be effective trainers.

Professionals need to realize there is a problem with the attitudes and methods of the banking system of training adults. All of the *dynamics* in the chapter on learning and teaching, are appropriate for the training of facilitators. (See "Learning and Teaching," chapter one.)

Often, it is more efficient and more effective to train farmers as trainers. Although farmers also have the idea that the lecture in the schoolroom is the only way people learn, that idea is more readily challenged and reconsidered when a person has had less formal education. The professional has a wealth of knowledge to share and so often forgets that the farmer also has a wealth of knowledge to share.

How can he remember well his ignorance, which his growth requires, when he has always to use his knowledge?
–Henry David Thoreau

Understanding the local context or reality

Many professionals have very different backgrounds from those of village people. Their whole social context is different. Although many agronomists and veterinarians come from rural backgrounds, it is often a wealthier one which permits them to study and complete an education. This difference in background makes the understanding of the social context of the villager very difficult, and sometimes impossible for the professional. The learner-centered approach has to begin from the context, knowledge, and reality of the village participants, and it is often quite difficult for a professional to begin there.

What an outsider can do:

✔ Learn as much as you can about the local community's social and cultural context **by living there with a family.**

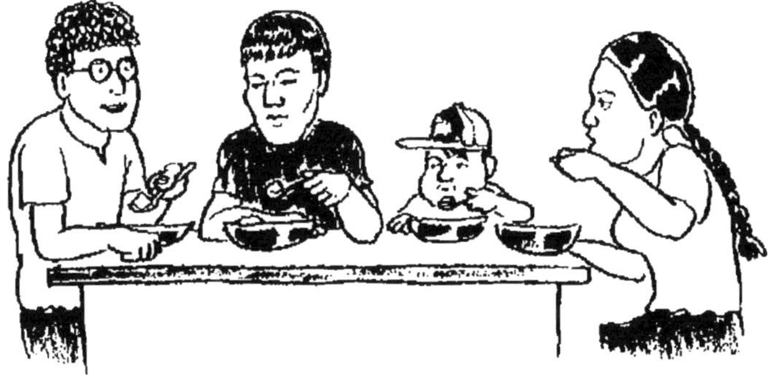

✔ **Recognize the difference** between yourself and the villagers and admit this to them. Admit that your understanding and knowledge base is different.

✔ **Ask for the villager's help in teaching you** about their knowledge and reality, and be willing to listen well and openly without judgment.

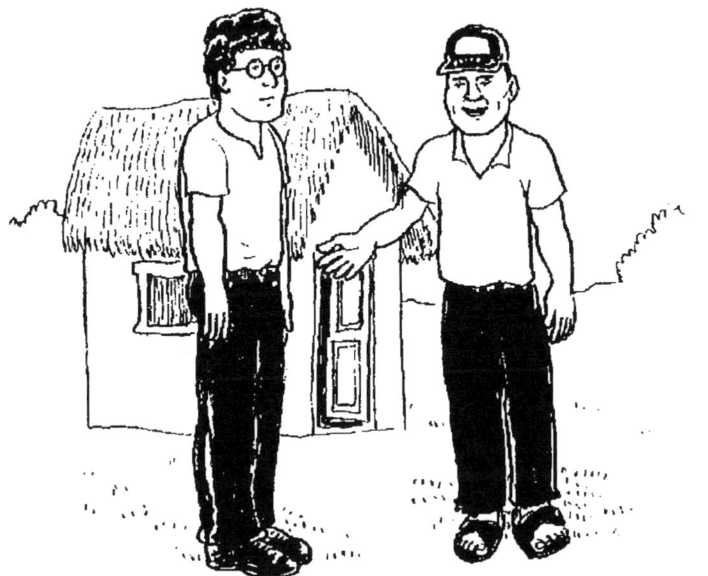

✔ Always begin the training with the knowledge and experience of the villagers, not your own.

✔ As soon as possible work yourself out of a job! Train local villagers to be facilitators and to take over your role. Begin by encouraging them to share their experiences and continue by sharing with them facilitation skills and training concepts. They will make great facilitators!

Local professionals

Often the best facilitators are people who are much closer to the people in the village. Look for facilitators who:

- Are from the same area as the training program, or close to it. If the training is for displaced people, try to find facilitators who are from the same area as the people being trained.
- Speak the local language well.
- Dress in a similar way to the people participating in the courses.
- Have the same cultural and social background as those who are participating in training.
- Have a similar educational background to those in the training.
- Speak with respect for the participants in the area.

Don't be closed to the idea that **a non-agricultural professional can be a great facilitator of agricultural production and marketing training.** Often young school teachers, technicians from other fields, sociologists, and communicators can be good trainers. They require a period of training in facilitation methodology and technical topics and some assistance in the process of workshop development initially. With this training they will be good facilitators. In some cases it is an asset not to have specific technical knowledge. This is especially true if the emphasis of the training is on using the assets and resources of villages to work toward a vision and to solve problems.

Village people as facilitators

Many programs encourage village people to train other village people through farmers sharing information on their farms. Often the same programs feel that village people cannot run basic community workshops or train CLWs. Initially, there may be difficulties in finding village people with the technical background and facilitation skills to train Community Livestock Workers.

It should be the goal, however, of every program to train facilitators among the villagers and to put the training into their capable hands!

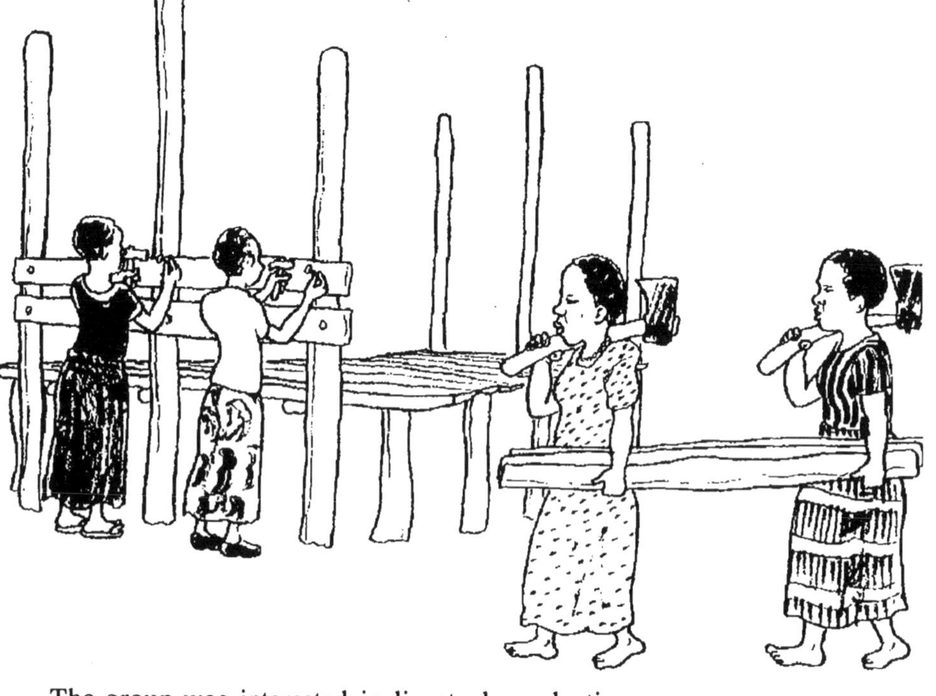

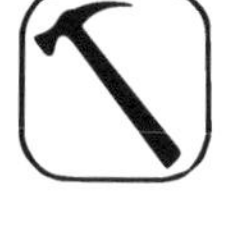

A story from Uganda

In the western mountains of Uganda a group of women from a village were invited to attend some training about the benefits of a village organization and building a strong active group. When they returned to their village they were very enthusiastic and organized training to share what they had learned with other women in the community. From that training, the women decided to form themselves into a cooperative group to work together toward their vision and to solve problems in their village.

They began to work together on several projects. Because the group was organized and was working well together, they received more invitations to send people for training in many different skills. They sent members to courses on accounting, crafts, sewing, and garden planting. After each course, the woman who had received the training would return and share with her fellow group members what she had learned. These trainings led to some very productive activities by the group.

The group was interested in livestock production, so they discussed how they could begin to raise livestock, and contacted a local institution to help them. The institution sent an extensionist from outside the area to work with the women in the techniques they would need to employ to start a zero-grazing system. The women enthusiastically put the system into practice.

Although the extensionist recognized the value of the opinions of the women with experience in the zero-grazing system and invited them to workshops for new participants, he never encouraged the women themselves to facilitate the training for the new participants.

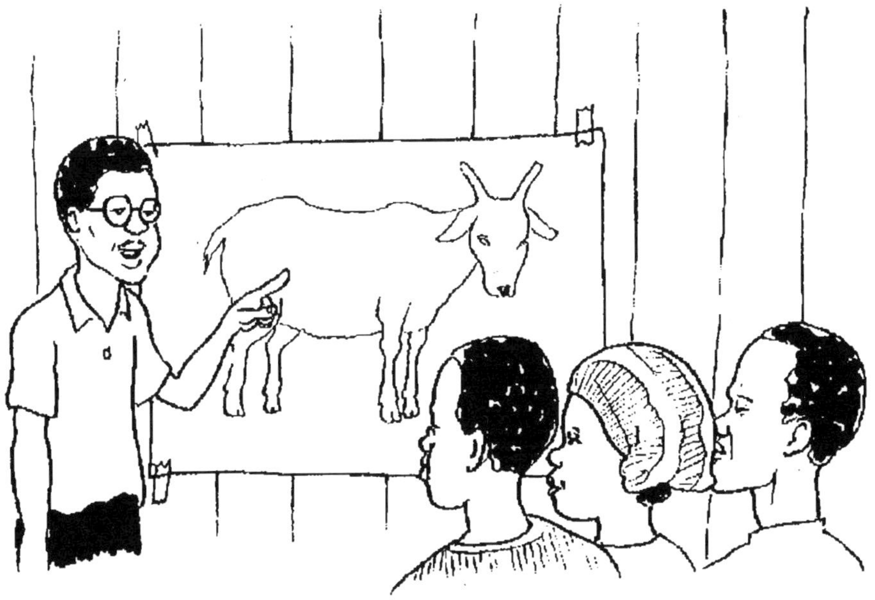

Now several women have successful zero grazing units and are raising goats very productively. There are more and more women who would like to raise goats in this way. But the extensionist has too much to do with the care of the sick goats, helping with artificial insemination, and many training sessions for new participants. The women depend extensively on the extensionist to provide all these services subsidized by the institution with the program.

By not using the women in the group as trainers:

- How has this affected their self concept?
- How has this affected their organizational capabilities?
- How does this affect the work of the extensionist?
- What could this program do differently?

Experiences from other programs with village people as trainers:

In Nepal, in the area of Surkhet, the United Mission to Nepal decided to use only village people as facilitators for a training program. The village people had a training course for several weeks to prepare them for the job. They were all people who were literate and with differing levels of education, up to secondary school. The effect in the communities where the project worked was very impressive. The local facilitators were able to begin from where the villagers were and to build on what they knew.

In Guatemala in the CAPS program and in the Philippines in a program called SEHRDEP, village people have been involved as facilitators in agricultural and livestock training programs for many years with very positive results. In Bolivia, the villagers who have become "animators" (trainers and encouragers of Community Livestock Workers) have put a creativity and energy into the training program which outsiders have found far more difficult to do. They have helped to produce many very effective Community Livestock Workers who work with a strong local organization where the animators participate as well. They have, in addition, applied their facilitation skills to other work in their villages and to strengthening their local organizations and churches.

Some things which village facilitators have shared:

- ✔ They often **need time off during the heavy part of the agricultural season,** especially harvest time, to work with their families on their own land.
- ✔ Sometimes when the trainer works close to home they **may not be listened to or respected by their own community.**
- ✔ **For village women to be facilitators, the project must have a real commitment to having women facilitators** - they need special arrangements if they have young children, they sometimes can't travel or stay as far from home, and they have more problems with family obligations. They also cannot usually travel alone. Teaching in teams is a way to overcome this difficulty.
- ✔ Some village facilitators prefer to work full time, others part time, depending on their own farm commitments.
- ✔ **Most people work as facilitators for between 3–5 years,** afterwards becoming a resource person to the project or community but returning to their farming and family activities. For most, this is because while they worked as facilitators, they did not have the time to apply much of what they learned on their own farm and they want to put it in to practice.
- ✔ **If village facilitators are married, it is very important to involve the husband or wife in as many activities and training sessions as possible.** As the village person becomes a facilitator they are learning and growing. It is very helpful if the spouse has the same opportunity, so they don't grow apart. The husband of a farmer trainer will also be enthusiastic about his wife's work and supportive if he understands it and is involved in it.

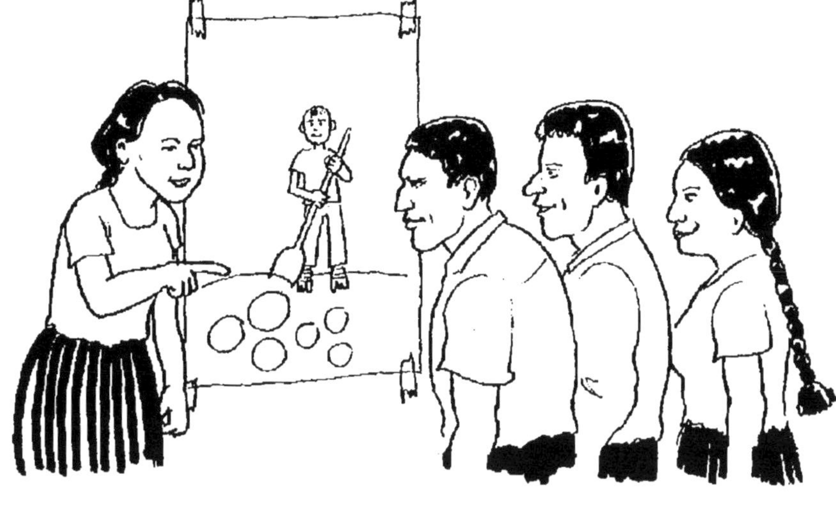

Payment of CLWs and trainers

It is important to recognize that when we talk of villagers as facilitators, we are not discussing a volunteer situation. If a villager works in their own community as a Community Livestock Worker, then the arrangement for their payment is between them and their village. If the villager works for an institution running a farmer training program in livestock care or training Community Livestock Workers, they are paid for their services, as an outsider would be.

Training of facilitators

The next five areas should be discussed with new facilitators as a part of their training process.

What are the characteristics of a good facilitator?

Ask the facilitators this question in a workshop and have them develop their list of characteristics of a good facilitator. Discuss together what leads to these characteristics. The group may come up with things like this:

Attitude:

a. **Trainers show no favoritism.** They allow everyone to participate without favoring males or females, treating all as equals and as adults.
b. Trainers **respect** the students and their opinions. They respect the farmer's ability to teach the facilitator and others.
c. Trainers must love what they are doing
d. Trainers must **respect local knowledge** and traditional ways of doing things such as medicine and management.
e. Trainers must understand that their knowledge is different, not better.

Actions:

a. Trainers wear **simple clothing** similar to what the people wear. If facilitators work in different ethnic areas they should dress as the people dress in those ethnic areas.
b. Trainers use **simple language and terminology**. They use a language closest to the first language of the people, especially in remote rural areas. Often there is the problem of mixed language groups in the training. This is an especially important factor for women participants.
c. Trainers are **excellent and active listeners.** They make good eye contact, show they are listening with body language, say "yes" to encourage participation, and make appropriate comments.
d. Trainers have a sense of humor; they joke and laugh with the participants.
e. Trainers bring the other participants into the discussion and to active listening – "Do you agree with what that person just said?"
f. Trainers must build the people's respect – do what they do, get involved in the doing – instead of just looking on.

Tips on good facilitation? See "Implementation," pg 137.

The roles of the facilitator in the change process

Sometimes the role of the facilitator is a confusing one because at different times in the process of looking for change, the role also changes. The facilitator can play several parts:

ROLE 1: A Catalyst

The facilitator may notice a problem or it may be raised by the community. The facilitator helps them to look seriously at the problem.

For the next co-op meeting, what do you think about the idea of a role play about what happens when people don't take care of their fires?
Good idea! This year many people lost trees and pastures.
My sheep burned to death.

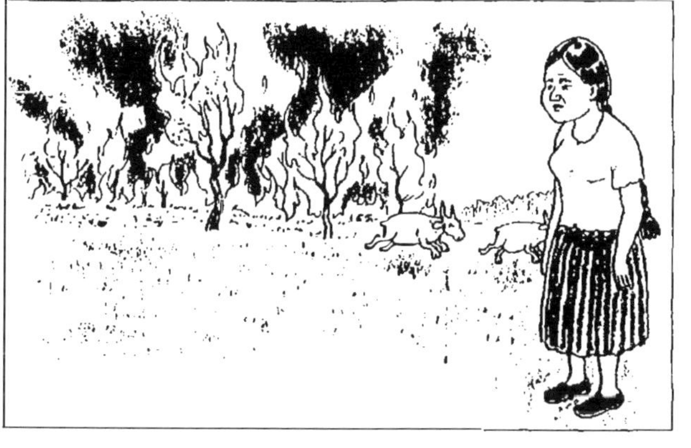

So, what did you see in the role play?
This happens here every year!
What can we do about it?
Let's learn about fire control.
Then we can meet in the community to decide how to enforce it.

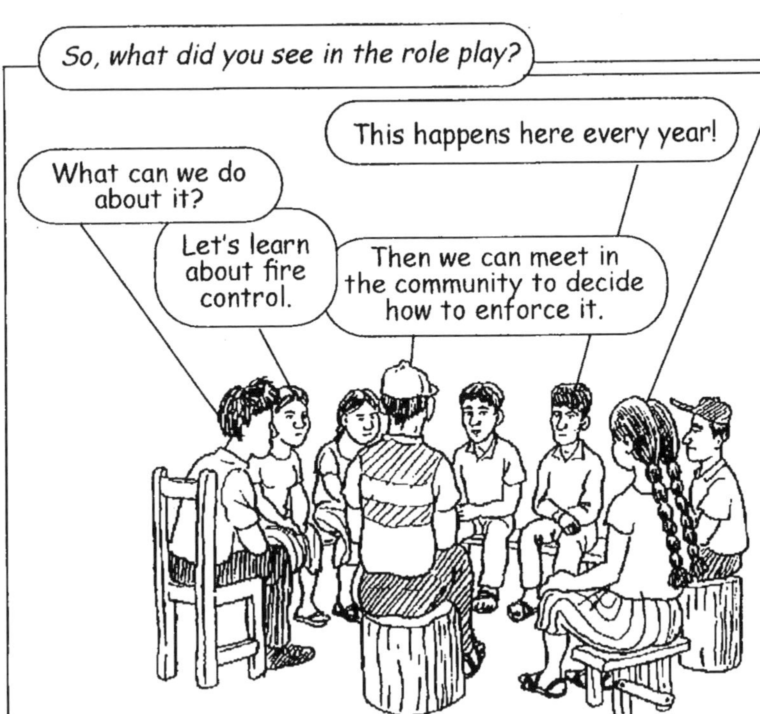

ROLE 2:
A helper in the process

Although facilitators don't give a solution to the problem, they ask good questions so people can think through and analyze deeply the problem. They also help organize and re-present the ideas of the villagers.

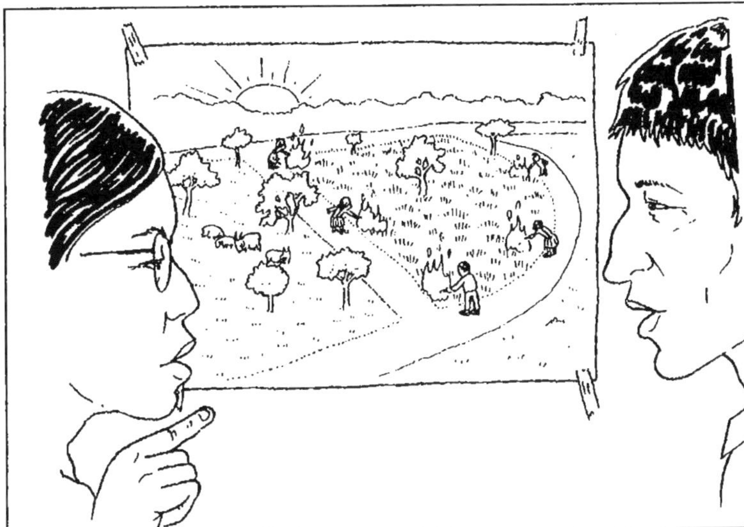

ROLE 3:
A resource person

When the farmers decide they want to take some action on a problem, they begin to share their knowledge about the topic with each other. Sometimes they need further information or outside information so they can make an informed decision. It is here that the facilitator will share outside technical information. Sometimes a member of another community may be invited to share what they have done, or an outside expert will give information.

With so many different roles, no wonder we get confused in our roles as facilitators!

The three roles of a facilitator

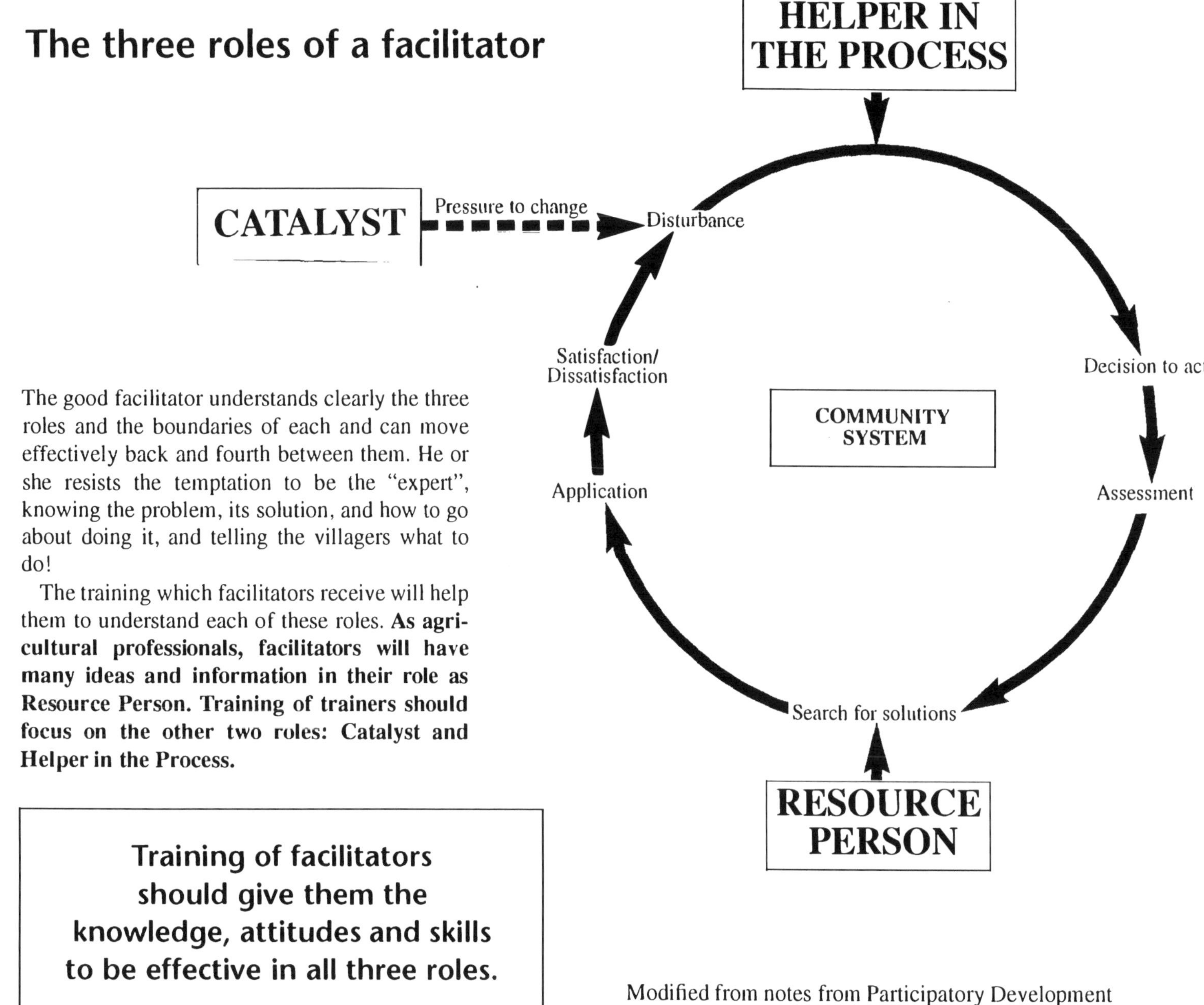

The good facilitator understands clearly the three roles and the boundaries of each and can move effectively back and fourth between them. He or she resists the temptation to be the "expert", knowing the problem, its solution, and how to go about doing it, and telling the villagers what to do!

The training which facilitators receive will help them to understand each of these roles. **As agricultural professionals, facilitators will have many ideas and information in their role as Resource Person. Training of trainers should focus on the other two roles: Catalyst and Helper in the Process.**

Training of facilitators should give them the knowledge, attitudes and skills to be effective in all three roles.

Modified from notes from Participatory Development and Education Workshop II PREMISE-AFRICA 1994

Training facilitators

These are some important topics throughout this book which should be included in the training process for facilitators:

The training of trainers is not completed in a single workshop! The best training happens through the experience of being a trainer and reflecting on that practice. Most programs which train trainers feel a series of workshops is necessary, with practice after each workshop.

Mentoring or apprenticeship gives the opportunity for the trainer to:

- Have a role model in training
- Be able to question and solve problems or difficulties together
- Reflect on their practice with an experienced trainer

New trainers can be given a series of tasks, or set their own goals after each workshop. The mentor provides the feedback they need to grow and asks questions to cause greater reflection.

Mentoring: the process where an experienced facilitator trains a new facilitator through exchange of ideas, consultation, and monitoring of the learning-by-doing process of the new trainer.

Looking at yourself and how you work in groups

A facilitator needs to analyze the question, "What kind of a person am I, and how do I work with others?" This will lead to better facilitation through self-awareness. This is true whether you are an outsider facilitator, a village trainer of Community Livestock Workers, or a Community Livestock Worker. There are several *dynamics* in the communication section to help self-awareness grow. The following *dynamics* and references to *dynamics* are very important for the training of facilitators.

Tip for the person who facilitates this training: These are *dynamics* which ask the participants to be very open and vulnerable. **It is important that an environment of trust and respect has been developed among the participants before these *dynamics* are used.**

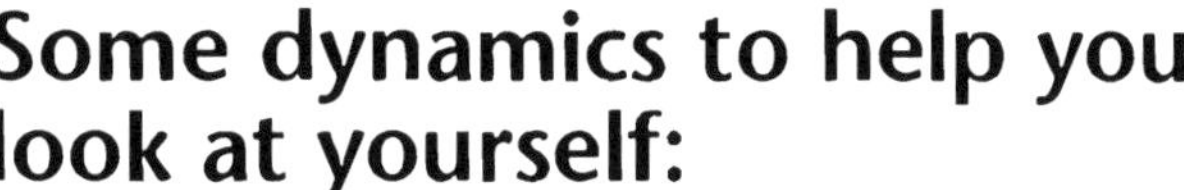

Some dynamics to help you look at yourself:

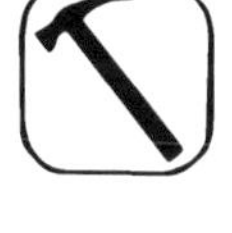

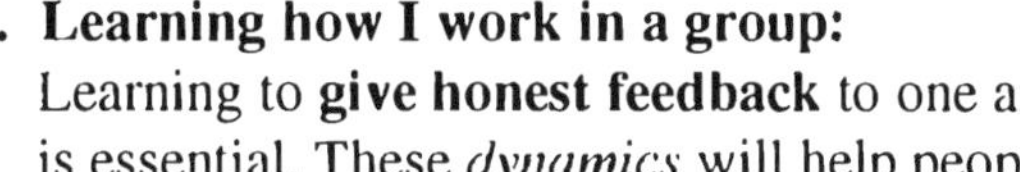

1. **Learning how I work in a group:**

   Learning to **give honest feedback** to one another is essential. These *dynamics* will help people explore how they work and relate in a group and about honest feedback.

   Please see:

   Which animal are you? "Communication," pg. 214

   "Feedback," pg. 208.

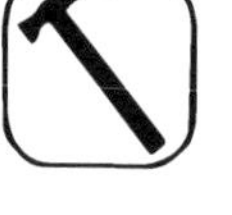

2. Knowing more about myself: **A letter from a friend**

- Divide into groups of four. Each person writes a letter to each of the other three in their group. In the letter each person should write to the others:
  - "What I like about you is..."
  - "One thing I have difficulty with is ..."
- Each person gives the letters to the people in their group that they are addressed to. Each person reads their letters in silence. The silence is very difficult.
- After the time for reading, people can ask each other questions, but only for clarification. Resist the temptation to defend or explain why you seem the way you are. Give some time to reflect on these letters in silence.

3. **Walking-talking partners.**

- In the beginning of a workshop, choose your own partners for walking and talking.
- At the end of each day you walk and talk and review what has been good or painful, what you think about yourself each day.
- In the beginning you go for several days with the same person. Later, new partners are chosen at random. This will help in reflection and feedback from a trusted source.

Source: Paul Daughtery, Oxfam UK Nepal

4. There are many other good exercises for self awareness in how we work together and cooperate in Hope and Timmel's *Training for Transformation* (See "References," pg. 330)

5. A practical way to look at your role in a group: During facilitator training, the facilitators must plan how they will do the cooking in **a shared cooking experience.** Then they can analyze what role they took in the group. Did I sit back, or speak up, or control?

Source: Uganda Change Agents Association

6. A **"process observer"** is very helpful in the above situations and in many other activities requiring group cooperation. The process observer is a person who is placed in the group, but not to participate. They are there to watch the process of the group. They need to understand they should not get caught up in the topic the group is working on. When the group activity is finished and the job has been completed, the process observer can share frankly what they saw in how the group functioned. Did someone take over control? Was there a democratic process? Who contributed and who didn't? Why were people not contributing? The process observer can be a great help in looking at how we act in group situations.

Source: Paul Daughtery Oxfam UK, Nepal.

There are several excellent manuals specifically designed for training-of-trainers workshops in participatory adult education. (Please see "Resources," pg. 330.)

You were controlling what everyone in your group did.
You're right! I really didn't give others the chance to talk.

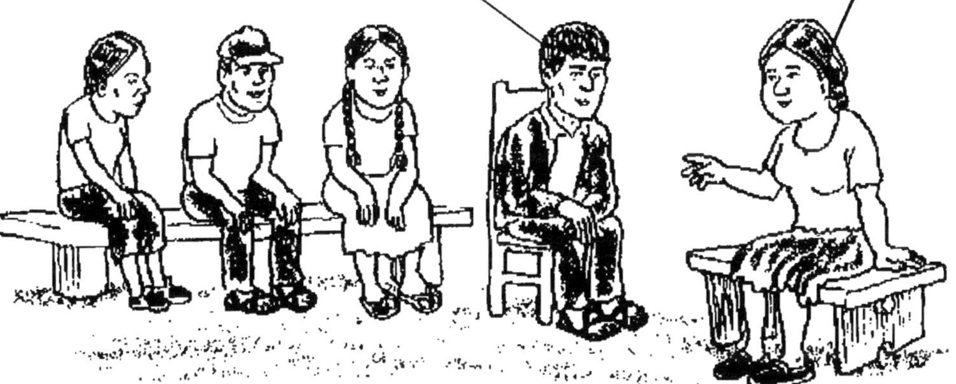

Some tips for managers of training programs

For some, the most important part of convincing trainers to use the participatory methodology is how the management of the program acts. If the management of the program is participatory it will make more sense to the trainers. Some managers are not willing to participate in the consensus process.

If a program has sent new trainers for training they have new ideas, abilities and skills in participatory training. They sometimes have a very difficult time in a traditional system. If they are younger or female on a male team their ideas may not be listened to on an equal basis. This causes great frustration for the new trainer who comes with participatory skills and new ideas. If the program wants to move toward a participatory approach, methods of integrating this person into the training team in a participatory way should be emphasized. They should often be asked for their ideas or opinions.

Some programs push their people to more education as a form of personal development. If this is desirable within the cultural context, it should be analyzed by the team within a program context. How will the new education be used to improve the work of the team and to improve the training program?

Section 2
Developing a Training Program

In these five chapters the full cycle of a training program will be mapped out. Each chapter is dedicated to one aspect of the training cycle.

The Training Cycle

A training workshop or program can be viewed from any one point as a cycle. For some reason, the community desires change. Together, insiders and outsiders assess the situation, plan a program, implement the program, and evaluate it. The results of the evaluation of learning may lead to the identification of new training needs and the cycle continues. It looks like this:

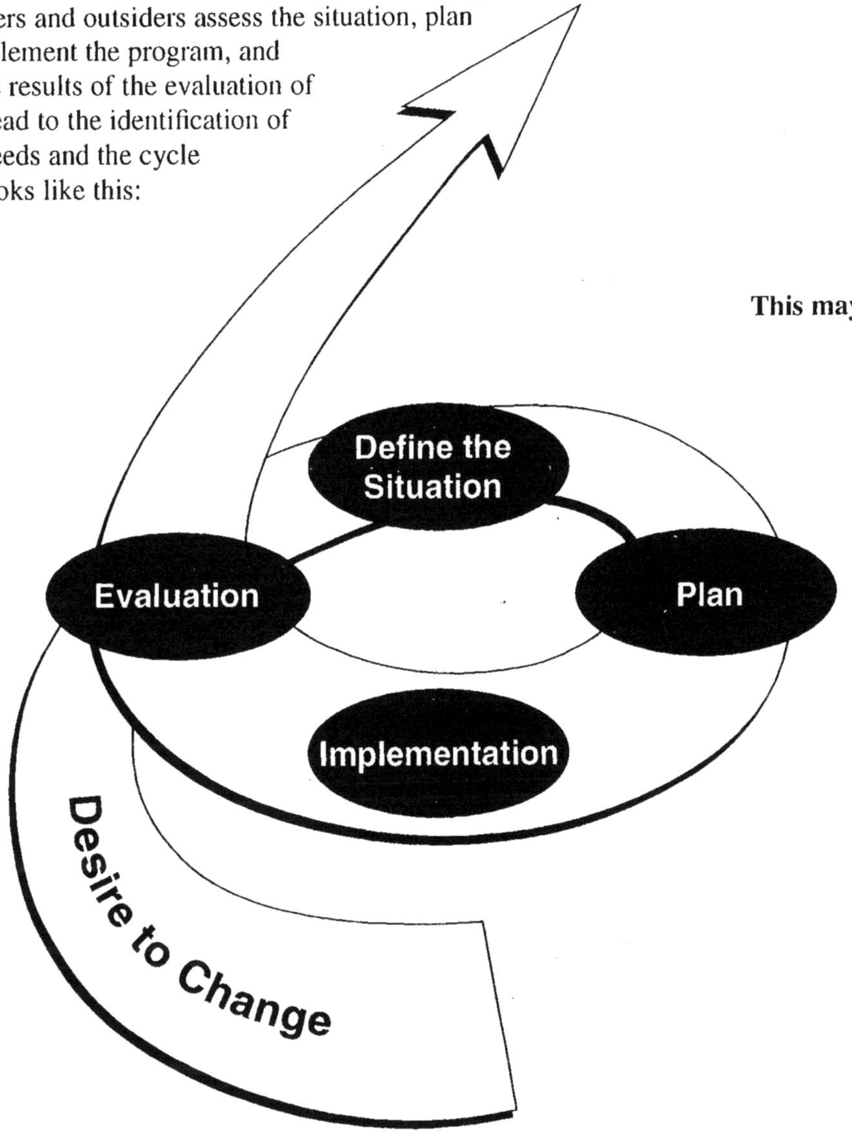

Define the Situation

Evaluation

Plan

Implementation

Desire to Change

This may look like an endless cycle but it's not!

On the contrary, if effective training is done, the need for dealing with a specific topic in a given community should be satisfied. However, the change initiated by the people as a result of the workshop will lead to a new situation in the community, one that may or may not require training.

Think of this process as a spiral rather than a never-ending circle. The spiral moves upward and forward as the training results in change toward the community's goals or vision.

Think of the training program in the larger context of livestock development or the even larger context of community life, and the applications are obvious. The same cycle applies for a development program of a community organization or institution.

For example on the program level:

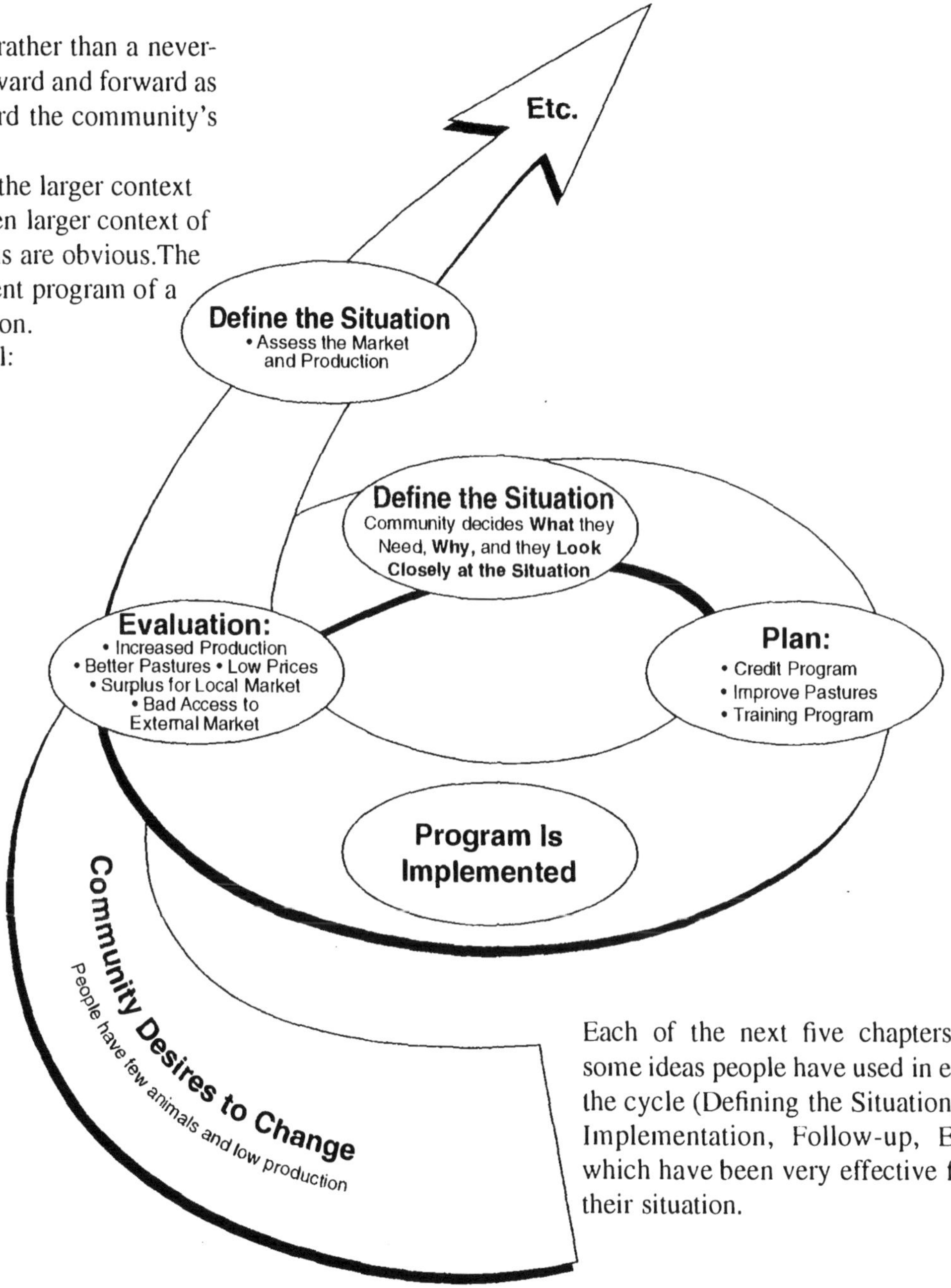

Each of the next five chapters will give some ideas people have used in each area of the cycle (Defining the Situation, Planning, Implementation, Follow-up, Evaluation) which have been very effective for them in their situation.

Chapter 4
Defining the situation

This chapter covers the following topics:

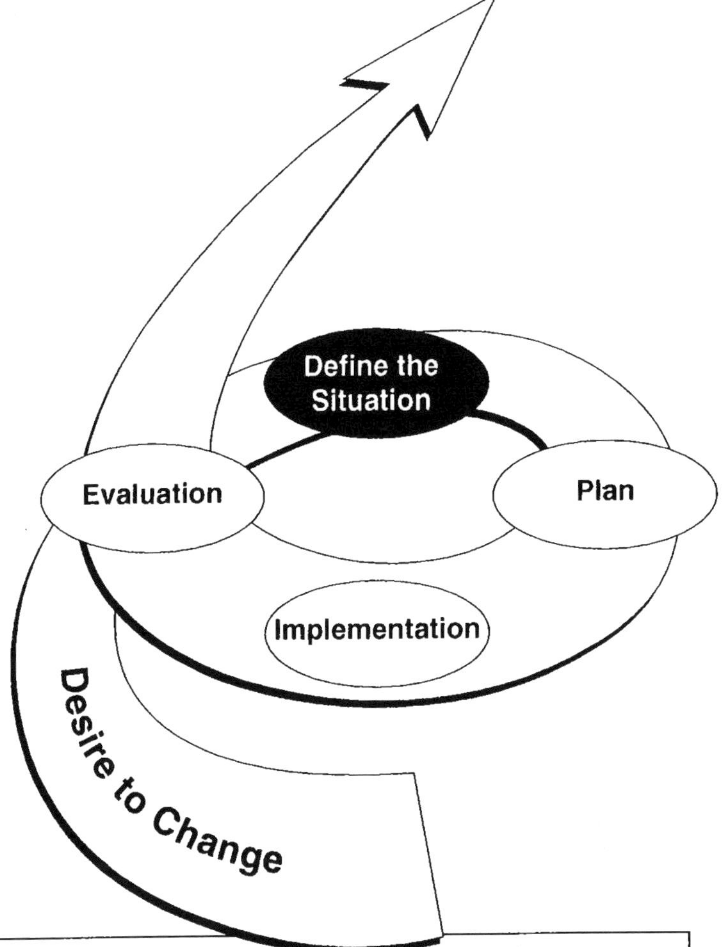

For an effective training program, insiders and outsiders need to understand how the community views the present, the future, and the steps to the future. This process of understanding is often called a needs assessment. But here we call it more broadly **"Defining the Situation."** Participatory training should always begin from what the people have and know and build on it. So the definition of the situation will be the springboard for the training program.

Why define the situation?

In the opening section, pg viii, is a story of the first community-level workshops by PROPECO in Bolivia. When the first training needs assessments were done, they were a series of meetings held with interested people in several communities. Generally more men came to the meetings than women. When the women were present they did not speak out. There was very little reflective dialogue about the need for the workshops. People had a desire for training and they requested it. The most important or vocal people in each community gave their opinions as to the training needs. The other people in the meeting echoed these thoughts. There were no participatory *dynamics* used to facilitate dialogue. The results were predictable. Only some of the information in the workshops was useful to the participants, even though each workshop was conducted in a participatory way.

After two years, an evaluation gave us much information about the appropriateness of the workshops. It also showed us how important it is for the people to define their situation before designing the training program. After the evaluation, each new workshop which was developed was based on a more involved assessment, such as the one described here. Later evaluations have shown us the impact of that change. Now the participants put much more information from the workshops directly into practice.

Some decisions to make:

After you read through this chapter you may ask, "How much time must we invest in this definition of the situation? This appears to be a very long process."

The time involved in defining the situation will be directly related to the size and length of the program. If a training program is being designed to benefit many communities, the assessment is worth an investment of several weeks of time. If one short workshop will be given, one meeting, several days before the workshop, may be sufficient. Remember, though, most training is related to a larger goal or vision. If that vision is not defined by the community people together with the outsiders, the training may be inappropriate.

Sometimes the process of defining the situation is more appropriately done at the very beginning of a program. Sometimes a more thorough assessment will take place when trust has been built between insiders and outsiders. But please, do not neglect to define the situation together simply because it appears to take too much time.

Equipping people for the future

The desire of most training programs is to equip people for the future.

For the training program to equip people well for the future, the program must be informed of three things:

1. **How the people see their current situation.**
2. **What the people want their future to be.**
3. **What the people feel are the most important steps to reach their desired future.**

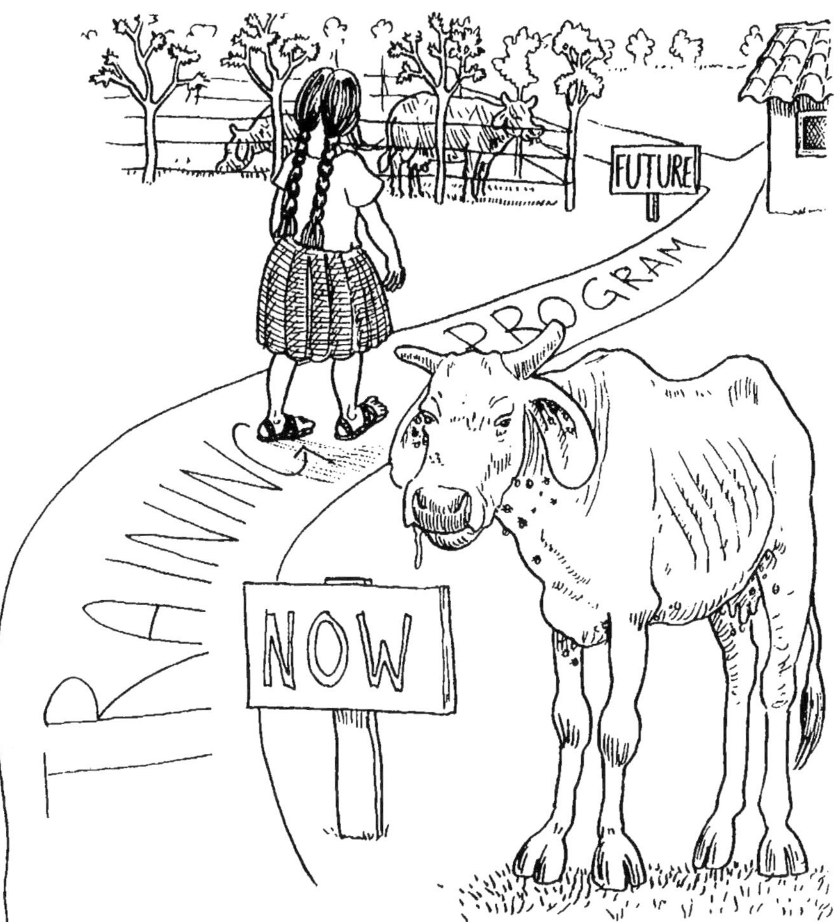

Redefining the situation:

In a participatory training program, the participants define and prioritize the topics for training. Because the participants are continually learning, their priorities for training will change. They are never static. This means we must continue to revisit the question, "What is the situation here?"

These are some places where the situation in the community is defined and redefined:

- A **community assessment** leads to the determination whether or not a training program is necessary. If it is...
- Then a **training assessment** defines the starting point for the training program.
- At the beginning of the training we look together at our **expectations** for the workshop and we adjust the content appropriately. Please see "Implementation" pg. 116.
- During the workshop there are times of **feedback and modifying** the workshop. Please see Chapter 6, "Implementation," pg. 134.
- The **closing evaluation,** the **follow-up** period and a **program evaluation** are points of needs assessments for further training. Please see Chapter 7, "Follow-Up," and Chapter 8, "Evaluation."

We will describe the process for a community and a training needs assessment here. It is important to recognize that this assessment can not be done once and then put aside. The purpose of participatory education is education for change. **The training process must be dynamic and responsive to the needs of the participants as they change.**

Types of situation assessments:

1. **Community Assessment and Visioning.** The community defines their situation, analyzes their current and relevant problems, and defines their vision. This will result in a community development plan for the future. The village makes an in-depth analysis of the root causes of the problems in their community and the resources they have to combat those causes. The villagers define their vision for the future. The outsiders describe what their program can provide. The community decides if and how the resources offered by the outsiders will be beneficial and necessary in helping the community to reach their vision.
2. **A Training Assessment.** The people who will be trained make decisions about what they want and the focus of the training. The training program is based on the analysis provided by the definition of the community's situation. Participants prioritize their training needs to assist the trainers in the planning of the workshops. Additionally, if Community Livestock Workers are to be trained, the community must participate in the development of the training needs.

Who should define the situation?

The situation should always be defined by the participants or community members together with the facilitators and organizers of the program. This may be the first time the community has ever assessed their situation in a participatory way, so patience is needed. Use the first assessment as a time of teaching how to assess as well. This way the community keeps the tools of assessment as their own. As their situation changes, they can use the tools at different times.

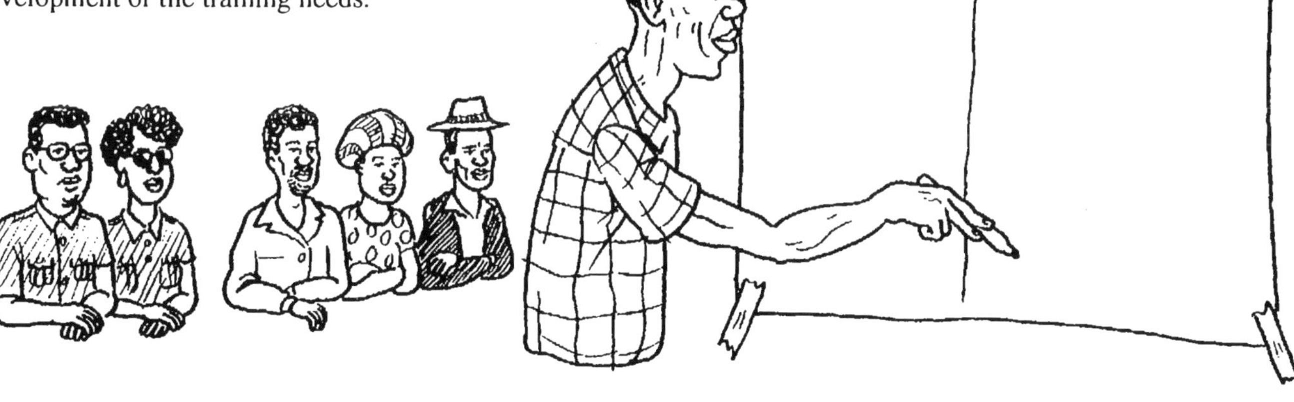

Why do a community-run assessment?

✔ It celebrates the community's local knowledge.
✔ It strengthens the community's confidence in their ability to analyze their own situation.
✔ It gives the community tools to continue in their development process when the outsiders are no longer working in the area.
✔ It puts the definition of the training program or workshop in the hands of the people who will use the training, making the training program more appropriate.
✔ It brings those who generally have no voice into the problem-solving process of the community.
✔ It leads the community to value their local physical, human, and social resources.

Three ways to define the situation:

1. In a an **outsider-based** assessment, outsiders decide:
   - What will be studied.
   - What the most important problems of the community are.
   - What data to collect and how to analyze it.
   - What the solutions to the community's problems are.

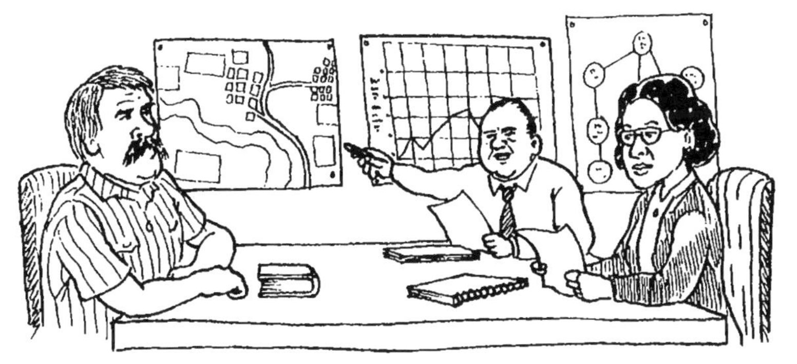

2. More recently in some **"participatory" assessments**, outsiders have collected the data together with the people in the village. Sometimes the outsiders will do some analysis of the data with the community. But the outsiders designed the study and made the final recommendations. In other words, the outsiders have maintained much of the control. (Some people use Rapid Rural Appraisal (RRA) and Participatory Rural Appraisal (PRA) techniques in this way.)

These studies reflect the outsider's point of view and generally do not include the reality or priorities of the community. The RRA is better than a completely outsider-based observation and survey but in either case the resulting training programs may be inappropriate or only partially appropriate, and the information may not be utilized by the people. Or the program makes people dependent rather than encouraging them to shape their own development.

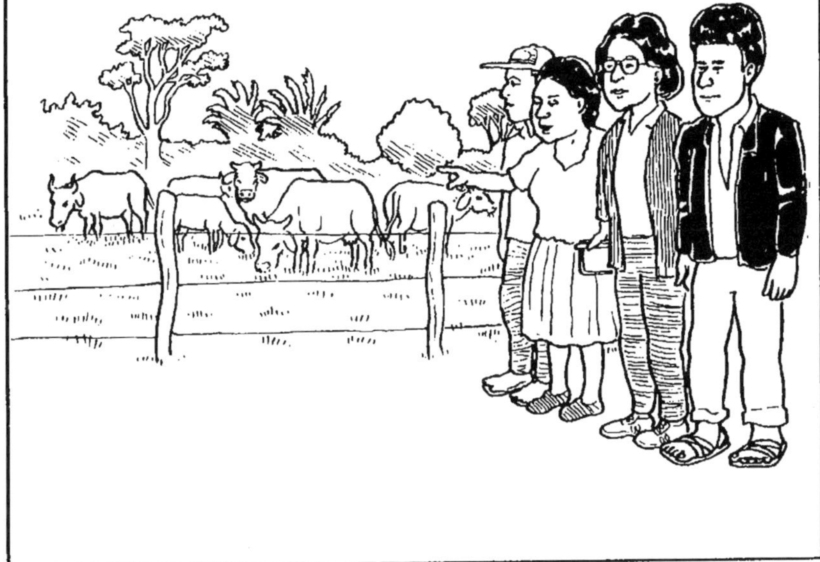

3. **In a community-based, participatory assessment** (also called Participatory Learning and Action (PLA), or Participatory Action Research (PAR), the village people and representatives from their organization are involved in every step of the assessment. Initially, as a program is beginning, outsiders work with the village in all phases of the assessment so that the training program, research, or other appropriate action can be planned together. (The techniques of PRA are intended to be used in this way.)

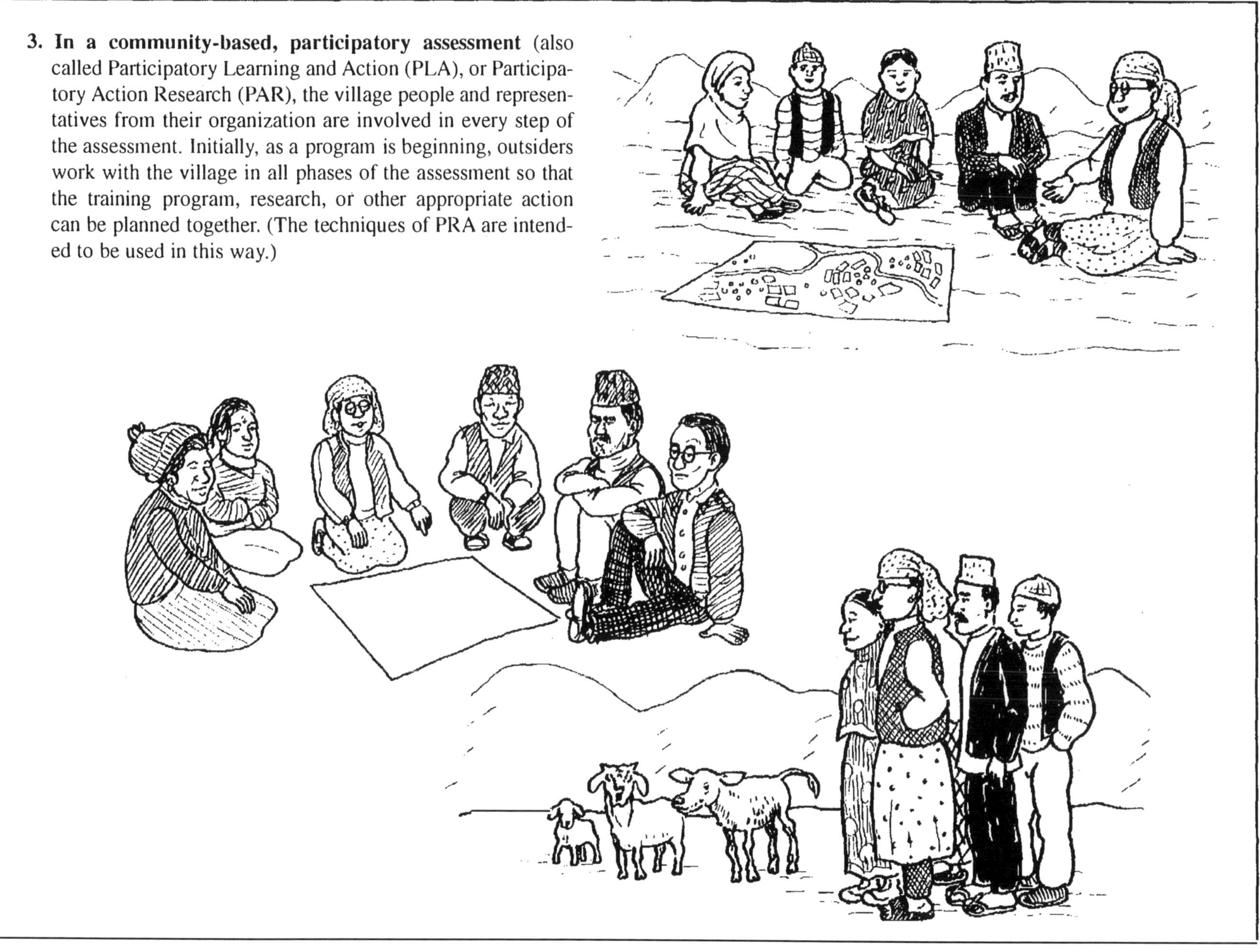

Dynamics to help facilitators examine outsider-controlled situation assessments

The first three simple but powerful *dynamics* that follow will help you when you are training facilitators and community assessment committees about defining the situation. They will help to open the dialogue about the importance of the community defining its own situation. One or several can be used. They were designed by C-CIMCA in Oruro, Bolivia. The fourth is a way to plan a training-of-trainers workshop to allow participants to discover this issue themselves.

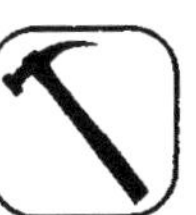

1. The Budget Plan

A *dynamic* to discuss planning **for** the community instead of **with** the community.

You will need packets of play money, a large chart as shown below, and markers.

● Divide into small groups of five or six people. Each small group receives equal amounts play money. Up front on the board is a list of types of projects and types of training appropriate for the area where these participants live.

(This is the chart on the board:)

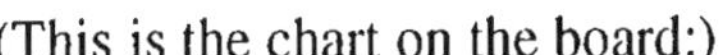

Group Names →	AMOUNT?				Group Names →	AMOUNT?				
PROJECTS	★	●	■	◆	TRAINING	★	●	■	◆	
Drill Well					Health Promoters					
Irrigation					Livestock Care					
Dig Terraces					Agroforestry					
Animal Credit					Well Maintenance					
Health Post					Irrigation					
Greenhouses					Home Building					
New Road					Nutrition					
Latrines					Organization					
Tree Nurserys					Leadership					
Credit for Crops					Other					
Other										

● Each small group is told they have their money in hand and must decide how to spend it. They can decide on the projects listed or others they want to add. They can budget as much or as little as they want. Each group presents their budget and it is marked on the chart up front. A discussion begins of the types of programs which are best as each group is presenting.

● A group may choose not to do a budget because they don't know what the community wants, or an individual may object in their group. The facilitator needs to ask what process happened in each group.

● From this activity springs the question: "On what basis have we planned? Do we know what the community wants?"

● This leads to a lively dialogue (sometimes with groans!) **about planning *for* the community instead of *with* the community.** In order to plan the vision and projects necessary, there must be a community-based assessment of the situation first.

2. This Is What You Need

A very brief but powerful dynamic to show how people feel and act when someone else makes a decision for them.

You need an aspirin, Paul.
No, I really don't.
Does anyone here have an aspirin for Paul?
I do. Here, Paul, take this aspirin, you need it.

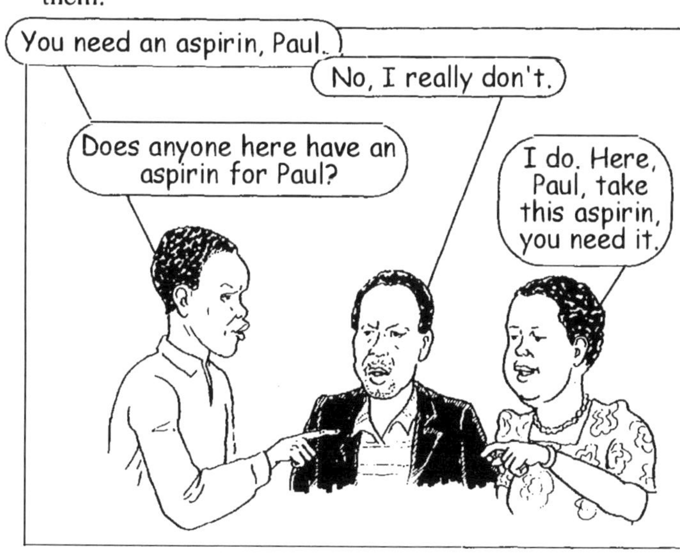

● You will need a volunteer to play the role of "Paul" below, left.

● The facilitator begins talking to the volunteer, telling him what he needs and how to solve his problem.

● Ask "Paul" how he felt when the facilitator was defining his needs and giving him the solution.

● Ask the participants where they have seen this happening. How did they feel?

● The participants can also say what could have been done differently.

● This is an example of **what happens when *outsiders* define the situation for the community.** The needs defined are often not the community's needs. The solutions offered are not the necessary solutions. Paul may say, "I'm not going to take the aspirin." This is also often the result of an outsider-based assessment: the people do not use the resulting project or training idea.

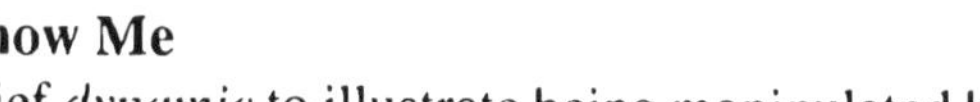

3. Show Me

A brief *dynamic* to illustrate being manipulated by a powerful or trusted person.

● You will need the circle of participants and whatever they happen to have in their pockets.

● The facilitator asks everyone to stand in a large circle.

● The facilitator says: "Take whatever is in the pocket of your neighbor on the right and show it to everyone."

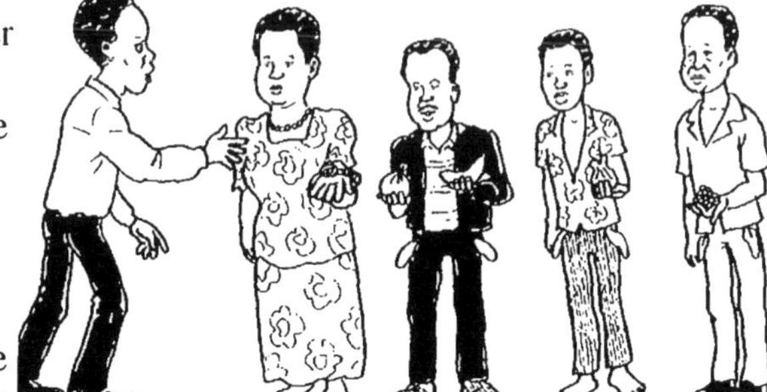

● Normally the majority of the people will do it. The facilitator encourages each to show what they found with much kidding and laughter. Generally no one will say, "Don't take my things" or "You don't have the right to do this."

● Now the facilitator says, "This is manipulation!" Analyze this together. Why are we so willing to trust outsiders and do what they suggest without thinking it through for ourselves?

● What are the weaknesses of a training program developed by a trusted, well-intentioned outsider?

● This is how manipulation takes place in the community. A village president or important person speaks for everyone without consulting the people. Or an outsider institution with good intentions tells everyone they should do something and they do it, respecting the expert knowledge. But in the end it may not be the best thing for them.

4. Within A Workshop Design

This is a way to design a training of facilitators workshop so the participant's own work throughout the workshop will teach them through reflection. It will demonstrate to the participants how their ideas about the farmers' needs are different from the farmers' ideas about their own needs.

● You will need a different assessment *dynamic* planned for each small group of participants.

● Divide the participants into random small groups. Each group uses a different participatory tool (such as a seasonal calender, mapping, ranking, etc. – see "Tools," starting on pg. 253). Each group uses the tool within their group to define what they feel the people in the community need. Then go to a community where your program is working. Each group can use their tool with the villagers so that the people define their current situation and their need. After returning to your workshop, put the two lists on the board, side by side. There will always be significant differences. Have the trainers discuss this issue as they see the differences themselves.

A community assessment or training assessment is not the same as a lengthy survey based on the needs of the institution. Many institutions need baseline information, or they want detailed information or studies of the area. While detailed studies serve the purposes of the institutions, they usually do not serve the needs of the community.

The Participatory Learning and Action (formerly Participatory Rural Appraisal, (PRA) tools really help a community to look *in depth* at their own situation. They can be used as part of the investigation or as learning tools in training sessions. They should result in community action.

However, many PRA's have been done that were never fully analyzed with the community or were never used by the community to plan a program. In these cases, the PRA has used the valuable time of the people without results. Such experiences will eventually sour people on the participatory approach when they see no results from their PRA work.

Ask yourself, **"Is the survey or investigation we are doing too complex to analyze together with the community?" "Can the information be used right away by the community to make a decision?"** These questions should help you to keep the assessment in perspective.

Steps to Defining the Situation

A *community assessment* can be an involved process. It can take several meetings over a period of weeks to accomplish. Each of the following five steps should be followed to do a complete definition of the situation in the community. With some of the steps, several ideas for *dynamics* are given. Use these or others which you feel are appropriate (See Chapter 12, "Tools"). If you are planning a training program (more involved than a workshop or two) to meet the changing training needs of an area, a *community assessment* will establish the vision and the directions of the training program.

A *training assessment* may be much simpler than a community assessment. If it is for a specific workshop, the participants can define their training needs in one meeting. All of the participants in a workshop should be contacted about their training needs prior to the workshop. This will aid in an appropriate design of the workshop.

If a training program is to be established to benefit an area of many communities (such as the training of CLWs), a much more involved assessment will be necessary. The vision and direction of the program should be defined with the village people. Once the vision is defined, the workshop sequences and topics can be outlined. This will usually require a series of meetings over time with the communities involved, the facilitators to be trained, and workshop participants.

Note: all of these steps assume you will use a participatory approach in facilitation. For tips on good facilitation see "Implementation" page 137. For information about the participatory approach see Chapter 1, "Learning and Teaching."

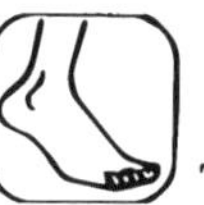

The steps for each type of assessment:

Community Assessment	**Training Assessment**
1. Identify the assessment committee and plan the assessment process with the committee. **2.** Define the current situation in the community. **3.** Analyze the situation and the current problems. **4.** Define the visions and directions for the future. **5.** Consider the available resources.	**1.** The assessment committee consists of the facilitators who plan the assessment. **2.** The participants define their current situation related to the requested area of training. **3.** The participants determine the goals or vision for the training program or workshop.

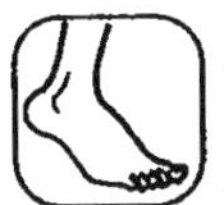

STEP ONE: Identify the assessment committee

The committee should be identified in a meeting prior to defining the community situation. The community, together with the outsiders, should decide who would be the most appropriate people. Usually a committee will be made up of both

- members of the community or organization and
- facilitators or members of the outsider institution.

Try to make sure that all the committee members are not important village leaders. It is good to think about including poorer people, women as well as men, and both older and younger people. The committee will not make the final decisions about the program, but they will help to motivate people, organize information and re-present the information to the people for their decision. We all come to situations with a bias and we should be aware of those biases. **Each member of the committee will have biases which they bring to the work of the committee.** Large numbers on a committee are cumbersome, so the size should be limited to four or five people.

The committee should plan the assessment.

- **Who** will participate.
- **When** it will be.
- **Where** it will take place.
- **What** steps it will follow.
- **How** it will work–which tools it will use to encourage participation.

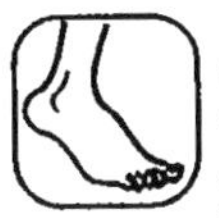

STEP TWO: Define the situation

In this step, people look at the current situation in their community. They define how the community is now and what the current problems are. In a *community assessment,* the results will be general for a whole community and will generate a community development plan. In a *training assessment,* the results are specific to a certain theme such as soil conservation or livestock production. The tools chosen to do this will depend on the purpose of the assessment.

Some *dynamics* for villagers to define their situation:

(See Chapter 12, "Tools" for more ideas–pages 253 through 262.)

1. Listening for important themes

A very good way for facilitators, Community Livestock Workers, and the assessment committee to grasp an idea of things which are central, important issues in their communities is listening. Whenever a group of people normally gets together they begin to discuss the issues which are important to them–the ideas and problems which excite and generate energy among the people.

Sometimes, if we ask people in a meeting or an interview what they think are the most important issues, they may not share their feelings because of the pressure of the group or the situation in the interview. So the facilitator, Community Livestock Worker, or assessment committee can try the following activities to help better understand the situation.

A. Listening where people normally gather

Go to places where people normally gather to talk and sit with them and listen to what they are talking about. This could be in front of a local store, at a tea shop, where the women wash clothes together, at a church before or after a service or during a festive gathering, or any other place people normally sit and talk. Listen for the themes which surface over and over, the topics people get excited about, and the ones they talk about in greater depth.

B. Listening while waiting for a meeting or a workshop to start

Ask people, "What are the problems you are having right now with your livestock?" Listen for the responses which are repeated several times and which generate a dialogue among the people present. What are the things they get excited or animated about as they talk and share? These are probably the most important and pressing issues. **Remember your own bias and do not lead the discussion!**

These important issues or themes are related to the deepest problems and issues the community faces. They are called *generative themes* because they generate energy among the people. When the community brainstorms about their situation, the assessment committee might mention these issues. This is especially true if there are some issues which have seemed to be present in informal discussions but which have not been shared in the community meeting. The village can then consider them and prioritize them with their already generated list.

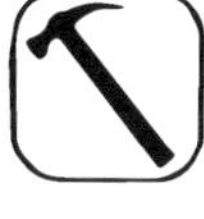

2. Brainstorming and prioritizing

Brainstorming is a rapid way for everyone to express their ideas in a safe environment. No idea is criticized. For more information on brainstorming turn to "Tools," Chapter 12, page 238.

A. Brainstorming on newsprint

- You will need newsprint and markers for each group.
- In a village meeting divide into small groups, men and women in separate groups. The facilitator asks all groups to answer the same question. If the community wants to look at current problems with livestock production, the facilitator asks the groups, "What are the current problems with livestock production in your herds?" Questions can be broad or focused but they must be clear to all the participants.
- By brainstorming, each group generates a list. Each group prioritizes their list, choosing the three most important problems.
- In the plenary, a list of all of the prioritized problems is made in large letters on newsprint. If a problem is repeated make a check mark at the side of that item–one mark for each group that mentioned the problem. Once everyone has shared their lists, you have a prioritized generalized list. Together with the community you can organize this list into categories.

B. Brainstorming with cards

- You will need lots of 5x7 cards or half sheets of 8 1/2 x 11 paper and marking pens for everyone.
- If the group is literate, a system of writing on cards can be used. If participants are preliterate, they can draw pictures to represent their problems and explain their pictures to the group. Everyone should be given a set of cards and a colored marker. Ask, "What are the most serious problems you have with your livestock production?" Or, "What are the most serious problems the community is confronting now?"
- Each person puts a different problem on each card. In small groups, each group discusses the problems. The group organizes and prioritizes their set of cards and each small group presents the top five or six needs.
- In plenary, each group tapes or sticks in some way their set of problems on a large paper or on a board up front.

The facilitator, with the consent and aid of all, moves the cards into categories, placing the repeat cards underneath one another. The group as a whole makes a decision as to overall priority of the problems.

C. Brainstorming with pictures on the ground

● You will need half-sheets of paper or cards and colored marking pens for everyone.

● In a very large gathering, this can be used to automatically prioritize problems:

● Each person draws a picture of the most pressing problem. As you go around the room and each person says what the problem is, their card is placed on the floor. Cards which describe the same problem are placed side by side. Cards which describe a different problem are placed in a new row under the first card. When everyone has shared their cards, there will be a large ranked table of problems on the floor.

● The dialogue which follows can discuss and confirm this ranking.

Source: Lina Maria Nivea, Colombia.

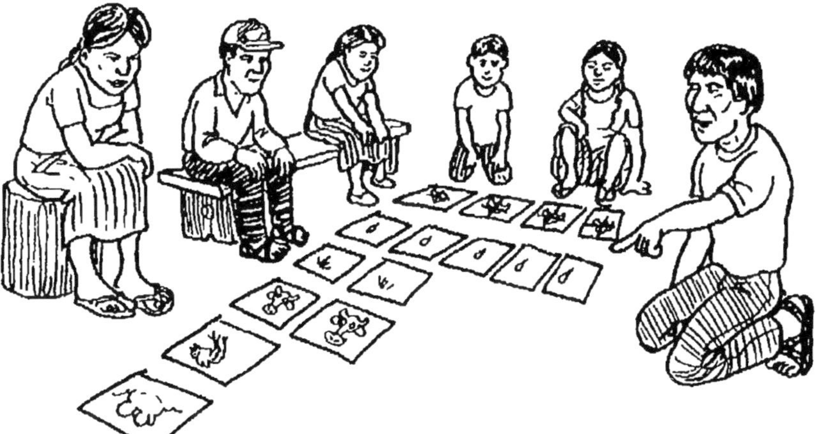

3. A walk through the community and fields

● You will need paper and pens for several people to record what they see.

● Insiders and outsiders together take a walk through the community or through someone's farm and herd. They talk together about what they see, writing down the things they observe and discuss.

● The facilitator can ask focus questions to aid this *dynamic*. Focus questions might be:

Why do you grow this?
Who works in this field?
How many people are in this family?

● They should not make decisions about the relative importance of these situations until everyone involved is together in a meeting. This walk can be used before a brainstorming session to get people thinking about their current situation.

4. Mapping

(See "Tools," pg 253.)

It is very helpful for villagers in small groups to make maps of the current situation in the village or on the farm. It helps people to have a concrete visual aid to analyze the current situation. For comparison, they can make a map of what the village situation was ten years ago. They can see change in one direction or another.

> Drawing a map together:
> From a mapping *dynamic,* villagers in Guatemala discussed how the trees had disappeared from the hill-sides surrounding their community. They discovered the effects of that change by looking at their current map. They could see decreasing production of their fields as erosion removed the topsoil and drought killed the crops. They also saw that, where there had once been natural springs, the land was now bare. They decided to attack this situation with a plan. Today the hillsides are covered with trees, the springs have returned, and production has increased.

5. Drawing and discussion

(See Chapter 12, page 249)

6. Seasonal calendars

(See Chapter 12, page 259)

7. Ranking the problems

(See Chapter 12, page 255)

Caution!

The tools of participatory assessment such as seasonal calendars, ranking, mapping, etc, can be used in a non-participatory or participatory way. A seasonal calendar can be developed with the help of local people but then analyzed by outsiders, who make the decisions. Or a seasonal calendar can be developed and analyzed by the community, along with the outside facilitator, and every-one can work together to make decisions.

When the analysis and decision making is done by the community, this helps them to see their current situation, evaluate it, and make decisions for action toward change. The learning process has already begun.

A note on gender roles

If a ranking *dynamic* is combined with a seasonal calendar (See "Tools," pages 255 and 259), the people will have an opportunity for a very good analysis of the gender-based roles of people in the family. This adds to the definition of their situation.

You can use ranking for the community to define who does which jobs in livestock care, crop production or forestry, and which are viewed as most important. (See "Valuing the Role and Participation of Women," Chapter 9). Then, a seasonal calendar like the following one can be used to view the distribution of work over the agricultural year.

Or, if the community has already made a seasonal calendar with the tasks in livestock care with rocks or sticks, they can add who does which job to the areas of each duty. For this they could use colored powder or seeds to represent the different people.

This allows the village to see who is doing the most work with the livestock and when they are most occupied. It can initiate many helpful discussions.

- It often has a tremendous impact on men who previously thought their wives did nothing or who didn't value the work their wives do.
- It can start a very good discussion and analysis of working together and carrying the load together.
- It can also help in the decision of who should attend workshops and when would be the most appropriate time to have them.

Seasonal Calendar

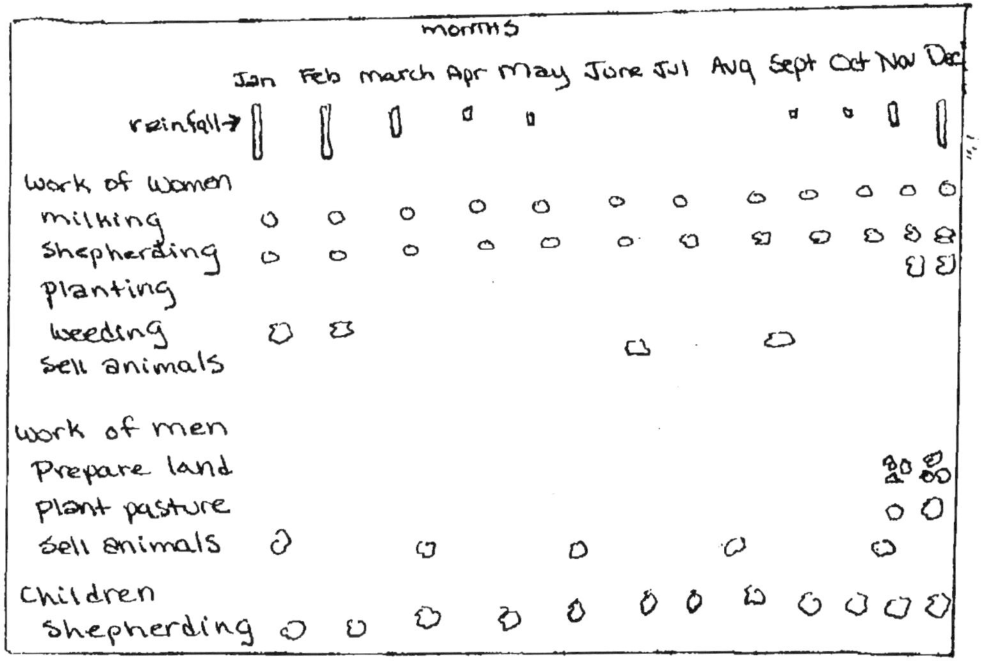

months

Jan Feb march Apr May June Jul Aug Sept Oct Nov Dec

rainfall→

work of women
milking
shepherding
planting
weeding
sell animals

work of men
Prepare land
Plant pasture
Sell animals

Children
Shepherding

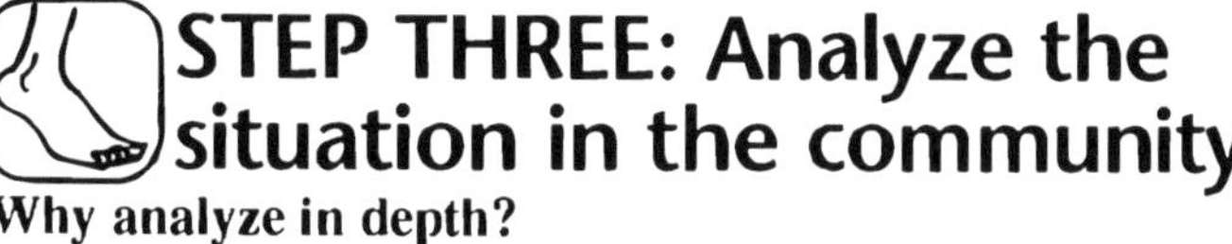

STEP THREE: Analyze the situation in the community

Why analyze in depth?

If the community has brainstormed a series of issues in the community assessment, they should analyze those issues in depth. This is necessary because it is easy to accept a superficial view of a situation and choose actions that may not solve the problem.

Be sure to analyze deeply to get to the root causes of the problems. Use the tool "The Process of Awareness" for community members prior to this in-depth analysis (See "Learning and Teaching," pg. 22.)

This type of analysis is for a community assessment, not a training assessment. In a training workshop, the in-depth analysis will become a part of the workshop as people look for solutions to these situations. The same method used here to analyze deeply can be used in a workshop with an agricultural theme.

A farmer has insect and weed problems in her crop. She applies more and more chemical insecticides and herbicides. But the problems do not stop. When she applies organic fertilizer she finds her crop improving. The first solution was based on a superficial look at the problem. The second solution focused on the root causes of the problem.

Divide to discuss

The more analysis that can be done in small groups, the better. In the plenary, fewer people tend to discuss than in small groups. A small number of people can control the outcome.

If mapping or ranking or another assessment tool has been used, the same small groups can be used to discuss the results in depth. Many times it is beneficial to divide these groups by gender, age or power and wealth. For example, a small group of young people will have a different view of the situation in the community than a small group of leaders. If the groups are randomly mixed, the results of the analysis will be highly influenced by the few more vocal and powerful people in the community.

Once each small group has analyzed the issues in depth, they each present their results to the plenary session of the whole community. The resulting plenary discussion will be enriched by the variety of viewpoints. During the plenary discussion the facilitator aids the community in reaching consensus about the root causes of their situation. See "small groups" in Tools pg. 236.

Consider the root causes

In analyzing the root causes of the problem the people may need to consider these causes:

- **Physical** (land erosion, earthquakes, mud slides, floods, etc.)
- **Economic** (subsistence, production, consumption, and marketing of goods and services.)
- **Political** (who makes local and national decisions, such as land rights, fencing, burning, markets, transportation, local organization etc. and how those decisions affect the people.)
- **Spiritual and Cultural** (values and beliefs of the community about farming or community life or raising animals and their management.)

Use the tools to analyze in depth

Many of the tools for determining the problem lead to a deep analysis. As people work to see and define the problem clearly, they begin to analyze the situation, as it appears on the map, the ranking chart, etc.

When brainstorming and prioritization has been done, a list of problems is defined. Return to the same small groups for the analysis of the top priority issues. A chart like this may help small groups to

In the example of mapmaking in Guatemala (pg. 70,) once the map had been made, the group looked it over for problem areas or areas they would like to change. They discussed this and reached a consensus. Then they envisioned a map of the future, what they wanted the village to look like in ten years. Then they discussed the steps to get to their future map. In this case the analysis of the situation was done together with the map, which defined the situation. No separate activity for analysis was necessary. The people did an in depth analysis from the reflection on their maps.

analyze these issues:

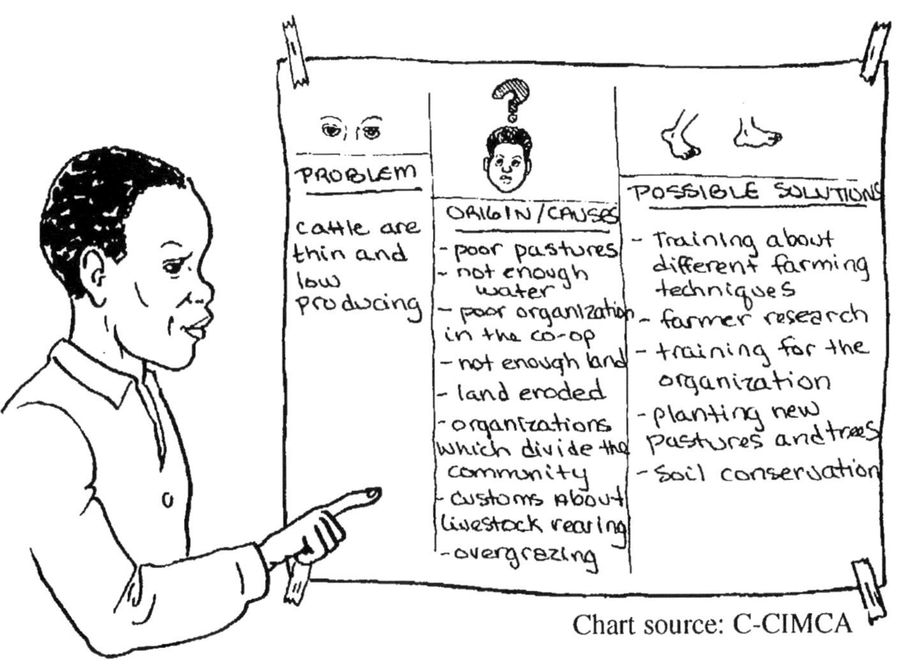

Chart source: C-CIMCA

STEP FOUR: Define the directions for the future.

Visioning: A process where a person, family or community thinks about and sets their vision for the future. They define what they would like their life, farm or community to look like at some point in the future. They also define the steps to reach that vision.

After analyzing the situation, the community participants identify what they feel are good solutions to their major problems. **The facilitator can assist by asking questions such as Why? Who? and How? to motivate people to think broadly.**

At this point in the community assessment, the committee can walk the village through a *visioning* exercise so they can determine what they would like their community to be like in the future, in five years or ten years. This will help people to see how the solutions they suggest can link to their future goals for the community. Individual farmers can take the time to vision how they would like their land and farm to look in five years and ten years.

> When people have a vision to work toward, they can make good decisions about the steps to reach that vision. If people focus always on current problems, they will often move from problem to problem without having a concrete direction in mind.

The role of the facilitator in this process is important. He or she needs to continue to ask open questions, probe deeply through asking why, and try not to bias or influence the results. (For tips on facilitation, see "Implementation," pg.137.)

Recording the vision

When the vision is defined, it should be recorded in some way by the community. If the vision was made through a map, the map in large poster form can be permanently displayed in the meeting room of the village. If the vision is a set of ideas, they can be displayed in poster form in a prominent place. This will provide incentive and encouragement to community members as they work toward the vision.

Returning to the vision

A vision is only useful for a community or organization if they refer to it regularly for decision-making and work to refine it. At the end of the first visioning process the vision may not be very clear or it may not be expressed in a way that everyone likes. Monthly meetings, monitoring of community projects, and annual evaluation sessions are all good times to review and refine the community vision. Whenever the community plans new activities they can check to see if the action will lead them toward or away from their vision. Having the vision posted in a prominent place will help to return to it time and again.

How community visioning is related to a training program

A training program which is designed to serve many communities should be based on the vision of the communities or region. Realistically, only very large programs have the time and resources needed to do community visioning with many communities and across a region. Working with communities to help them establish their vision may be one of the topics for a training program.

If your training program begins before the communities have established their vision, the goals of the training program may be more outsider-influenced than community-influenced. In this case, visioning would ideally be a part of the training program. Once the communities establish their vision, the goals and objectives of the training program should be adjusted to fit the community vision.

The family farm vision and the community vision are related to establishing a training program in these ways and others:

- The goals and objectives of the training program are based on the vision the community is working toward.
- The specific training topics will come from working on each step of reaching the vision.
- If the community decides they need a CLW, they will vision the role of that person in the community (See "Community Selection of a Community Livestock Worker," pg. 35). Once the role is defined, they can identify the training needs.

In a **training needs assessment** for a training program some visioning is also necessary. It is important that the community or participants define their goals and objectives for the training program.

The community has a stated vision or issues which they want the training to address. What do they hope to accomplish by the training? These things the community wants to accomplish are their broader goals for the training program.

Sample goals for a training program:

- Every livestock producer will understand how to design and start using a sustainable system for their farm.
- Our community will have three Community Livestock Workers trained and assisting us in livestock production.
- We will know how to treat our animals for the most common and serious diseases which affect them.

On the next pages are some *dynamics* which could be used in a community visioning process.

Examples of *dynamics* for visioning

These are some sample *dynamics* which can be used for visioning. Generally one *dynamic* is used to initiate the dialogue. From that dialogue the participants reach consensus and define their vision.

1. Determining what our values are:

As was stated in the Opening Section (pg. xi) the individual's or community's values are at the root of their vision. In most cases it is helpful for the community to think about what their values are before they set their vision.

● First, help people think about what a value is. One way to do this is to ask a series of questions. The first set of questions can be answered in the whole group. They can be used as a warm-up. The second set of questions can be answered in small groups.

● **Questions for the whole group:**

1. What food do you like?
2. What is your favorite thing to do?
3. What would you like to change in your community?
4. What qualities do you look for in a friend?
5. What makes you happy?

● **Questions for small groups:**

In small groups answer the following questions for yourselves. Share some of your personal values with your group members.

1. What is the most important thing you want your children to remember?
2. What is the one thing you do not want your children to have to experience?
3. What makes you mad?
4. What are the qualities of a good spouse?
5. If you found $10 how would you spend it?
6. What have you done to help someone?
7. If you were to meet the president of your country, what would you say to him?

● The plenary analysis of this exercise will help people define what values are. Once people feel comfortable understanding what values are, they can define the values the community organization holds.

Source: Kindervatter 1991.

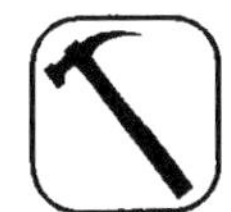

2. Brainstorming about and analyzing the future:

● What do you most value in life: for yourself, for your family, for the community, your production, and your organization?

- What are the values we hold as a community?
- What are the principles we want to live our lives by?
- What quality of life do we desire as a community or family for ourselves and our children?
- What family goals or community goals are we working toward, with our livestock production and on our farm?
- When this child is ten years old (pointing to a baby) what would we like the community to be like?

For more about brainstorming see "Tools," pg. 238.

● All of these are good questions for small group work or for family work together. Can each family define what they are working toward? Can each small group define what the community is working for?

● In the plenary, present the results, discuss, and analyze them. Make a chart of family goals and community goals for future reference. This chart can be used to question the proposed solutions or community actions to see if they will help to reach the family and community goals. To help start the brainstorming they can play "The Road to Our Vision": pg. 276.

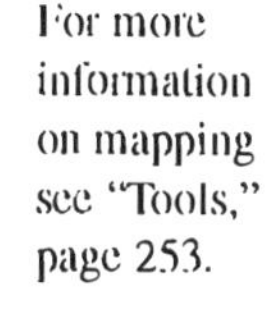
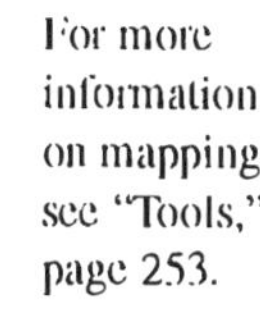

3. Mapping:

This is a good tool for visioning whether or not it is used to help the community analyze their situation.

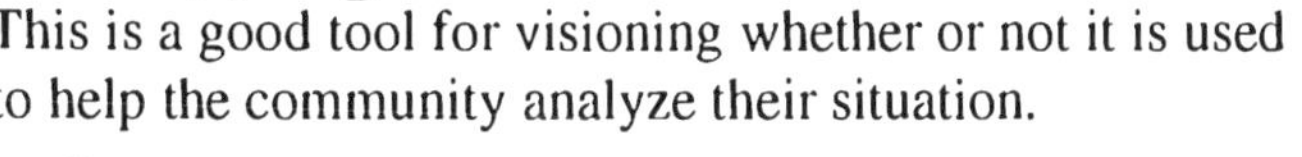

- Divide everyone into small groups. Each group draws a map of the village the way they would like it to be in five years or ten years. They highlight the things they would like to see changed. Please note: mapping can also be used for a family to set their vision for their farm in the future.

For more information on mapping see "Tools," page 253.

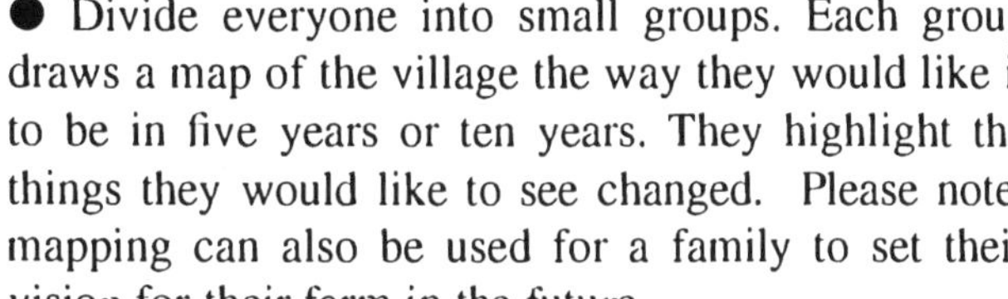

- Encourage each family to make their map for their family farm on a piece of paper. At the end of the session

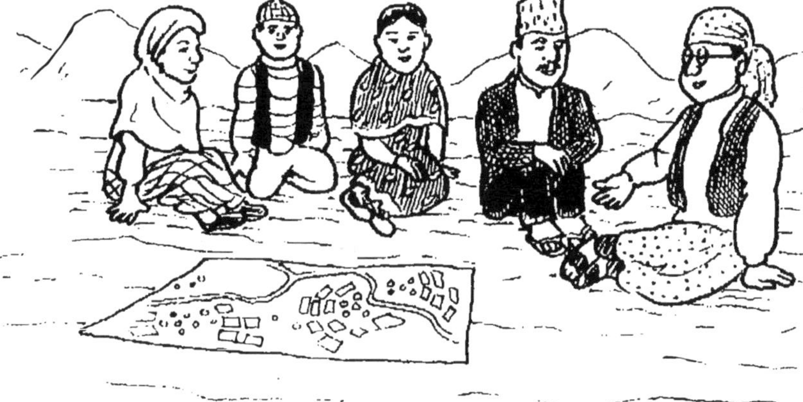

they can take the map home, put it on their wall, and refer to it for planning each day.

- Each group presents their map to the whole.
- As the discussion unfolds, the facilitator writes the things the people want to change on a list. These things to change are then converted into objectives.
- Once a village has a list of objectives, they can make a plan to reach those objectives.
- As the village looks at where they want to be, **they can identify appropriate solutions for the problems or issues previously defined.**

Note: this dynamic is time consuming and should not be rushed so that people really can look in depth at where they want to be in the future. For this reason, it may be more appropriate to use this visioning in a workshop where the villagers can then plan the steps to reach their vision. Or it could be planned for a separate community meeting.

As the community group works together, they will be defining solutions to the problems they have previously discussed. They will prioritize those solutions based on their vision for the future.

The maps produced in this *dynamic* should stay with the community. They can display them on the walls in a meeting room alongside the written vision. The community may decide to make one consolidated map of their vision, once they reach a consensus about their priorities.

4. Clarifying the vision

Writing a vision which is clear to everyone is important so that it will inspire everyone in the community. But writing a clear vision is also difficult! Here is a short game to play which can begin a discussion about clear and unclear goals and visions.

- The facilitator reads a series of questions. At the end of each question she asks the participants to raise their hands if they think the vision is clear.

Some sample questions:

1. Betty wants everyone in the community to work together and to be united. (NOT clear)
2. Peter wants to have a better life. (NOT clear)
3. Mary wants her children to finish elementary school. (Clear)
4. Ruth wants to fix her house with the help of her friends before July. (Clear)
5. John wants the community leaders to help the people more. (NOT clear)

6. Alice wants to work with her community to have clean water within the next several months. (Clear)
7. Greg wants the leaders to build a recreation center this year (Clear)
8. Paula wants more money (NOT clear)
9. Josephine wants to take a course in repairing small electrical equipment this year to find a better job. (Clear)
10. Jose wants his family to be happy (NOT clear)

● After playing this game give people the opportunity to write a clear personal vision. Be sure they understand the long term nature of a vision and don't write short term goals. Small groups can help each individual to reflect on the clarity of their vision.

● When personal visions have been clarified, small groups can determine the vision of the large group.

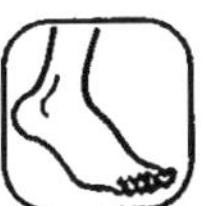

STEP FIVE: Consider the available resources

Once the vision and the possible steps to reach the vision have been decided on, they can be analyzed together to determine the best plan of action. In order to plan, the community must examine the available resources. First they look at the resources they have in the community, then at the resources necessary from outside the community. This is true whether they are planning for their community vision or for the vision of a training program.

Resources can be divided into categories to help people think about them. Heifer Project International suggests the resources be considered in the categories of *People, Place,* and *Productive Resources.*

A. People:

This includes the people living in the community and the outsiders who work there.

This category will also include the grassroots organizations of the community and any outsider organizations or businesses who work there.

Here are some questions to help the community think about these resources:

- Is there a group of motivated people who want the training?
- Is there a community organization that can implement the activity?
- Is there strong community leadership?
- What outside organizations are present in the community?
- What skills could the outsiders bring to obtaining the vision or implementing the training program?
- Are there social, religious, economic, class/caste, legal, and/or political conditions which might affect the activities?

B. Place:

These are the **natural resources** in the community. They include the land, water, trees, hills, swamps, etc. This category also includes the **infrastructure** of the community. It includes roads, schools, health post, store, training center, etc.

Here are some sample questions for people to think about the place:

- What are the natural resources of this community?
- Where are they located in relationship to the houses and buildings?
- Where are family-owned land and forest, community-owned land and forest, government-owned land and forest?
- What are the boundaries of the community?

And for a workshop or training program:

- Is land available for planting and maintenance activities during training?
- Is there a place to hold training sessions? (school, church, community room, training facility)
- Is there a place for people to sleep if CLWs come from other communities?

C. Productive resources

These resources are the wealth of the community. They include the **monetary resources** such as livestock, crops, artisan products, things made by the people, equipment, etc. The productive resources also include the **skills, knowledge, and experience of the people.** They would include pottery making, carpentry, masonry, weaving, a health promoter, a Community Livestock Worker, etc. They also include the knowledge of farmers in livestock and crop production.

Some questions to help the people think about these resources:

- What types of work do people in the community do?
- Which people have received special training which they use to serve the community?
- What crops are produced here?
- What livestock is produced here?
- What community labor is available to reach the vision?

And for a training program:

- Who are the people who treat the animals when they are sick?
- Are there animals available for practice sessions in training?

It is important for the community to identify and value these local resources. So many times a community feels they can bring nothing to the accomplishment of their vision. They often feel only the outsiders can bring solutions and resources. When the community sees the value in their local resources, they see the possibility for resolving their own problems and moving toward their vision. Once the community values their resources, the outsider's resources are seen as only part of the solution.

In this analysis of resources, some difficult situations within the community may become apparent. They might include a trained health promoter who no longer serves the community. Or there could be an institution which has committed to accomplishing something and has not done it. The community does not need to solve these difficulties at this time but they should be written down so that they can be discussed, planned for, and negotiated later.

A *dynamic* to analyze resources:

● Divide into small groups. Each group is given a resource area:

- **Natural Resources** (land, water, trees, hills, swamps, etc.)
- **Infrastructure** (health post, school, store, etc.)
- **Work** which people in the community do (health promoter, carpenter, mason, butcher, weaver, potter, etc.)
- **Organizations** (mother's club, parent's organization, water committee, etc.)
- **Institutions** which help (church, NGOs, government, etc.)

● Each group makes a map of these things, their locations, and who they affect. Or they can draw a diagram which shows their connections to the people's houses.

● Each group will present their drawings in each category. The facilitator asks, "Are there any others in this category?"

● As the community analyzes the information presented in the plenary, they will value and appreciate their local resources. They can then make the links to the necessary resources for implementing a training program or for implementing their vision.

Source: Lina Maria Obando Nivea.

What can the outside institution contribute to the program?

This is a time for the outsiders to share frankly with the community what their institution can do and what their stake in the program is. If community members have identified water resources as their most serious problem and the outsider institution works only with livestock production, they need to be frank. In the community needs assessment, it may happen that the community will decide their priorities are for needs which the institution cannot help with. Then the community can decide if the work of the institution is within the realm of what they would like to work on right now, or not.

If the community has defined their vision, the outsider organization can see how their program does or does not fit into the community vision. It is important for the community to look at their own resources before the outsider organization suggests the resources they have available. This will help to prevent the situation of the community accepting outsider resources just because they are offered.

NOW THE COMMUNITY HAS DEFINED IT'S SITUATION! MOVE ON TO THE NEXT STEP TOGETHER, PARTICIPATORY PLANNING.

Chapter 5
Participatory planning

This chapter covers the following topics:

The seven steps of planning a training program

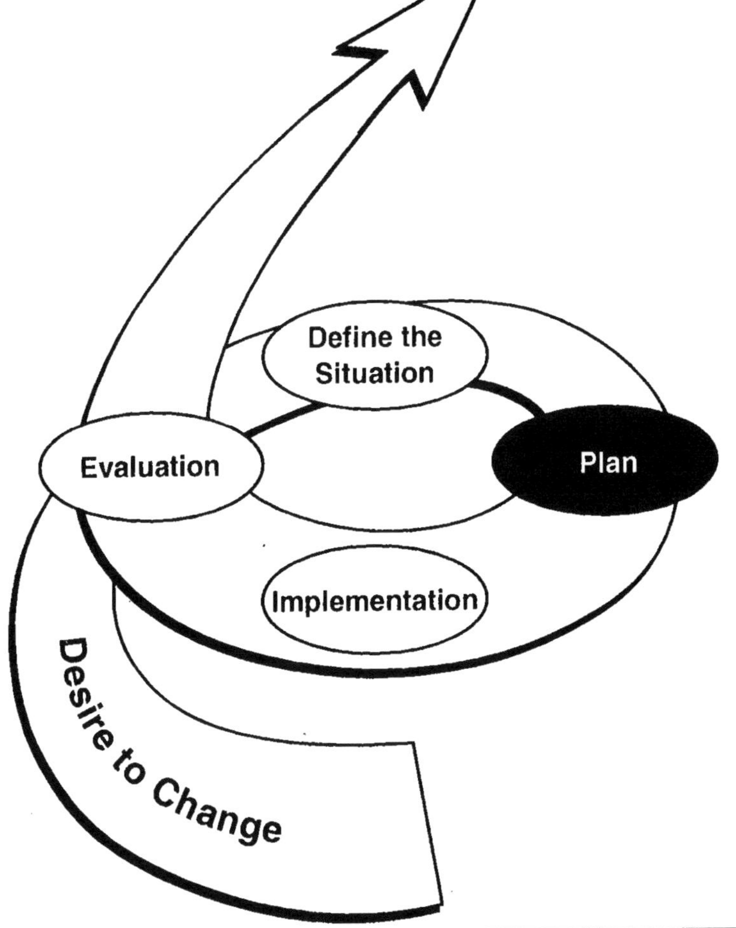

The training assessment has been completed by the community together with the facilitators of training. The situation may have been defined through several means; during the community livestock selection process in the community, during meetings with the villages, during small group meetings and visits, and/or during a meeting with the participants in the training. If a good analysis of the situation has been done, much planning will already be available, and some of the decisions will have been made by the communities and future Community Livestock Workers. Now the planning stage of the training program begins.

A *dynamic* to illustrate the importance of planning

Tamali's taxi:

This is a role play where a group of people gets into a taxi owned by Tamali. The taxi begins on it's trip and several mishaps happen. First they run out of gas and Tamali goes off and gets some. Then a tire is leaking air and he continually has to get out and fill it up. Then they take the wrong road because he says he knows where he is going and they get lost. He wants to be paid but the people don't want to pay him because he hasn't taken them to where they needed to go.

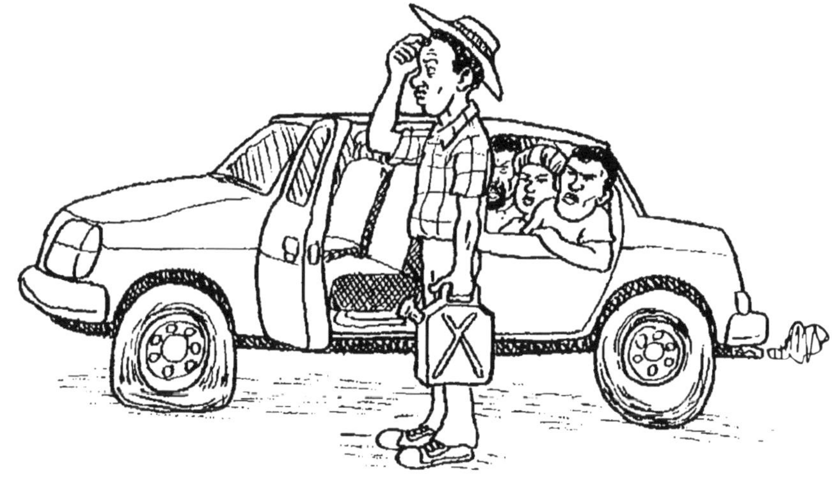

This is a great way to start a discussion about planning. What happened here? Does this ever happen in real life? Why did it happen? What could he have done differently?
Source: Valorie Shean

The seven steps of planning

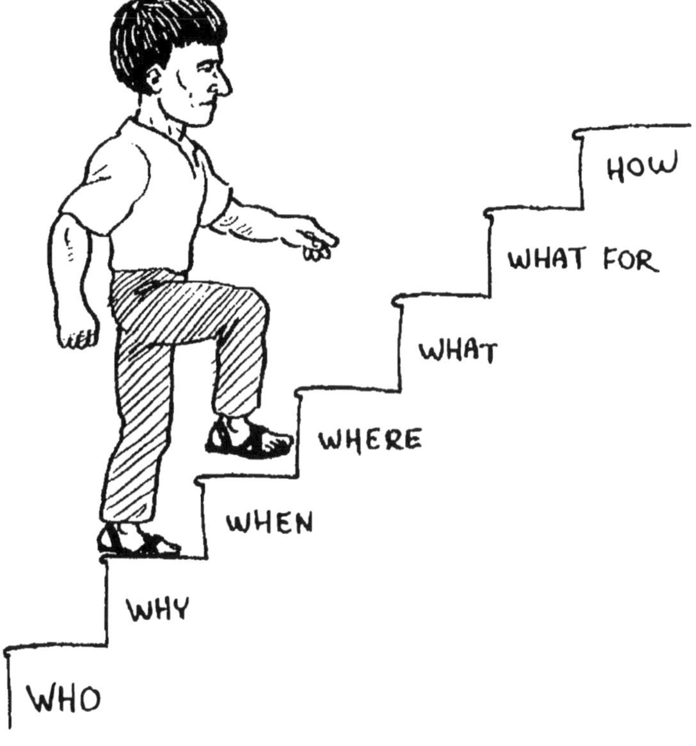

For the planning for a workshop, course, or program we can use the seven steps of planning to assist us.

Each workshop should be developed or adjusted to the experiences and needs of each new group of students. It is important that a **plan be flexible** so that as the workshop proceeds and the participants identify their needs more specifically, the plan can be changed.

STEP 1. Who?

This step defines who should participate and who should facilitate. Since the participants will define the content, we first need to know who the workshop is for.

We have already talked about:

1. The selection by the community of **community workshop participants** (pg. 29)
2. The selection by the community of their **Community Livestock Workers** (pg. 35)
3. And the selection and training of **facilitators** who are appropriate for participatory training (pg. 39–51)

How many people should participate in a workshop?

Consider this situation:

When many people are in a workshop, the banking system of education usually results. This is because people will not discuss and analyze problems in a large group. Consensus in solutions to problems is very difficult to reach when there are many present. So the trainer usually resorts to a lecture.

Also, if there are too many participants, hands-on practice of technical skills like examinations and vaccinations or social skills like leading a meeting and teaching is almost impossible. There aren't enough hours, facilitators, or animals for individual practice and coaching. If people don't get the opportunity to practice it with their own hands, they may never do the skill, so is it worth teaching?

Generally **between 15 and 20 people is an optimum number** of people for a participatory training workshop.

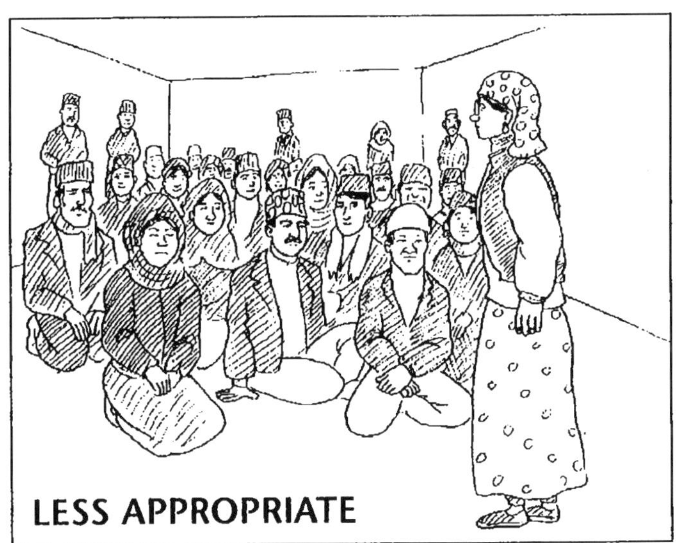

LESS APPROPRIATE

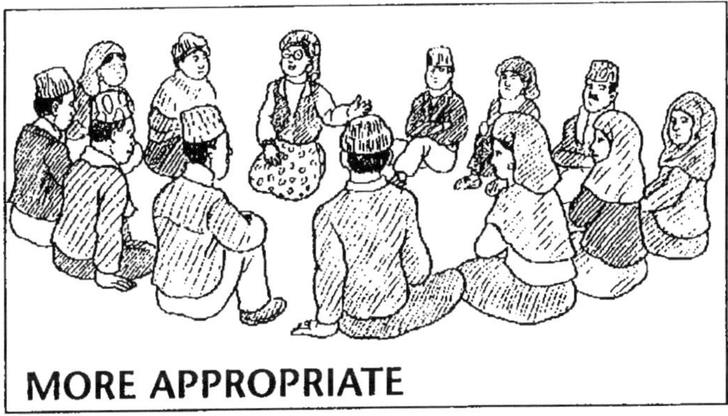

MORE APPROPRIATE

Everyone can easily see each other's faces and hear each other speak. This encourages sharing of ideas and group analysis and makes the discussions exciting. Even this group is too large for many discussions and must be divided into small groups for in-depth discussion and practice.

Who should facilitate?

A team of facilitators is always a good idea. They can encourage one another, give ideas for improvement of each others' training, and plan together as the workshop is changing.

There should be one facilitator for every 7 participants in a small group. In a highly hands-on practical program, where there is much practice with animals, participants need the opportunity for coaching. If the group is too large, one or two will be interested and engaged and the others will be bored.

So if you have 20 participants in a workshop, you should have three facilitators.

A note on the participation of men and women:
If you have men and women in the workshop, there should also be men and women facilitators.

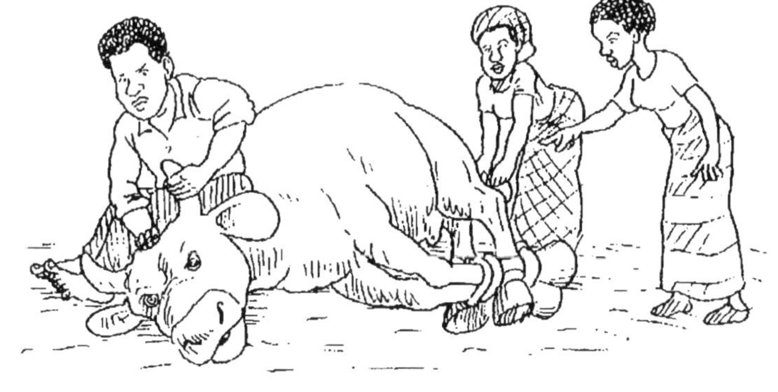

Women especially need to be coached and encouraged by other women to try the new skills and to speak out. Many village women feel they cannot perform animal care skills or planning skills. Once they see village women facilitators practicing the skills with ease, they are encouraged to try with positive results.

Training should always take place in the first language of the people. If, for some reason, a trainer is used who does not speak the language, there should always be a co-trainer who is fluent in the language. This allows people to deeply question the concepts and to fully engage in the training.

STEP 2. Why?

You may be working with the village on one of several different types of training:

- A topic to be considered at a village meeting,
- A one-day or half-day workshop,
- A training workshop for all farmers, a group of farmers, or a group of children,
- A training program to train Community Livestock Workers.

For each of these a similar planning process will be used, although it must be more in-depth for a longer program.

The assessment will have defined:

- The **problem or situation** which exists in the community,
- The **vision** or where the community wants to be in the future,
- The **resources** available to reach the vision or solve the problem,
- The **goals** of the community in relation to this problem and the training solution they have chosen,
- Clear and concrete action **objectives** for the training course or program.

These goals and objectives should be clearly written before proceeding with the planning.

The reasons for the training program or workshop will have been defined as the situation of the community is defined. It should be clear for all involved why the workshop is happening. The men and women involved in the training will know they need to deepen or strengthen their knowledge, skills, and attitudes about the topics to be covered. They will also be aware of the training needs in their own organization or community.

STEP 3. When?

In planning for the right time four things will need to be decided, based on the community assessment of their situation:

Right time of year for content: If you are teaching about pasture planting and management, do it during pasture planting season so you can practice in the course. Train for pest control during the pest season. This is especially true for village courses on specific topics. People don't have any desire to learn how to dig wells during the rainy season, and by the time they can apply the information, they might need a refresher on techniques.

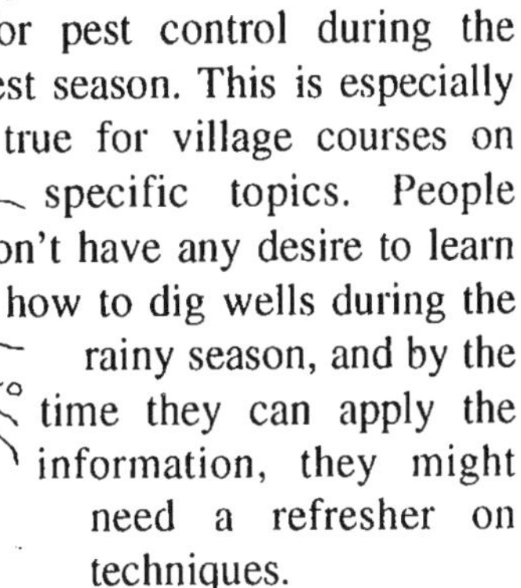

Right time of year to have time to attend: As the seasonal calender of tasks is developed with the community, they identify the best times of year for training (see "Seasonal Calender" in "Tools" pg. 71, 259). In Bolivia, farmers always want training when it is raining. Sometimes this must be balanced with the opportunity for practice with animals. Pastoralists in northern Kenya are always dispersed during the dry season, so workshops are planned for the rainy season when people and animals are together. With the agricultural calender of your area, people may have more time during some times of year for training. During planting and harvest they may be too occupied to participate in a workshop.

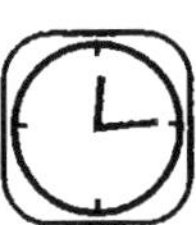

Right time of the day to have time to attend: The most appropriate time of day for a workshop may be different for men and women, this is due to different work responsibilities. Women may want to have workshop hours early in the morning and in the evening. They may need from late morning to mid afternoon off for cooking and childcare. For any workshop, it is important the participants set the hours of the workshop on the first day.

Setting the times of the workshop, see "Implementation" pg. 121.

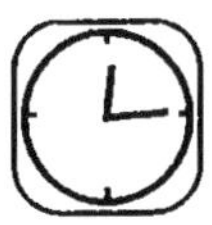

Right length (days and hours) for the workshop: How long can adults sit and think? How long can the workshop be when it includes women who have many responsibilities in childcare and cooking? A workshop planned for many community members will have a different schedule than that of a workshop for specialists like CLWs.

Community workshops

These workshops are for anyone in the community who wants them. They might be for men and women on animal husbandry and disease prevention as well as for pasture, tree, and water development. Flexibility in scheduling is very important. **The villagers should always be involved in the decision of how long the workshop should be.**

- **Half-day or one-day workshops.** These are designed to cover one topic in depth. There is usually a classroom session with discussion and practice with animals, planting, or trees, etc. Depending on scope and available time there may be just a practice session with a dialogue. These can be a very effective use of time if the village has identified one specific issue they want to address. There should be a coordinated, overall program so the training is not just "hit or miss." The overall vision should be analyzed with the village and the facilitators.

• **3-7 day sessions.** These workshops allow for the development of a system, or a cohesive idea of care or management. They are short enough that women can attend, but long enough to develop a set of related ideas.

Interestingly, when we began the training program for villagers in Bolivia, we asked the villagers how long the workshops should be. They decided that 4-5 days would be a good length. When the training team began to plan and shared with other outsider "experts" the length of the workshops, these experts were uniformly negative. The experts said villagers can't or won't go to workshops longer than half a day. The workshops have had great popularity and are continually requested by different communities. The "experts" don't know what to think. Could it be the method of training and the villager-chosen content made the workshops exciting, appropriate, and worthwhile enough for the men and women farmers to devote 4-5 days?

Training Community Livestock Workers

These are programs to train village specialists.
There are several different approaches:

• A series of **many very short workshops**
In these programs the CLWs receive training one day a week for as long as they work in their communities. It allows close relationships and continuous skills development in the atmosphere of the real problems the Community Livestock Workers face. It may be impractical for CLWs who must travel long distances to a workshop. It may also be difficult to develop certain topics which require continuity in the training process.

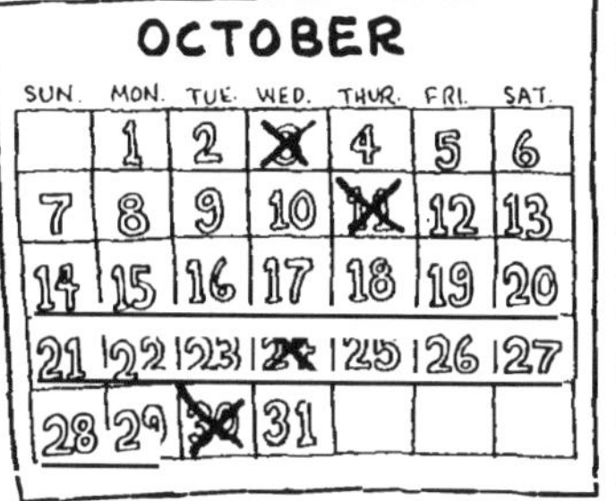

Some programs which initially have 1-2 -week sessions or a long 2-3 -month session will use this type of training for follow-up and continuing education.

• A series of **one or two-week workshops** with practice time in the village in between:
In this type of program, participants have the opportunity to practice in their communities during the 1-2 months between workshops and to bring their real problems to the workshops for exploration and analysis together. This enriches their study and builds their skills and problem- solving abilities. CLWs who must travel a long distance to come to workshops may find this system difficult. Most women are able to participate in this type of workshop, whereas most find a longer workshop difficult to attend due to their other responsibilities.

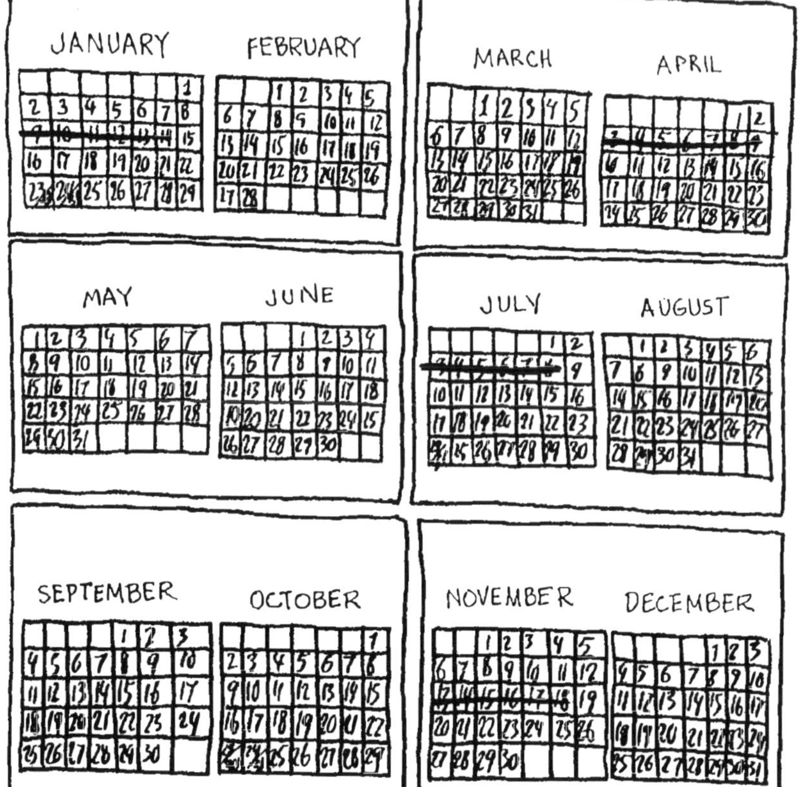

- **One long continuous workshop**

These workshops are more difficult for many farmers to attend, especially for women who have many obligations at home and on their farms. The workshops do allow for greater development of topics, and for building on previous sessions. Many times only young single men will attend these programs. They often view them as an opportunity to learn a skill which will help take them out of the community.

Make sure that in your planning of workshop length you **plan enough time for:**

- **Field trips** to visit a family who has applied a technology successfully on their farm, so that the farmer can train the participants;
- Opening and closing ceremonies;
- **Evaluations and feedback**–daily, weekly, and at the end of the workshop;
- Icebreakers and introductions;
- **Revisions** and review based on learner feedback;
- Practical applications and hands-on practice.

STEP 4. Where?

The best community-based, participatory workshops for farmers or CLWs take place in or near their communities. Men and women farmers want training to be physically close to save on costs and time of travel. In the community, the village becomes the classroom as real village problems are analyzed and activities done under conditions similar to those in the participant's home community.

The **advantages of community-based** workshops:

- CLWs and trainers see a greater variety and greater numbers of cases.
- Community members, not just trainees, are motivated about animal production and health.
- There is more interaction between the learners and the community in real-life situations
- Participants are able to practice with organization and communication topics in the community with community members.
- Night sessions with puppet shows or videos or cultural nights can draw the whole community into an analysis.
- Community-based training is generally less expensive than center-based training.
- It allows outsider trainers to feel and experience the local context.
- It allows bonding with village families where participants and trainers eat and sleep. There is exchange between the families and the CLWs each evening about workshop content and community problems.

Some **limitations of community-based** training:

- Often there is not adequate space for sleeping and eating together, a training room or, a place to prepare and review for the next day's topics.
- Sometimes it is difficult to find cooks who can cook well for large groups
- Audiovisual equipment can be difficult to transport and use (no electricity).
- There are too many animals to see them all. Most programs make a schedule and limit the number of animals seen per day.
- In some villages there is no place for playing sports together. In center-based training this is one of the things that builds camaraderie. However, in workshops with men and women, some sports can be difficult. In the village, appropriate games can be played together.
- An important aspect of bonding, learning, and working together happens outside of the classroom during eating and relaxing times. Often in community-based programs the trainees and trainers may be spilt up to eat and sleep. This does not facilitate the develoment of the camaraderie which center-based training develops. But it also helps prevent an "us" and "them" mentality.
- If the workshop is in their own community, there is a temptation for participants to return home to complete tasks. Holding the workshop in another community will alleviate this problem.

Many times training centers are built on the outskirts of towns with their own land and animals so they can be self-contained. This effectively takes participants outside of the community reality. In the traditional banking system of training, the teachers want the students to be away from distractions so they can concentrate on the lectures. In participatory training the desire is for flexibility and developing a consciousness of the community situation.

If center based training is necessary because of circumstances, it is very important to **plan field work in the community during the week.** This gives the opportunity to have practice sessions with the community and helps to bring the village setting into the workshop.

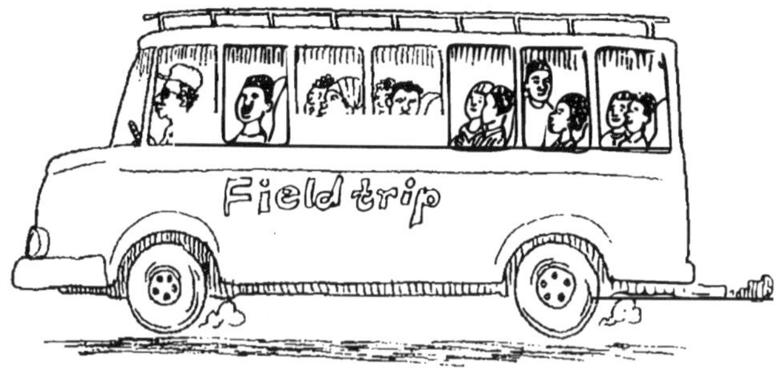

When technical high school or college training programs want to develop service professionals who are open to the needs of the community and to empowering community members to solve their own problems, they locate their training centers in communities. This is inconvenient for the instructors and the institution but develops community-oriented professionals who have not been isolated from the community reality for the years of training. These programs have dynamic relationships with the community where they are located. The students learn from the wisdom of the community people as well as from their other professors.

The workshop place:

When planning the workshop make sure there is a room large enough for participants to sit in a circle, with adequate lighting for group work. If there will be small group work, be sure there is room for each small group to work. Make sure there is

✓ **adequate seating,**
✓ **good food, and**
✓ **comfortable places to sleep with men separate from women.**

STEP 5. What?

This is **the list of topics to be covered throughout the workshop.** It includes the **knowledge, skills, and attitudes** to be taught.

The topics to be included in the training were identified by the training needs assessment, by talking with the people who will be trained, and by discussing with the team of facilitators. The participants have informed the training program of their training needs. The facilitators add the topics necessary to accomplish those needs. For more on content see "Implementation," pg. 122.

STEP 6. What for?

These are the **objectives of the workshop.** They tell you what the participants will have achieved by the end of the workshop.

They are like a road sign telling you what you will find when you reach the end of the road:

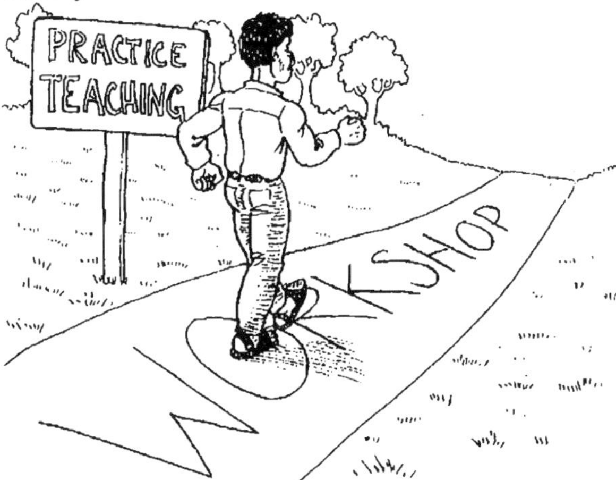

In the case in the picture the objective would be:
By the end of the workshop, the participants will have designed a training topic and practiced teaching their own topic so that they can teach in their community.

Workshop objectives should be **SMART**
Use this to check out the objectives you wrote:
S pecific - Do they say exactly what the learner will accomplish?
M easurable - Is there a way to measure the result?
A ppropriate - Are they relevant to the people and the place?
R ealistic - Can they be achieved?
T imely - Is there a time frame within which they will be finished?
See if the above objective fits this:
S pecific - participants will have "designed...and practiced teaching."
M easurable - they will complete one design and one practice teaching session.
A ppropriate - the CLW's will have to teach in their community in the future.
R ealistic - enough time has been planned for everyone to practice.
T imely - Training and practice will take place "by the end of the workshop."
Source: Rod McKean

Please notice there is a **first half of the objective which gives the activity to be accomplished and a second half which tells why the activity will be done.** These two halves are bridged by the words, "so that." Those words help us to remember to put in the "why" of the activity. Without the why it is an activity to be done and not an objective to be accomplished.

Why bother to spend time on SMART objectives? Isn't this just an exercise, a waste of time? This is important to community and **participant ownership** of the program. These road signs point to the results of the workshop. If the community has decided where they are going with the training program from the beginning, the participation will be dedicated and engaged. **Without engagement there is no learning!**

If you have a good set of objectives when you begin a program, you will be able to evaluate the success of that program at its end. **Because the objectives can be measured we are accountable to achieve them.** The participants will be able to see what they have accomplished during the time they have spent in the workshop. They will know they have learned because they have accomplished the objectives.

STEP 7. How?

This is the actual structure of the workshop program. It includes the learning tasks which will be done, and the materials necessary to do it.

Use these steps:

1. Choose the high-priority topics.
2. Decide the sequence of the topics.
3. Balance the program.
4. Teach the essential.
5. Use appropriate tools.
6. Make a skeleton plan of the week.
7. Make the plan flexible.
8. Make detailed lesson plans for the first few days.

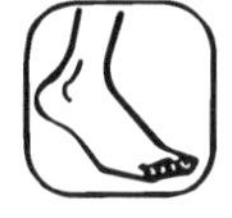

STEP ONE: Choose the high priority topics

From the participatory training needs assessment you will have a list of the most important topics to be covered. You may have already done a ranking exercise with the community of participants and have the information about relative importance of the problem (see "Ranking" pg. 255). A more in-depth ranking can be done with the Community Livestock Workers and training team to decide the relative priority of each topic.

A *dynamic* for prioritizing topics

- A simple way to prioritize with the training team is to make a chart on a piece of newsprint or a blackboard.
- For each topic which has been suggested, the group discusses:

  How Common: How common is the problem? Does it happen often or once in awhile?

  How Serious: How serious is the problem? Is it life-threatening?

  People Concerned: How much are people concerned and talking about it?

  Able to Teach?: Is it possible to teach about it in a way people can practice it?

  Change with the CLW: How much can a Community Livestock Worker do about the problem if it is taught?
- **The resulting chart may look like the chart at the bottom of this page.**
- The group comes to consensus and for each topic they rate each area from 1 to 5. For example, broken bones may not be very common, so they receive the rating 1. But they are often very serious, so they receive the rating 4.
- Pluses or numbers can be used if the chart is made on paper. If the chart is made on the ground, use rocks or sticks or anything small and solid.
- The "People Concerned?" column is filled out from the

PRIORITIZING TOPICS FOR A TRAINING WORKSHOP

PROBLEM	How Common?	How Serious?	People Concerned?	Able to teach?	Change w/CLW?	TOTAL
Thin Animals	++++	+++	++	++++	+++++	18
Diarrhea	+++	++++	+++	++++	+++	17
Cough	+++	+++	++	++++	+++	15
Disorganization	+++++	++++	++	++++	+++	18
Broken Bones	+	++++	+	++	++	10
Erosion	++++	+++++	+	++++	++	16
Worms	+++++	++	+++++	++++	+++++	21

ranking done during the community assessment.

- The last column shows the importance or priority of the topic for training and is the sum of all the other columns.

Tips:

- This chart is very useful in planning with farmer trainers and Community Livestock Workers. In some situations it may be too complicated and involved to fill out the whole chart when CLWs are trainers. People may get bored in a large group. To prevent boredom and increase participation divide the trainers into small groups and have each small group consider a section of the chart.
- The topics can be put into categories (for example, diseases, nutrition, organization, etc.) and the categories considered separately.
- Or the ranking can be done by voting, with each person placing rocks to show how important each topic is.
- With communities, a chart with only the first two columns can be used so they can define their priorities.

Once the chart is completed, it will give the training team an idea of the relative importance of each topic. In the planning of the workshop, **topics of greater importance should have more time dedicated to them.** Topics of lesser importance will be removed from the workshop schedule or given less time.

STEP TWO: Choose the sequence of topics

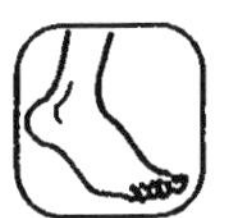

If you are designing an extensive training program, you now have a long list of prioritized topics. For a short workshop the list will not be as extensive and will not require categorization.

PART 1: Put the topics into useful categories

Here is an example from the list of the CLW training program in Bolivia:

MANAGEMENT
- Land erosion control
- Appropriate agroforestry systems
- Pasture management
- Housing & management
- Breeding and selection/Castration
- Shearing
- Administration of financial resources
- Cost analysis/Credit/Writing a project
- Use of manure
- Integrated farm system
- Record keeping

PREVENTION
- Parasite control
- Vaccination
- Nutrition
- Sanitation and hygene
- Care of the pregnant female
- Newborn care

CURATIVE
- Scientific method
- History and physical exam
- Diagnosis and treatment
- Concentrations of medicines
- Good and bad uses of medicines
- Wise purchase of medicines
- Traditional medicines
- Record keeping
- What antibiotics are for
- Common disease problems
- How to use your manuals

ORGANIZATIONAL/SOCIAL
- Participatory investigation
- Visioning/Goal-setting/Participatory planning
- Evaluation
- Gender and the life of the woman in the family/community/organization
- Awareness raising
- The leaders and their roles
- How to teach
- Popular education and the role of the CLW
- The organization and it's importance
- The group statutes and bylaws
- How does an organization function well?
- Accountability
- Group dynamics and functioning
- Marketing
- The intermediary
- District, regional and national structure and function
- Networking–linkages

SPIRITUAL
- Working together well
- How the spiritual life is related to daily life
- Customs and traditions which are harmful and helpful
- The characteristics of a good CLW
- What are our values?
- How do we apply our values?

PART 2: Decide if there is a natural sequence of topics.

Once you have the topics in categories, you can determine if there are some things which should be considered before others and plan the sequence accordingly. The logical reasons for the sequence may differ from place to place and will depend on the overall content of the program.

Whatever your team decides is the logical order, be intentional, not random, about the sequence of topics taught. Wherever possible, each new topic should build on topics previously learned in the workshop.

In a long workshop, or a series of workshops, you might teach this sequence in technical topics:

- Scientific Method then
- Physical exam then
- Use of antibiotics

You may want the CLWs to understand how to do a physical exam and make a diagnosis before they begin treatment of specific diseases.

In organizational topics you might use this order:

- How to run an effective meeting and
- The roles of the officers of an organization and
- How to teach before
- Organization of a vaccination campaign.

Within the categories of topics you have made, put the topics into appropriate sequence.

PART 3: Decide if you will have a 'homework' sequence:

Sometimes the only homework learners have after a workshop is the accomplishment of the goals they have set for themselves at the end of the workshop. But assigned homework is a good way to absorb and practice the learning that has taken place in the workshop.

The 'homework' should have a logical sequence, just like technical topics. If you decide to include 'homework', make a draft of the series of homework assignments.

An example from Bolivia follows on the next page.

Goal setting: How and when to set goals, see "Follow-up" page 149.

An example of 'homework' sequence from Bolivia:

In Bolivia, the communities decided that they wanted their CLWs to be able to organize the community for training, vaccination and worming campaigns. The training team decided they would give a series of 'homework' assignments to the CLWs so that they would be proficient community trainers when the series of workshops finished.

During each workshop the CLWs designed and practiced their next 'homework' task.

This is a sample set of homework assignments. (in a series of one-week workshops with two months between each workshop).

After the first workshop: **Practice training–** They developed training materials and facilitated a training session in their community.

After the second: **Participatory investigation–** They facilitated their community's defining their situation.

After the third: **Consciousness raising–** They used their own puppets to raise the community's consciousness of the problems and solutions that had been defined through the participatory investigation.

After the fourth: **Vaccination campaign–** Together with the community, they organized and implemented a vaccination and worming campaign.

After the fifth: **Organizational support–** They worked with the village organization on their specific goals, which varied from writing their visions, goals, and statutes to carrying out a project such as digging livestock wells for all those who raised livestock.

In this way the homework assignments were sequential and built on one another, and they also developed out of the experience and needs expressed by each village and their Community Livestock Workers. Please note that these assignments were not all defined at the beginning of the initial workshop and were adjusted according to the expressed needs of the CLWs and their villages.

PART 4: In a CLW training program consider dividing by animal types:

The program in Bolivia divides the workshops **by species,** which is one possible approach.

For example, in one area the people decided their need was for information related to the husbandry and treatment of these species:

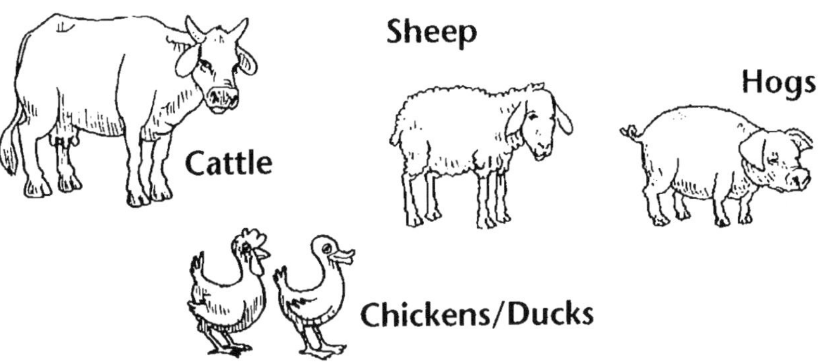

In the training program developed to meet this need there is a separate workshop centered around each species. A final workshop on Veterinary Principles caps off the series. This workshop brings closure to different topics, concentrates on areas pertinent to all species, and helps the CLWs to be careful and cautious, and to refer to other professionals.

Some reasons to divide by animal types:

- **To reinforce the information:** If you teach how to diagnose a problem with cattle in the first workshop, for example, you can reinforce the lesson and point out the difference in diagnosis for each species in successive workshops. When a disease like rabies is discussed in the cattle workshop, point out how it occurs in goats and horses. Later, when the goat workshop is taught, you have an opportunity for review.

● **To simplify the information:** Dividing complex management principles like pasture systems or care of pregnant animals by species helps make the species differences clearer in people's minds. For example, to talk about livestock pasture systems all at once could be very confusing. But beginning with a pasture system appropriate for cattle, and then discussing the appropriate systems for each species in successive workshops, helps to clarify and reinforce the principles of pasture systems.

In Nepal, a training program uses a mixed-species approach and works with different diseases and management areas as its focus. First, trainers talk about parasites in general. Then they discuss which species have problems with which parasites. Then they discuss all the treatments (local and outside) for all species. The facilitators feel the CLWs have a greater understanding of the overall problem this way and a broader perspective of the disease problem.

What is important is to design the program so that it makes sense to the participants and is organized and sequential.

STEP THREE: Balance the workshop and program

As we begin to fill in a plan for the training program we need to think about balance in the program.

A. There should be a balance of topics which relate technically to production and socially and spiritually to the organization and the person.

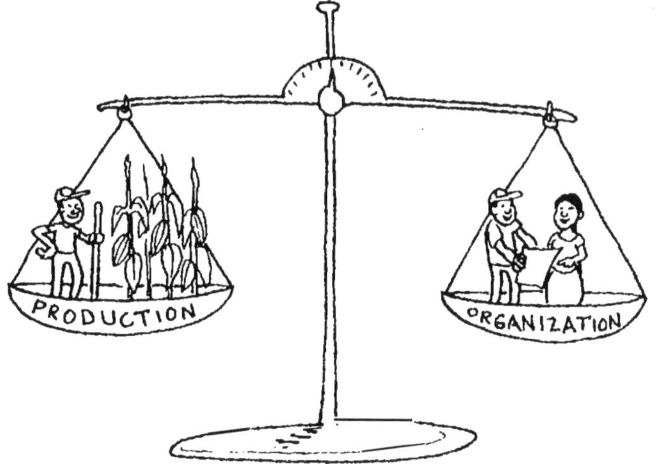

The training program may give the people an awareness of a need to vaccinate and the skills necessary to vaccinate. But if the cost, distance from the source of the vaccine, or cold chain require community coordination and cooperation for a successful vaccination campaign, people still may not vaccinate. CLWs need many social and organizational skills to be effective in their work.

Add up the hours planned in each of these areas and consider whether they are appropriate based on the people's needs and concerns. Adjust by removing some and adding others or spending more or less time on the things which are out of balance.

B. There should be a balance of classroom discussion and practice, hands-on work, and play.

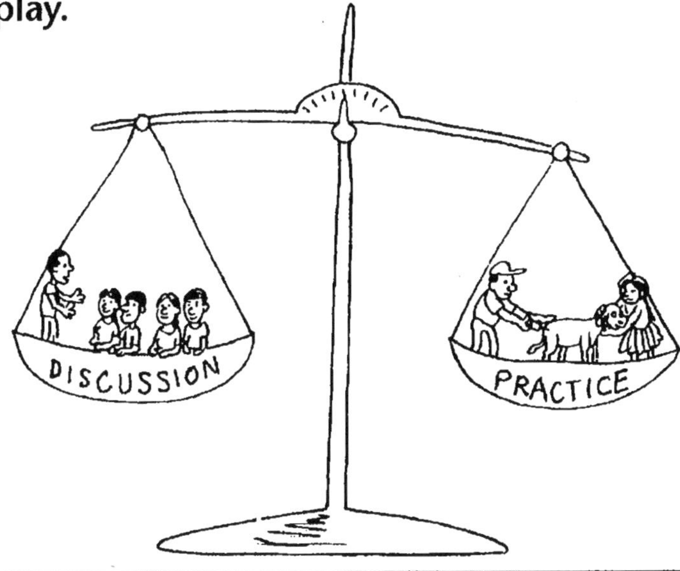

LEARNING BY DOING IS IMPORTANT!

We know that we learn:

20% of what we hear

50% of what we hear and see

70% of what we hear, see, and discuss

90% of what we hear, see, discuss, and do.

Please see the section on practice in "Tools," page 240.

As you look at your overall plan, is too much time spent in discussion in the classroom? Is there some way you could shift some of the activities to practice? How much of the classroom time can actually be practice (practice teaching, or doing a puppet show or role play)?

A program in Nepal makes appointments to see local animals throughout their workshops. They arrange the appointments in advance. When the time schedule has been set for the workshop, they post the appointment schedule on newsprint in a prominent place in the community. This brings in community people who want to come and watch the treatments.

C. There should be a balance between husbandry topics and treatment topics.

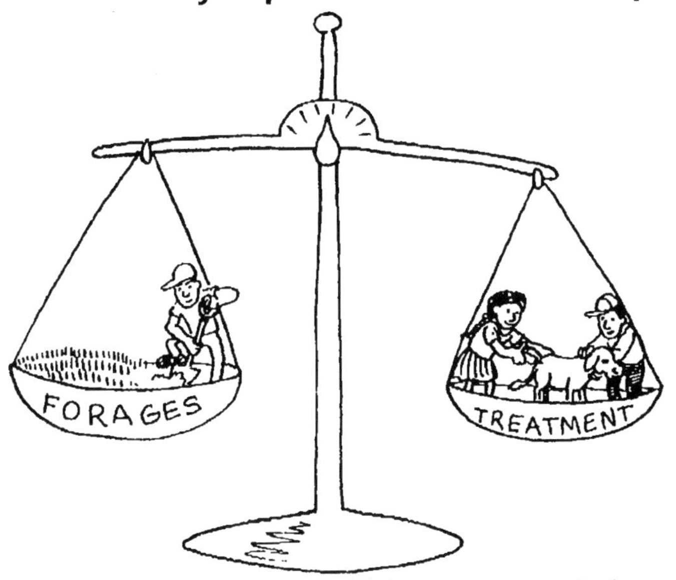

Many livestock production training courses taught by professionals include only management and prevention topics. The professionals feel it is the role of the professional to do all diagnosis and treatment, even when there is no professional care available in the village! This is organizing a workshop from the outsider's point of view.

Villagers go to workshops to become Community Livestock Workers because they see their animals sick and want to know how to cure them. Therefore it is important they gain knowledge and confidence in recognizing and treating diseases. Sometimes, however, CLWs leave workshops having been taught nothing they didn't already know about curing animals. When the CLWs return to their villages without new curative skills, members of the community lose confidence in their ability to give advise in other areas as well.

Moreover, recognizing that the villagers will be far more interested in curative medicine than in prevention or husbandry, we need to respect their expectation and plan to include enough curative topics early on. This can include local medicines and their use as demonstrated by the Community Livestock Workers. It can also include a discussion of how things like the use of water, good food, and proper care of the sick animals are important treatment tools. In addition, Community Livestock Workers should be taught history taking, physical exams, and diagnosis early on so these skills can be perfected as the workshops progress. Curative medicine and preventive medicine can be linked in the workshop. It is just as important to include the preventive topics to give the Community Livestock Workers the tools to fight disease and increase production in their villages.

D. There should be a balance of types of learning activities.

Getting to know each other

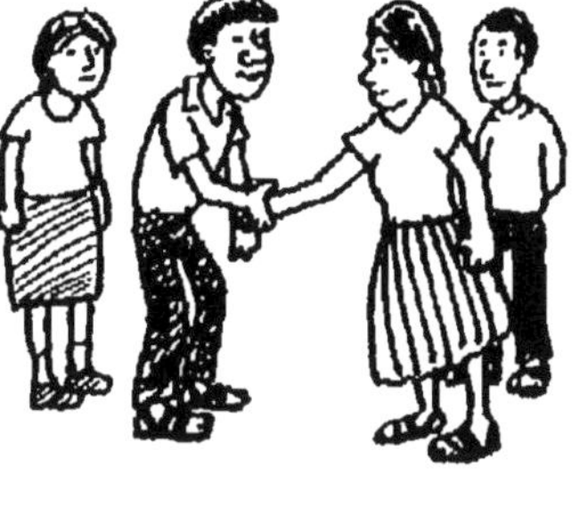

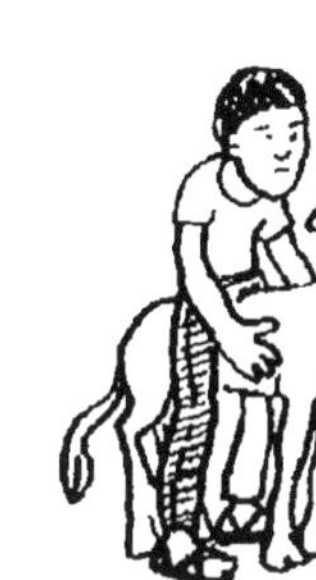

Animal diagnosis and treatment

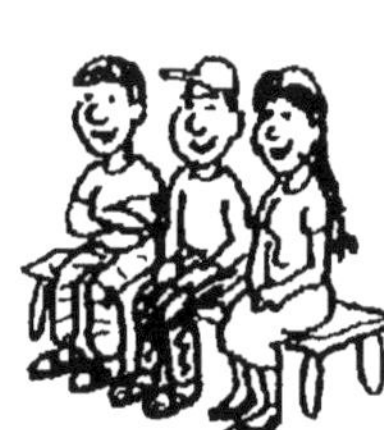

Community theater

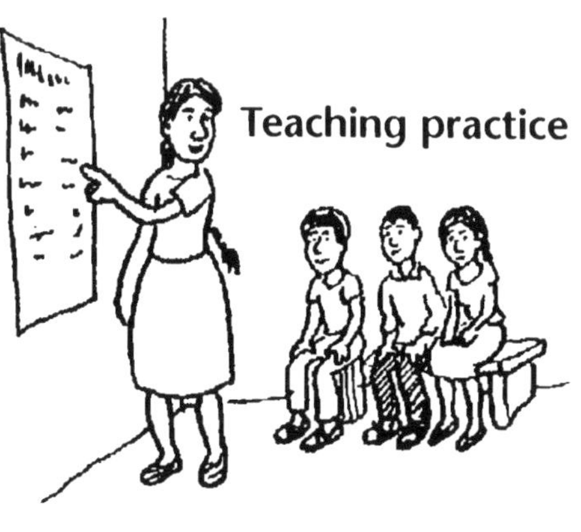

Teaching practice

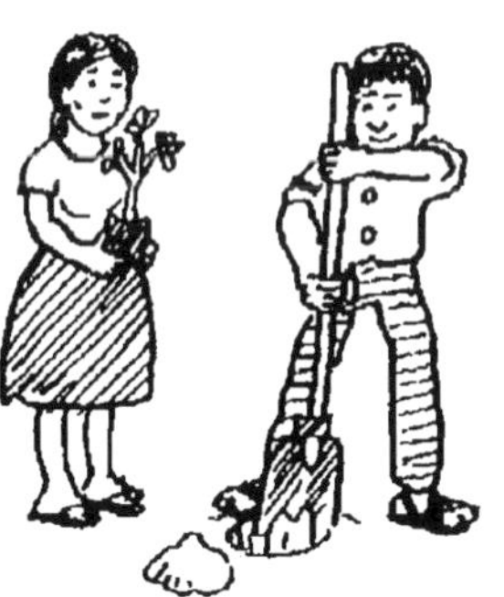

Planting agroforestry systems and other productive work

A note on women's participation:

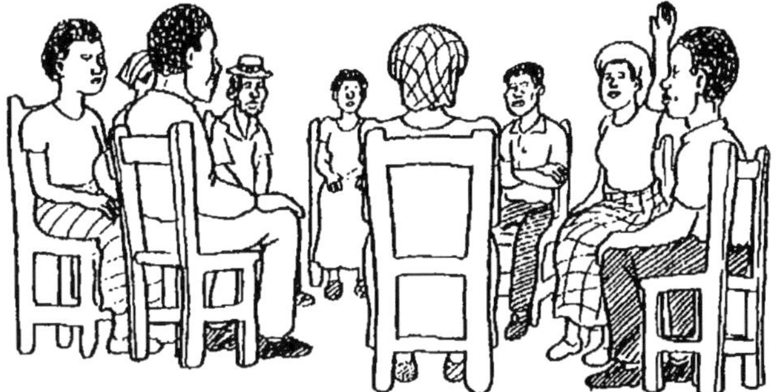

Many livestock training programs recognize the important role women play in the production of livestock yet they repeatedly have difficulties with few or no women participants in their training courses.

If we want women to participate, the conditions must be appropriate.

✓ Consult with the women of the village to find out when and for how long they would like training.

✓ Ask them what topics would be most important and helpful to them and include them in the workshop.

✓ If necessary, conduct preliminary workshops to raise the awareness of both men and women as to the women's potential and abilities. (See "Women" pg. 196).

✓ Hold the training program in the first or heart language of the women.

✓ If women are pre-literate, make sure all training materials and *dynamics* do not depend on writing for learning. Avoid all writing in the workshop.

✓ If training CLWs, encourage women with nursing babies to attend by providing for child care. Some programs hire a local woman to care for the babies while others cover the costs of the food and travel of a child-care person to come along with the mother (an older sister or cousin).

STEP FOUR: Teach the essential

Shoot for the essential!

The vast amount of knowledge which exists in animal husbandry and health management makes it very important to think well in advance about:

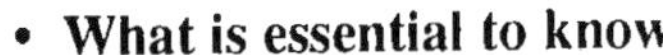

- **What is essential to know**
- **What is useful to know**
- **What is nice to know**

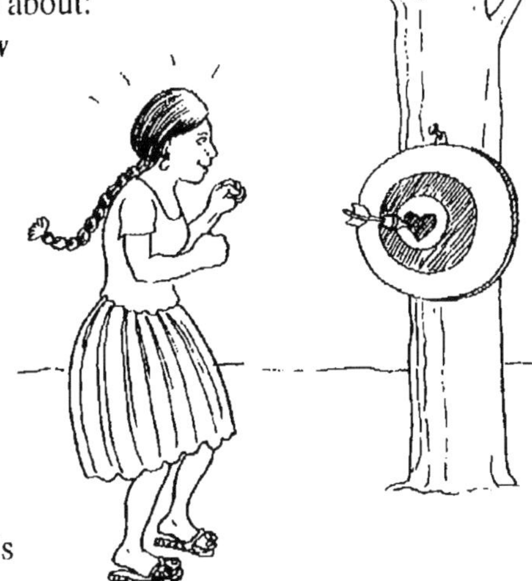

For example, trainers may want to present:
Detailed discussions of anatomy and physiology
Long descriptions of diagnosis and treatment
Discussions of rare conditions and diseases
Analysis of protein and carbohydrate content in feeds
Parasite life cycle drawings.

These things are nice to know about but waste participants' time. They may also bore the participants if they don't see how they relate directly to their situation. Memorizing facts and figures for an exam are banking system techniques. Many instructors have been taught this way so they also want to teach this way.

Start from where people in the workshops are starting; build on what they have and know. Think about what is essential. Before you put anything into the plan ask yourself:

- Why am I teaching this topic?
- Is it the best use of people's time?
- How will it help the Community Livestock Workers do their job?
- How will it help farmers improve their production?
- Is there a more effective way I could teach it?

How do we know what skills to teach?

Analyze new skills to decide whether they need to be taught. Here are some questions to help the facilitation team in that analysis:

1. Identify the job related criteria:

- How often and when is the skill performed?
- Is the skill important to beginning the job?
- Can this skill be learned later on, on the job?
- What tools, equipment and supplies are needed to perform this skill (is it appropriate for the village?)
- Try this test with two skills, – vaccination and artificial insemination – for a first-time Community Livestock Worker in your area.

2. Identify learning-related criteria:

- How difficult is this skill to learn?
- How much time is needed to get to a level of good performance?
- What tools, equipment, and supplies are needed to learn this skill?

3. Identify teaching-related criteria:

- How difficult is this skill to teach?
- What, and how many resources are available to teach this skill
- If we do not have the equipment, should we teach theory only?
- Do we have a trainer with expertise in this skill – if not, is training available?
- Is it a skill some trainees will know and will be able to teach others?
- **Should we teach this skill? When?**

Source John Collum

Stay away from a body-systems approach in training CLWs

The common way to teach veterinary students is by a body-systems approach. Everything in the digestive system from the mouth to the anus is taught. Then the whole respiratory system is taught, then the cardiovascular system. This may not be the most appropriate for the community.

People need to see the importance of things and their relation to real life before they want to learn about them. CLWs will want and need to know about the most common and serious diseases in their area first. For example, in a systems approach you would teach about ulcers in the stomach before you would teach about diarrhea. Yet because diarrhea is much more common it is something the Community Livestock Workers must know about as soon as possible.

Use a problem-focused approach. As each condition or disease is discussed, it is related to a real-life situation or problem. Sometimes it makes sense to talk about all the things which cause cough in all animals, at one time (as in a systems approach) to help people distinguish between the different diseases when they are examining a coughing animal. But often, it may be best to talk about the diseases which cause pneumonia in calves when you talk about calf care and diseases and the learners are practicing preventive care. Then you can talk about the diseases causing cough in cows when you discuss adult animal care and examine an animal for cough.

Stay away from the teaching of anatomy as anatomy

Anatomy and physiology is a dangerous subject! It will bore and confuse the students, and it may make them feel stupid.

Talking about anatomy brings in the use of lots of big Latin words. It isolates the participants from the trainer and ensures they do not understand! **Make sure you use common words for body parts.** Always encourage participants to question and challenge big words. If you continually use big words, participants will think they are the most important things and will return to their village wanting to impress people by using them. They just perpetuate a gap created by the jargon of animal health and production.

For example:

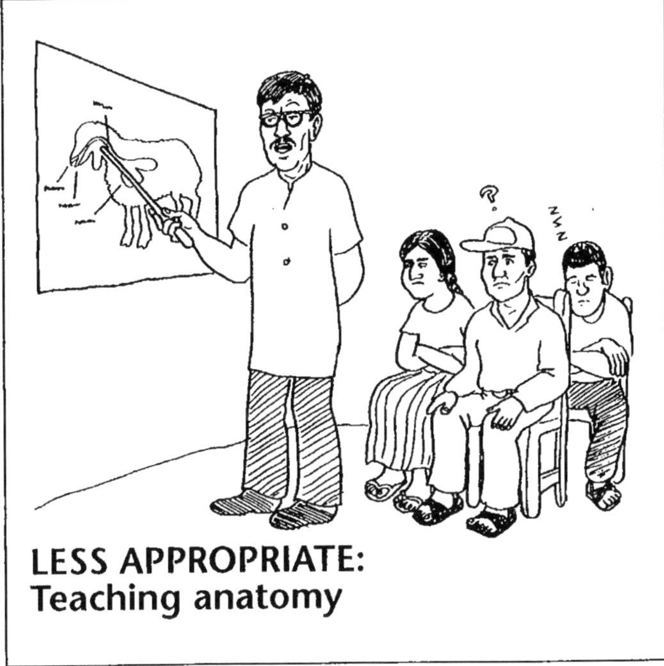

LESS APPROPRIATE:
Teaching anatomy

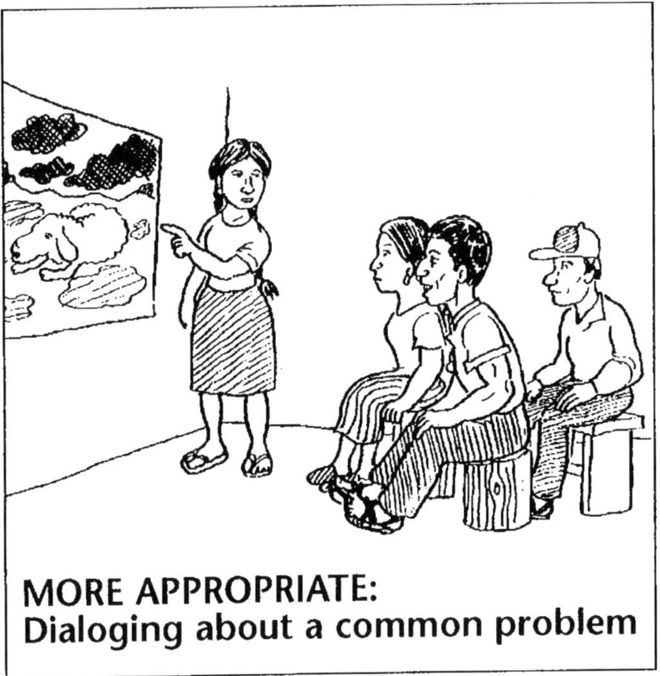

MORE APPROPRIATE:
Dialoging about a common problem

Often, after we have talked about a disease or problem in class, we will have the opportunity to do a necropsy of an affected animal or see the changes caused at slaughter. This makes a great time to review what has been talked about and see which body part is affected.

Use local names for body parts

Many times village people will have different names for the different body parts. It is good to use a necropsy opportunity to discuss together the names of different body parts and to come to an agreement about what everyone will call them. Because village people do their own slaughtering, they are all familiar with body parts. Use the locally used names for body parts after everyone has agreed on what they are.

Teach a CLW how to facilitate

Many Community Livestock Worker training programs have an expectation that when CLWs work in their villages they will teach there and share what they have learned. Almost all communities in their selection process of their Community Livestock Worker say they want their CLW to teach the community what they have learned in training.

How can Community Livestock Workers teach if they have not learned how to teach or facilitate a group? For suggestions of dynamics for teaching CLWs how to teach please see "Training Facilitators" pg. 45.

STEP FIVE: Use what is locally available and appropriate (medicines, concepts, species, and tools)

Many programs which introduce a new technology imply that the old technology is not worthwhile.

There are many traditional practices in agricultural and livestock management which can be encouraged and shared through training. These practices are less expensive, more appropriate to the local conditions, and friendly to the land and the people.

Some examples of traditional practices:

- Using animal manure and urine for fertilizer,
- Composting crop residues for fertilizer,
- Contour ridges or terraces on sloped land,
- Locally adapted and culturally appropriate animals, crops and trees,
- Planting trees for their many uses,
- Encouraging diversity on the farm,
- Traditional livestock management for parasite and disease control,
- Traditional medicines and pesticides

Plan time in the schedule for the discussion and use of local treatments. Allow time for people to share local treatments they know to be effective, and time for the preparation of those local treatments.

Listening to the farmers

History shows that traditional small farmers had very diverse farm systems with mixes of crops, fodder, and animals. Scientists said monoculture systems where one crop or animal was raised were better. Development professionals taught this.

Then all of the problems of monoculture systems developed: crops attacked by pests, resistance to chemical treatments, weakened genetic potential of purebred animals and hybrid crops, poor performance of breeds and crops not suited to the local conditions, land degradation, very high costs. Now many scientists recognize the value in the old system of intercropping with different plants and trees and the vigor in the mixed genes of plants and animals. So now many development professionals are teaching diversified farm systems as if it were a new idea.

Wouldn't it have been much simpler to listen to the traditional farmers in the first place? It would have been easier to go to them, respect what they were doing, and learn from them about diversification on the farm.

In many parts of the world, it is extremely difficult to have "modern" medicines available all the time in the village. Many programs have done an admirable job of helping Community Livestock Workers to have a small stock of medicines available for their use. But there are many, very effective local treatments. Sometimes only one person or a few people know that treatment. These treatments are less expensive, readily available, and easy to use.

By teaching only medicines and tools from outside the area we imply that the local medicines have no value and often make villagers reluctant to use them. By including the local medicines in the workshop we are building self esteem of the participants and respect for traditional medicines. Not all traditional remedies are helpful or good. That is why it is so important to schedule time to share the medicines and tools, to teach one another how to use them, and to reflect on good and bad traditional medicines and tools.

See "Traditional Knowledge" pg. 221.

STEP SIX: Make a skeleton plan of the week

Now you are ready to outline the weekly plan of your training workshop. It is a good idea to have the first weeks more extensively outlined and detailed than the later weeks so there will be some flexibility in the scheduling.

An example of a weekly plan which we use is shown on the following page. The larger the sheet, the more details can be included. We usually make a large sheet on the wall for the initial plan and then make small copies for all of the training team.

As you begin to fill out the weekly plan, think about the timing of different activities:

✔ **Determine the best time of day for activities.**

- Early morning when it is cool is best for castrations and hard physical work.
- Mornings are best for serious discussions and classroom time.
- Afternoons are best for the majority of practical activities or action activities because people get sleepy after lunch. You can include role plays and active small group work here as well as making training materials. Consider the time of day for working with animals as well. Right after lunch may be too hot, but in the later afternoon may be best.
- The evenings are good times for videos, films, and slides with discussion which may include the community, or for puzzles and debates among the participants. They are also good times for role plays, puppet shows, and talent nights for community awareness and for fun.

✔ Plan to use **the rhythm of the community** for the rhythm of the workshop. The schedule should reflect the times when people normally wake up, eat, rest, play, work and do other activities.

✔ Leave **enough time to practice a new skill and to discuss the experience** because we learn by watching and discussing someone else's practice and by reflecting on our own.

✔ Allow time to have the participants **plan the "what's next" steps** at the end of the training, What is their next step in action?

✔ Plan time for the **opening session of warming up and sharing expectations.** Also plan time for checking back with participants during the workshop – at the end of each day to see how it is going, and at the end of the workshop to evaluate and plan change for the future.

This checklist continues following the plan on the next page.

Community Level
Basic Sheep Workshop

MONDAY	TUESDAY	WEDNESDAY	THURSDAY
Welcome Icebreaker Expectations	Devotion Review/reflect Hair and wool sheep Management when on pasture	Devotion Review/reflect Diseases to vaccinate against Pink eye	Devotion Review/ reflect Worms
BREAK			
Agenda Schedule Work groups	Separating males How many ewes per ram?	Goiter Photosensitivity Over eating disease	Lice, ticks, flys, etc
LUNCH			
Agroforestry systems for sheep	*Practice* Care of the newborn Corals and housing	*Practice* How to vaccinate	*Practice* Deworm *Reflection on practice*
BREAK			
Practice Pastures Salt/mineral Fat or thin? *Discussion of new skills*	Restraint Selection Feet trimming *Reflection on practice*	Oral rehydration liquid *Reflection on practice* Checking back	What's next? Goal setting Evaluation Closing ceremony
DINNER			
The Community Organization (with the community) Checking back	Types of education (with the community) Checking back	Cultural Night	

✔**Include a variety of activities** so you don't spend extended periods of time on one kind of activity.

✔ Plan to **include review sessions** and exams. These are very important for feedback and continued learning.

✔**Plan visits with the community** for different activities when people are most likely to be home.

✔Think about how frequently each activity should occur. Some activities like physical exams, diagnosis, and treatment will need frequent periods scheduled for them. Other activities should be included once or twice a week.

✔Follow a logical progression of activities from beginning to end. Right away participants need to be involved in learning knowledge, attitudes and skills related to diagnosis and care for animals so they build on this as the workshop progresses. They also need to dialogue about education and learning and teaching early on so they will be effective communicators in their villages. Putting on village puppet shows and awareness raising take place later on as participants gain more confidence and skills.

STEP SEVEN: Make the plan flexible

Make sure that your weekly plans leave enough room for changes to the schedule. There may be animal health emergencies or other real life training opportunities which can be included in the workshop. This will cause another class to be canceled or moved. A class which was not well understood or was poorly taught, may have to be repeated in a different way later. So it is wise to leave extra time in the schedule.

The same workshop should not be repeated in village after village, since it gets boring for the villagers and the facilitators. We have developed a set of resources and a basic curriculum in our program which is adapted and adjusted for every workshop. There are several things which are done.

An example from a community forestry program in Nepal:

The program knows from past needs assessments and workshop experiences a number of needs which come up repeatedly in villages. They have lesson plans prepared for these topics as well as resource information in a file which has been prepared over time and through experience, and which they continually revise and improve. They also make a loose workshop plan for the week of training. Then, to see if the plan is appropriate they visit the community and do the following:

Three days before the workshop:

- Observe and listen for important themes.
- Have discussions and informal chats with families and individuals.
- Hold a community meeting for a training needs assessment, asking the community these questions:
  - What are the problems in the community?
  - What are the resources?
  - What are the community interests?

With the results of the training needs assessment they revise the workshop schedule.

The first day of the workshop:

- Discuss the participants' expectations and prioritize them.
- Give a practical skills test: How are the learners now pruning or planting or grafting? This is to see where

Continued on next page

they are at the beginning of the workshop.

The first night of the workshop the training team compares the participants' expectations to the planned workshop. They revise the workshop if anything comes out in the expectations section they had not planned for, or if they see a need to emphasize certain skills.
Source Helena Vesterinen, RDC Nepal

The workshop plan needs to have built-in flexibility. The training team must be able to prioritize, add and remove topics, and adjust the timing of the workshop schedule according to the needs of the participants. If the team is not flexible, the result is a workshop with far too many topics to cover in too short a period of time. Some people try to stuff it all in, but that just lowers the overall quality of the workshop. If people are too rushed for time they turn to more lecture, less dialogue and less practice. The resulting workshop is not appropriate.

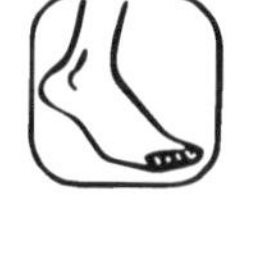

STEP EIGHT: Make detailed lesson plans for at least the first few days:

A. Do a task analysis where necessary

Once you have decided to teach a new skill, a task analysis will help you to decide **how to teach the new skill.** This process breaks the task down into its steps with all the knowledge, skills and attitudes necessary to accomplish the new task.

Example:

Task	Knowledge	Skill	Attitude	Resources
Transplant seedlings	How to transplant	Tossing seed	Be careful	Seeds, water, tools

This is a simple task without multiple steps to be followed. A more complicated task may have several steps to complete, as shown on the next page.

The task: Castration:

	Stages of the Task	Knowledge/ Skills Needed	Attitude Needed	Ways to Learn	Resources
1.	Find out community interest	Ability to listen well and explain	Caring & concern	Group dialogue, role play, interview	Village people Time
2.	Decide if castration is possible at this time	Understanding of seasons, customs, and people	Respect Details are important	Group dynamics, Discussions about customs	Village people Large paper Markers
3.	Help people learn the importance of castration in management	Breed Improvement Castration pros and cons Teaching skills	Respect Patience Enthusiasm Care	Observation, Books Discussion Practice teaching using dynamics	Manuals, Puppets Large paper Flannel board
4.	Get the materials needed	What local materials are available, What others at low cost, Where to buy	Details are important Be exact	Trip to vet shop Check equipment	Equipment Tetanus vaccine Disinfectant/Razor
5.	Examine the animal	History and physical exam knowledge and skills	Be complete Respect	Have students do the history and exam Discuss reasons not to castrate	Rope Thermometer
6.	Demonstrate castration	Restraint, Rope use, Clean technique Castration technique	Be careful, Patience Be thourogh Do not be hurried	CLW's do restraint Explain each step Ask questions	Equipment and vaccine for castration
7.	Discuss problems, care and questions	Facilitation skills and listening	Respect Desire to learn Enthusiasm	Manuals, Discuss with experienced CLWs	Manuals
8.	Everyone practice castration	Coaching skills Good questioning	Be exact Be thorough Be careful	Have CLW's assist each other	Equipment and vaccine for castration
9.	After care	Teaching skills Encouraging skills Home visits	Be encouraging Respect	Practice, Puppet shows Role plays, discussion	Materials for dynamic chosen eg puppets

A task analysis is not necessary every time for each task. This sample task analysis would not apply to every community. This technique can be used in the beginning to help train new trainers and CLWs so they can see the steps to accomplishing the task.

This also helps them to remember that **just teaching a new skill does not mean the person will have the attitude change required to implement it.**

B. Write the lesson plan

For every topic, a lesson plan should be developed. As a facilitator you will be well organized and you will feel more relaxed if you have a good lesson plan to work from. A good lesson plan will also help you to evaluate your effectiveness as a facilitator.

There are many different ways to write lesson plans with greater or lesser detail. The basic lesson plan we use in our workshops supplies the Objective, the Method for teaching, the Materials needed, and the Time the lesson will take. You can use more or less detail in your lesson plan. Remember to make the plan flexible. We use the following chart:

OBJECTIVE	METHOD	MATERIALS	TIME
By the end of the session participants will have practiced designing and using open questions	**Warmup:** Brainstorm. What is an open question? **Dialogue:** Divide into small groups. In each group a facilitator will ask a series of questions. Decide which questions are open questions and which are closed questions. Tell the others in your group what you see as the difference between open questions and closed questions. **Practice:** The facilitator will ask each person in the group a closed question. Tell how you would make each question an open question. Each person designs an open question to invite dialogue. Share your question with your group. **Dialogue:** Look at the chart of the four open questions. In your group describe how you have seen these questions used in the workshop so far. Why are open questions important for learning? **Conclusions:** With everyone together share the open questions which each person designed. Share each groups' conclusions about the importance of open questions for learning. Make a list from the participants ideas titled: *"Why open questions are important."* Define together when a facilitator should use open questions.	List of mixed open and closed questions. List of closed questions. Chart: the four open questions	1 hour

For more information on open questions please see "Ask Open Questions!," pg. 132.

For another sample lesson plan please turn to: "A Community Livestock Worker Selection Process," pg 35.

C. Include a framework for every lesson

An old speaker's axiom is:
Tell them what you are going to tell them.
Tell them.
Tell them what you told them.

The new speaker's axiom:
Discuss what will be learned.
Dialogue and learn.
Discuss what was learned.

Every lesson needs a beginning, middle, and end to ensure good communication.

BEGINNING

An orientation to the topic with brainstorming or a brief description of how it fits into the workshop.

MIDDLE

- **Dynamic** or motivator – to pose the problem and
- Discussion, **dialogue** and analysis/including details and needed skills.

–OR–

- **practice or learning tasks** and
- **reflection** on the practice.

–OR–

a combination of dynamic, dialogue, learning task, reflection

END

Review of conclusions, and **closure** – the determinations of the group are put in summary form up front on a large sheet of paper or blackboard (where appropriate in literate groups).

Look at the lesson plan on the previous page to identify the framework within the Method section of the plan.

D. Write the objective.

Most people are taught to write their objective first in the lesson plan. However we often write the objective last. Generally, the process of task analysis and lesson planning clarifies the objective. You may write a tentative objective before you analyze and plan. But the objective will often be clearer after you plan the lesson.

You and the participants must know the objective of each topic in the training session. Each specific learning objective is an action objective. At the end of the session, students and trainers know the purpose of the lesson was accomplished if the participants performed the action included in the objective.

Training objectives like program objectives should be SMART!

S pecific: Does a clear action verb say specifically what people will do?
Measurable: How will you know if you have done this?
A ppropriate: Will the group support this objective?
R ealistic: Can it be accomplished in the workshop?
T imely: Does the objective include a time frame within which it will be accomplished?

Example: By the end of the session all CLWs will castrate an animal.

E. Reflect and revise

Keep good notes on what worked and what didn't; update the lessons as necessary.

Other considerations in planning

Checklists:

Checklists or TO DO lists are very valuable in organizing and managing a training workshop. A list is made of all of the items left to do before things can be started and the resources or materials needed to do them. A checklist is for the training team and Community Livestock Workers who generated it. Don't try to use the same checklist for successive workshops because each workshop situation will be different.

Checklists are usually most useful for those who have made them. It is hard for someone else to use my checklist. If the checklists are predeveloped, they are a recipe handed to the trainer, and they do not allow for input from the trainer or the community.

If checklists are used as an aid in planning, and they help facilitators prepare for the beginning of the workshop, they are excellent. From your lesson plans and workshop plans, lists can be made of the things necessary to buy or make or get ready for the workshop. If you are prepared for the first days of the workshop, you will relax and listen and enjoy the learning process as a trainer. If you are not prepared, many things could go wrong!

Funding:

In the planning process, it is important to plan how the workshop or program will be funded.

Training costs money. For this reason, it is not available for many poor people. But many outside institutions have taken on the whole burden of the cost of a training program.

In many cases an institution running a livestock production program combined with training, credit and extension activities has evaluated the program at the end:

What benefits have you received from this program?
We received animals which we paid back.
We also received small trees, pasture seeds, and wire.
Also, the agronomist visited and gave us advice.

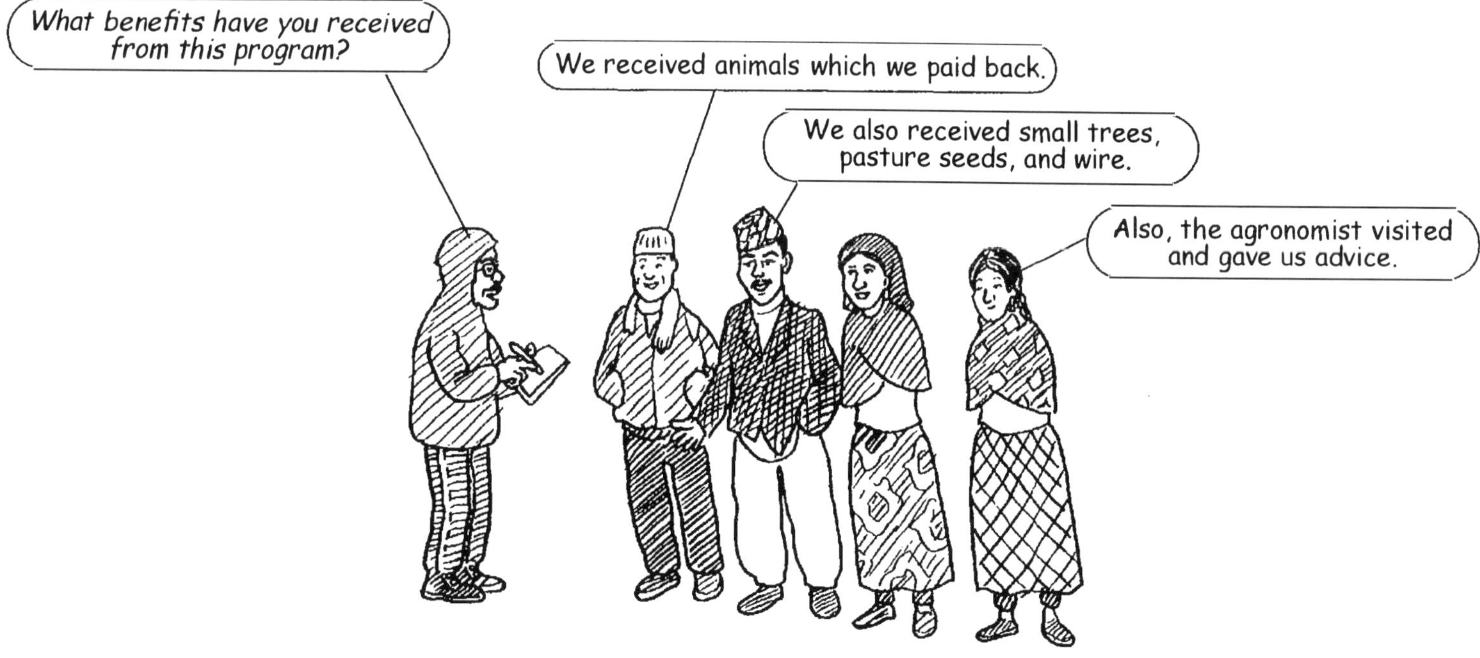

Most villagers do not list training as a concrete benefit of the program, partially because they do not see the costs involved and feel it is just something the institution is supposed to do.

Some programs pay for absolutely everything – travel, food, lodging, and all the costs of training. They even give a daily wage to those attending! The long-term success rate of these Community Livestock Workers in their villages is not good. People with influence fight to be included and often use the training as a stepping stone to leave the village.

If the training program is a village-based training program, and it works with the local village organization, the cost of the program should be clearly defined by villagers and outsiders together, and a decision made initially as to who will pay for different aspects of the program. What resources are available in the community for the program and which ones need to be obtained from outside should also be defined.

In the training program in Bolivia villages who send Community Livestock Workers pay an inscription fee which covers part of the costs of the manuals they receive. They also agree to take care of the Community Livestock Worker's farm or children while she or he is away in the workshop. The Community Livestock Worker or the village pay transport to and from the workshop.

For community-level workshops the villagers who participate pay the costs of their own food and the food of the trainers. They also provide sleeping places for the trainers and animals for practice.

In one community, the community built a mud brick enclosure to be able to have training workshops there.

Sharing the costs of the program between the community and the outside institution creates a relationship of mutual esteem. If the funding is all from outsiders, the outsiders will control the whole program. It is advisable that a good portion of the costs of training come from the local villages or organizations involved.

Chapter 6
Implementation

This chapter covers the following topics:

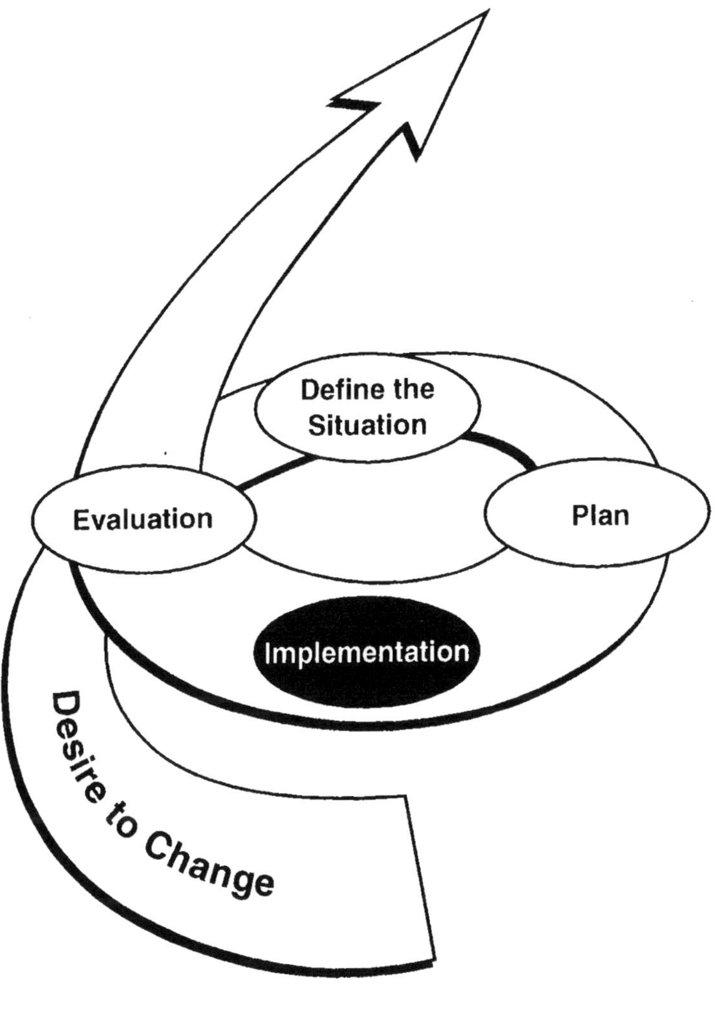

Training takes place all over the community, not just in our workshop!

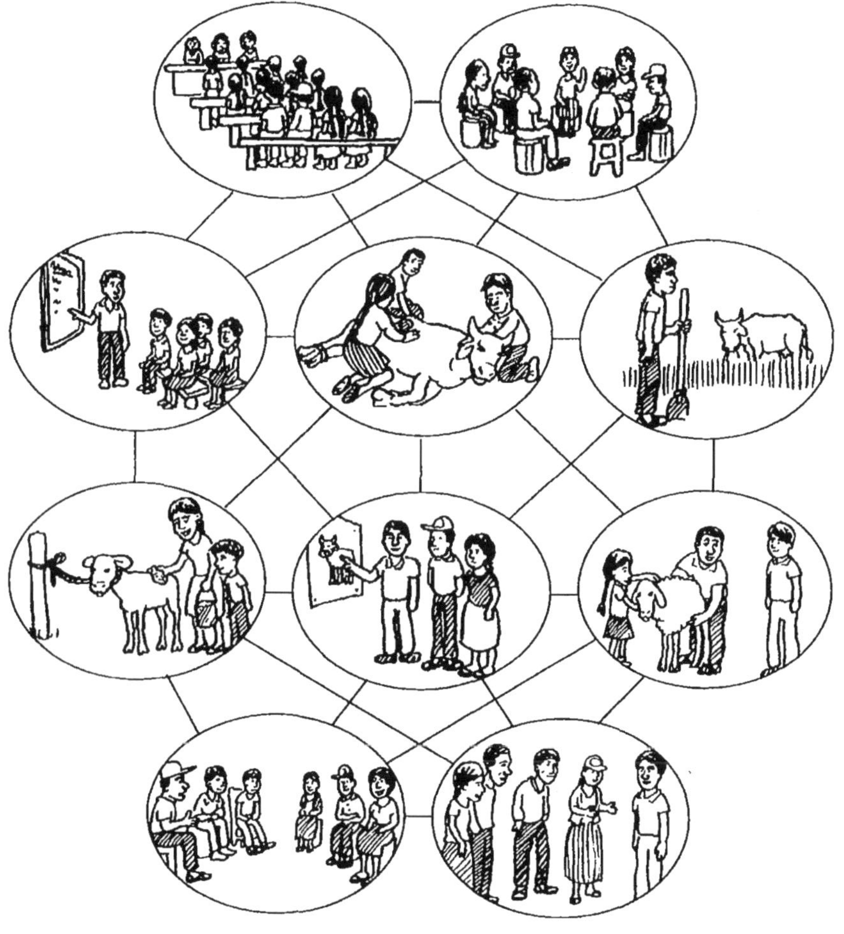

Education is not just something which happens in the classroom. It is learning from others, and from our own experience of past successes and failures.
–Julius K. Nyerere

Ideas and experiences are exchanged in community and association meetings, or when parents teach their children, during a reflection on experiences, through informal discussion, and in working together.

As we begin to put our training plan into action, we should think about how participants become engaged and involved in their learning process. We must build ways of involving the participants into the program. There are many ways this happens in participatory training. One of the most important is in a **shared responsibility by the trainer and the participants for the outcome of the workshop.**

If there is involvement, there is commitment.

These things help to encourage involvement:

- Shared responsibility
- Shared experience – learning from each other
- Analyzing – drawing our conclusions together
- Equality – there is no big or small
- Mutual respect
- The trainer facilitates rather than teaches
- Planning the action together
- As a group we see – analyze – then act.

Getting ready

You will be happier and more relaxed if you get as ready as possible before the workshop.

- ✔ Arrange the details of living and studying space.
- ✔ Make sure food and babysitting care for mothers with small children are available.
- ✔ Make sure your training materials are ready and you have all of the equipment you need, like lots of large paper, markers, masking tape, pins, chalk and a blackboard, medicines, syringes, manuals, pencils, notebooks, seeds, small trees, etc.

It is best if the workshop participants can be a part of the preparations. For example, in the community-based training workshops for any community member in Bolivia, the participants organize all the food, housing, and animals for practice. If benches are needed trainers and participants can make them together. If you are doing some last minute materials preparation the night before the workshop and the students arrive, let them help get the materials ready. This is part of the shared responsibility. It is good to work together, the trainers with the participants. This will be the first time that the facilitators have the opportunity to demonstrate that they see the participants as their equals.

Arranging the classroom

How you as facilitator set up the classroom from the first session of the first day tells everyone what the workshop will be like.

If the seating arrangement is like this:

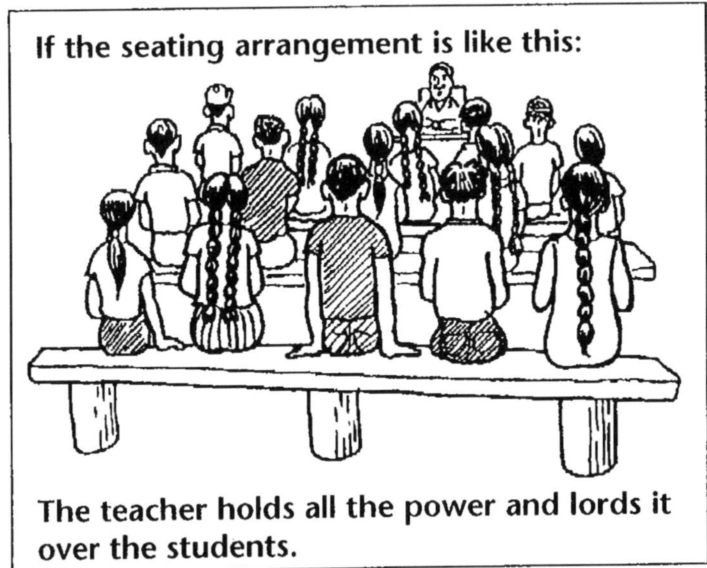

The teacher holds all the power and lords it over the students.

If the seating arrangement is like this:

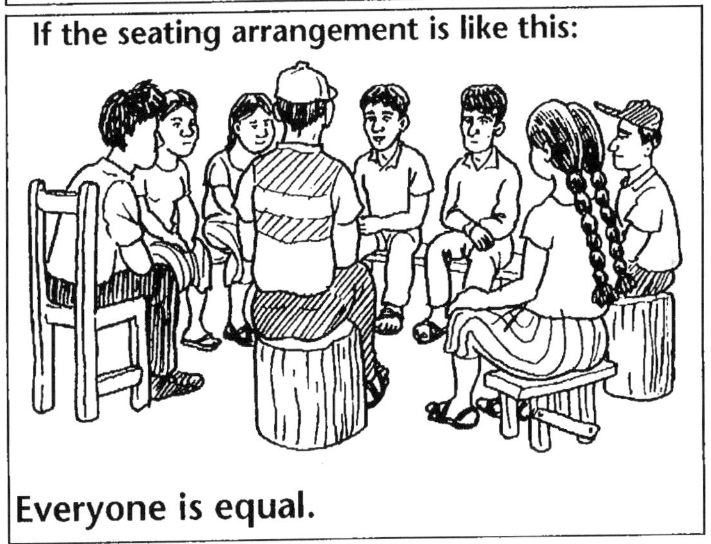

Everyone is equal.

All opinions are of equal value. The facilitator is not better than the participants, he or she is a learner as well. People feel a sense of safety in talking to one another. Everyone can see the other person's face when they talk. This makes for better direct communication and better understanding.

Sometimes it is necessary to work in a workshop with tables.

Here are two ways to arrange tables in an inclusive way:

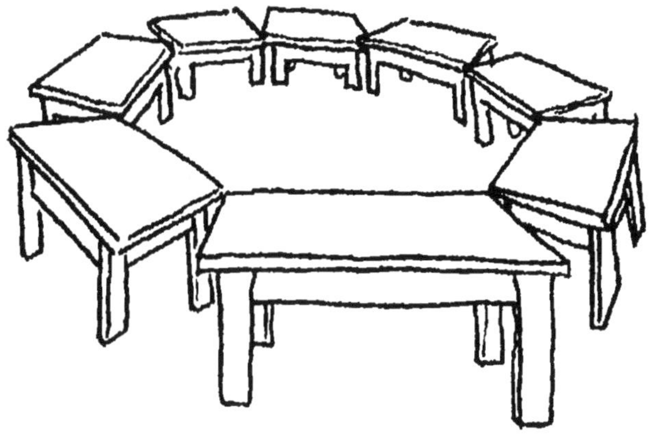

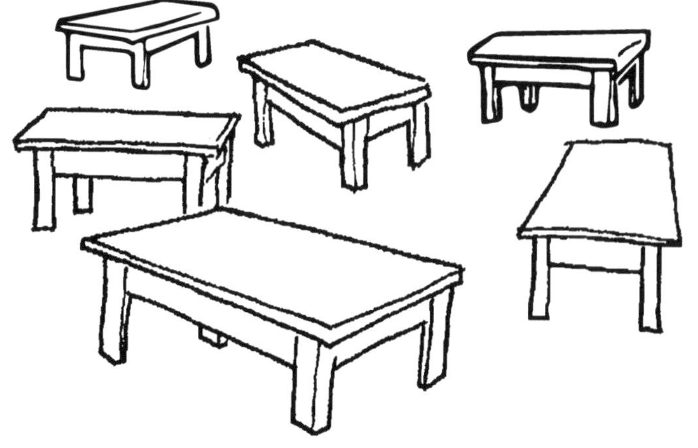

Whenever possible, use the plenary to come together in a circle.
If the local tradition is to sit on the floor together the facilitator should sit on the floor with the participants, not on a chair above them.

The first day

So, how does the first day start?

Many participatory workshops begin in similar ways to set the atmosphere and get everyone working from the same place. Look at the box on the right.

A sample start up schedule:

A. Opening and introduction of the program
B. An icebreaker for introductions
C. Sharing of expectations
D. A look at the course plan
E. Workshop work groups
F. Setting the rules and timing of the workshop
G. First activities on the main topic

A. The opening of the program

In many cultures people expect to have a ceremony when a workshop begins. This ceremony usually serves the purpose of defining how important the workshop is to officials and how important the instructors are. **It automatically creates an atmosphere of separation between the instructors and the participants if it elevates the instructor.**

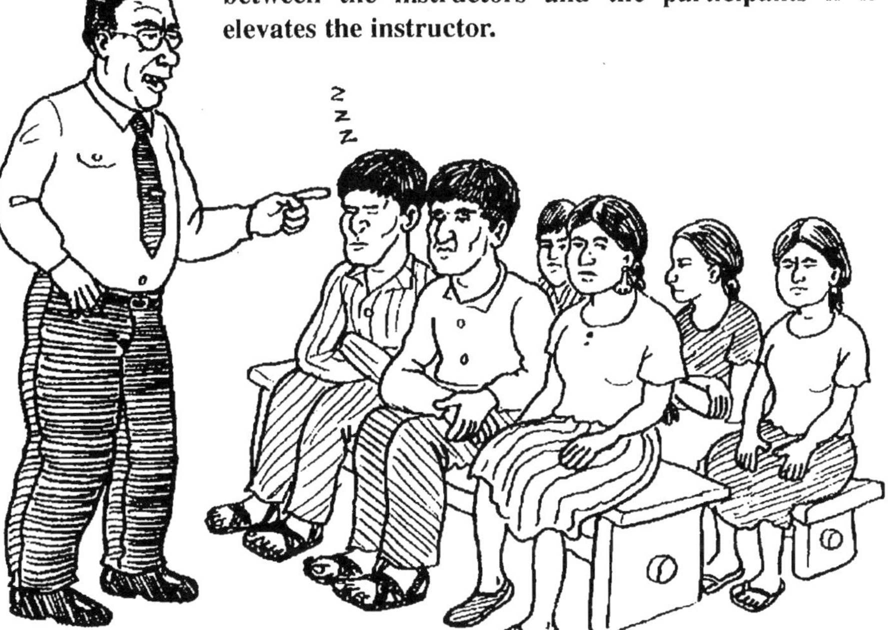

It is true that the credibility of a facilitator should be apparent to the participants. The participants want to be confident in the workshop content, especially if it is very different from what they have previously experienced. So an opening ceremony can give that credibility. It can also show the support which the local village organization has for the program, a very important factor in working together and in the village ownership of the training.

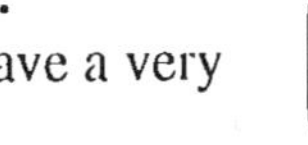

Some suggestions for opening ceremonies:

- Either eliminate the opening ceremony or have a very short one.
- Hold the opening ceremony the night before the workshop.
- If you have an opening ceremony, expect the special guests to be late.
- Hold the ceremony on the second or third day of the workshop.
- Use a culturally appropriate *dynamic* which includes everyone. One example: A candle lighting ceremony. Each participant lights a candle from the person next to them. The "opening candle" is the last candle lit.

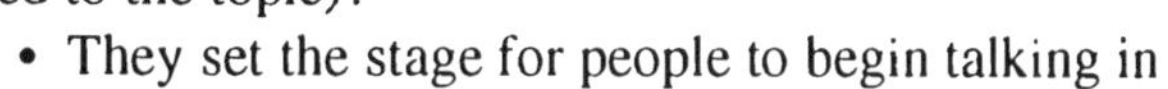

B. Use an icebreaker or a warm-up

Why do we use icebreakers or warm-ups (learning tasks related to the topic)?

- They set the stage for people to begin talking in the larger group.
- They help people start to get to know each other in a friendly, open way.
- They create a relaxed and fun atmosphere for learning.
- They should be used to start the next step of a workshop. If the next step is setting expectations, use the warm-up to begin sharing them. If it is later in the workshop, or with a group whose members know each other well, use the warm-up to start working on the topic in a fun and creative way.

For several ideas for icebreakers and warm-ups see "Tools," page 263. Many of the reference materials have other good suggestions. See "Resources," page 330.

It is important that the facilitators join in the warm-up with the participants. This is where the tone of equality is set. **Facilitators must also have name tags with their first names in large letters, just like everyone else.**

No titles here

If the facilitator is a professional, there may be the desire on the part of the participants to give them some title of importance, such as Doctor or Engineer. It is very important in the introduction time to state that there are no titles here, that we are all equal, and we go by each others first or commonly used names. This sets the stage for open sharing.

A stupid waste of time?

Is it silly or stupid to play games with adults? "I didn't come to play games, I came to learn" one participant said as he stomped out of the workshop. It can be stupid to play games. If the game in some way mocks the participants or trivializes the topic or the process of learning, it will destroy the learning potential of adults. But hostility to games is not common–most adults find them fun and tension-releasing. The games also set the tone for the whole workshop. If we want to have a creative, problem-solving environment, people need to be able to relax, feel they are among friends, and trust each other.

Joy and laughter should honor the learning taking place, and will help people to learn more. Laughter and learning go together. **If we are laughing we are learning.** If this subject comes up with participants, use the time to dialogue about why we use games and laughter in participatory training. In some cultures it will take longer than the warm-up time to establish this environment of trust and laughter. Be patient.

It could be that by "wasting time" at the beginning to establish relationships, you save time in the end!

C. Sharing expectations

One of the ways we can all come to agreement about the purpose and aims of the workshop is to set the expectations for the workshop together. This can be a very simple exercise or a very involved one. If people are new to the participatory methodology, they may find an expectation sharing process tedious. Normally it is best to keep it fairly simple as people will want to move on to some specific technical topics. But, since it is the setting of expectations which defines the direction of the workshop, it is very important that they be shared.

Why do we share our expectations?

- To mutually agree on the purpose and direction of the workshop,
- To give the workshop participants shared ownership in the outcome,
- To adjust the workshop plan according to participant expectations,
- To enhance the evaluation of the effectiveness of the workshop at the end.

The expectations are displayed in a prominent place on the wall throughout the workshop. They are printed in large print on large paper. The expectations can be compared to the scheduled workshop. If the facilitation team has done a good job of assessing the needs of the participants before the workshop, the expectations should fit the workshop schedule. If there are expectations which the facilitator knows will not be met in the workshop, they should be discussed. It may be appropriate to schedule further training, or a visit or meeting to fulfil other expectations.

At the end of the workshop, schedule a time to go over the expectations once again. The participants can use their list of expectations to measure the effectiveness of the workshop.

Four *dynamics* to share expectations:

1. Icebreaker

As a part of the icebreaker and introduction, pairs can introduce one another and share the other person's expectations. These are written on a large piece of newsprint. If there are duplicate expectations these are noted with a slash for each duplicate. The resulting list is briefly discussed and put on the wall in a prominent place to be checked by the participants at the end of the workshop. This way they will see if their expectations were met.

2. Hum

This is called a hum because when the pairs are all talking the room hums. This is a technique often used to quickly discuss a point in a workshop. It is essentially the same as the above dynamic except that the facilitator asks participants to form pairs with their neighbor. No ice breaking dynamic is used. Each pair shares their expectations for the workshop in 2–5 minutes with each other. Going around the circle each pair shares one expectation without discussion. They are recorded on large newsprint. The second time around the circle each pair shares another expectation. The list can be briefly discussed. It is important that facilitators participate as well.

3. Small groups

It will be useful to have small groups formed to serve as work groups later in the workshop. Form a set of small groups now. You can form small groups in many fun ways.

See games for forming groups in "Tools," page 266.

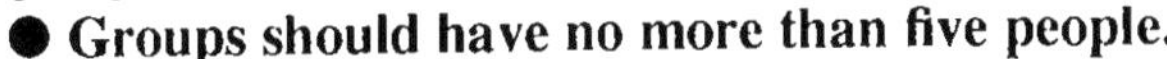

- **Groups should have no more than five people.**
- Each small group meets together and brainstorms a list of their expectations. Then, they need to prioritize their list and list the top five expectations of the group.
- Go around the room asking each group to share one top expectation. Continue going around the room until all of the top five expectations are shared from each group and a list has been made on large newsprint.

4. Cards

- For a literate group, expectations can be shared with cards. The cards are the size of a half-sheet of regular paper and can be of paper or of lightweight cardboard. Make sure there are plenty of cards available.
- Each person gets 2–3 cards and on each card writes one of their expectations.
- Each person shares his or her most important expectation card and tapes it to the wall.
- The facilitator puts the cards which are the same together, consulting with participants.
- Once each person has shared one expectation, ask, "Is there anyone with a different expectation from one up on the board?" Any other expectations can be shared this way.
- A final list of expectations can be made on newsprint. A discussion takes place to ensure all the expectations are there. If there are some expectations which might be impossible to meet, these should be discussed and an agreement made by the participants about them (perhaps they will have to be dealt with at a later workshop).

D. Sharing the workshop plan, topics and objectives

At this point, after the expectations have been shared, the rough outline of the workshop should be shared. It helps to have an outline on large newsprint. If you need to revise to accommodate the expectations, share that information with the participants. Tell them that as revisions are made they will be informed. Ask if the plan meets with their approval. Once the workshop plan is approved, it should be posted in a prominent place for the rest of the workshop. In a literate group a list of topics and objectives for the workshop can be shared. If there are any questions they can be answered. The lists of topics and objectives should be posted on the wall throughout the workshop.

E. Organizing the work groups for the workshop

For every workshop we organize all participants and facilitators into work groups. They will handle many of the tasks of management and organization of the workshop process.

Why organize into work groups?

- To give ownership and control of the workshop to the participants,
- To teach the participants how to work effectively in groups,
- To give participants experience in running different aspects of the workshop,
- To have effective decision-making bodies.

This can be a critically important aspect of participatory training. In many workshops, although the dynamics of participation are used, the facilitator still holds ultimate control. It is sometimes very hard for a facilitator to give up control! It means the participants may decide to do something the facilitator would not normally do, or something the facilitator thinks is not in the best interests of the participants. But what does "participatory" mean? Shared responsibility! If there is involvement, there is commitment.

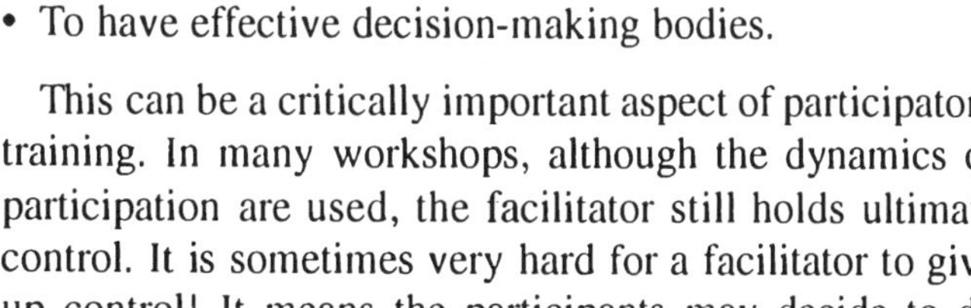
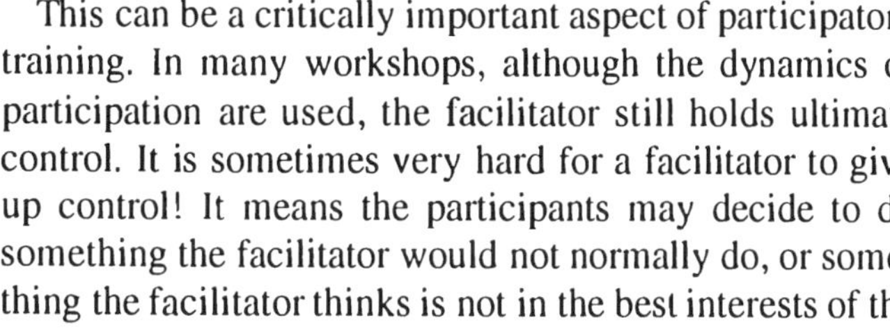
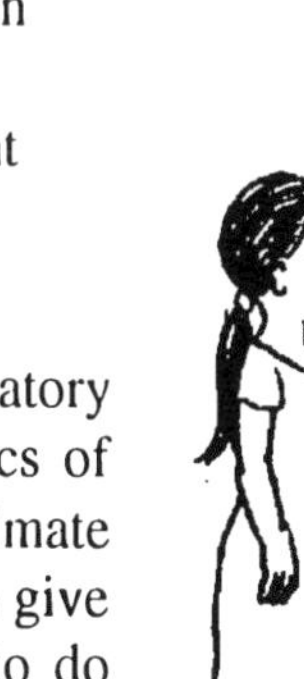

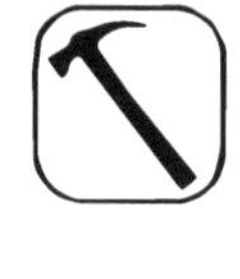

One way to organize work groups:

- Brainstorm a list of all of the duties in running a workshop.
- Divide the duties into appropriate categories.
- Divide the participants into small groups of five to six people.
- Make a large chart of the jobs for each group each day, and post it on the wall.
- Each day there is one team per job. Every day the teams change jobs.

One list of possible jobs:

Reporters–They listen to the news, find out what is happening in the community, and record what has taken place during the workshop. The following day they begin the day by presenting a people's newspaper, drama, or picture and informing everyone about the events of the previous day.

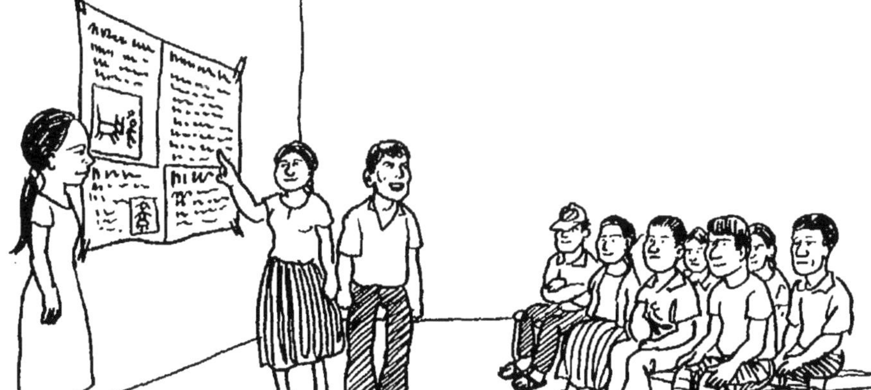

Motivator–organizers–This group keeps the attendance, oversees penalties for lateness or falling asleep, thinks up games or activities to motivate the class when they get sleepy, and keeps the time schedule of the day. This is also the group who says if there is something not going well in the workshop or brings problems to the participants' attention for solution.

For example, a workshop was planned for a week when a local one-day festival would take place. Workshop participants were aware of this when they began and decided to forgo the one-day festival. During the workshop they realized the village was on a path to the central marketing area, and that many people would be passing by. This may disturb the workshop. The participants decide if they want to reorganize the schedule, change the place of meeting, or have class anyway and use the time to involve the community.

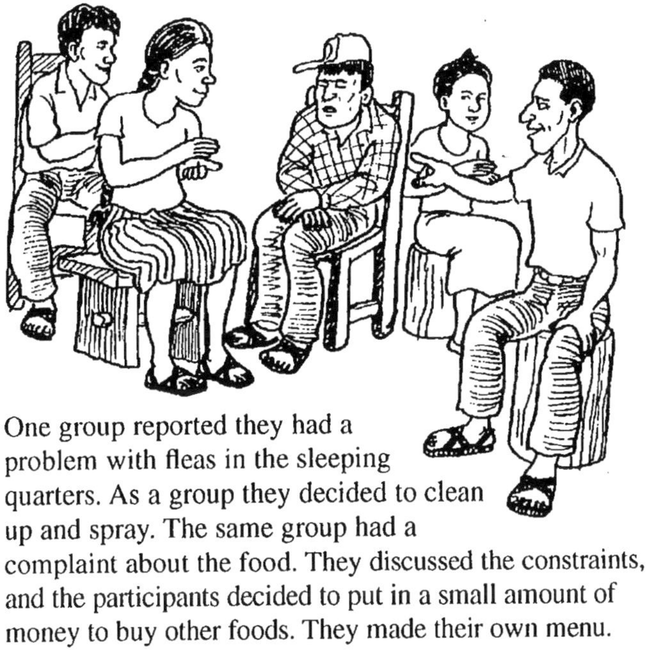

One group reported they had a problem with fleas in the sleeping quarters. As a group they decided to clean up and spray. The same group had a complaint about the food. They discussed the constraints, and the participants decided to put in a small amount of money to buy other foods. They made their own menu.

Cleanup crew This group is responsible for daily cleanup of the classroom, sleeping area, and bathrooms.

Reviewers This group starts each day with a review of the previous day's training content.

Food and debate group This group addresses any difficulties with the food or food service, and organizes meal times. They also run the debates at night after a video, slide presentation, or popular theater.

Make a large chart so everyone will know what their group is doing each day.

An example: Each group chooses or designs a symbol for the group.

If you have used cards with symbols on them to set up the group, it is an easy matter to make a wall chart of this with the cards from the people in the groups. So instead of words, the symbol is there for each activity each day. Put this wall chart in a prominent place.

ACTIVITIES	MONDAY	TUESDAY	WEDNESDAY	THURSDAY	FRIDAY
Reporters	☆	✿	✌	✎	✂
Motivation	✂	☆	✿	✌	✎
Cleanup	✎	✂	☆	✿	✌
Review	✌	✎	✂	☆	✿
Food/debate	✿	✌	✎	✂	☆

Once the work groups have been established, you need to give them 15 minutes to decide how they will begin to work together. They can elect the officers they need and begin taking on their work function.

In Uganda, the Uganda Change Agents Association has the goal of training all the people in its programs in **bookkeeping and business management.** They feel these tools are very important in the running of a transparent village organization. Their workshops run for two weeks and they have a series of four of them. For all of the workshops, a group has responsibility for the day-to-day financial management of the workshops. They spend the whole first day on business matters of the workshop and on setting up the work groups, menus, and work plans. They divide the participants into groups based on the following activities:

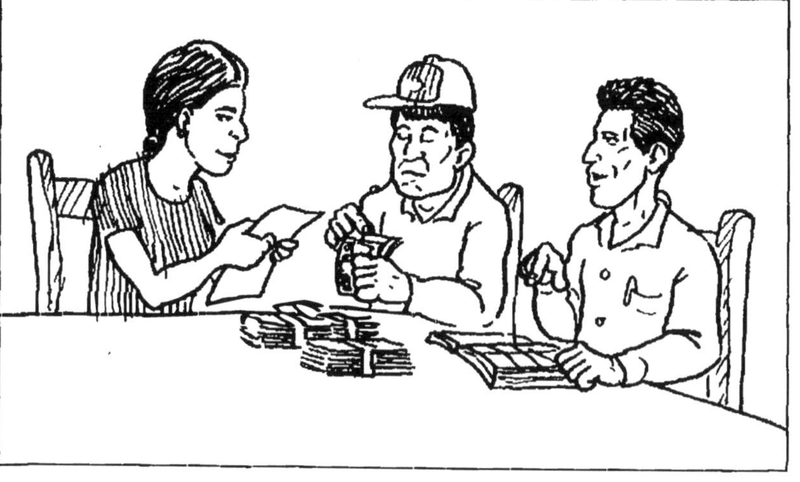

Cooking: brings supplies from purchasing to cooks and supervises meals and an inventory of utensils at the end of the day.

Cleaning: cleans up all common areas

Purchasing: prepares the daily purchasing list, gets it approved, gets cash from bookkeeping group, buys food and stores it, reports purchases to the whole group, etc.

Entertainment: deals with any entertainment functions. (Since this group will be purchasing on the next day it has to prepare for that responsibility as well.)

Bookkeeping: collects money, keeps cash, gives cash to purchasing and gets back balances, prepares a daily balance sheet, does daily budget analysis, makes daily financial report to group.

The workshop includes two business meetings per day for reports and taking care of the business of the workshop. At the beginning of the workshop a lump sum is divided among the participants. They must then decide their budget; how much they want to spend on food, on the cooks' salaries, on their travel, etc. From their allowances, they make daily contributions to cover the workshop costs.

After eight weeks of running such a system, they are quite proficient in the transparent operation of the business side of an organization. Not every program will allow such an in-depth study of business and organizational management, but imagine the strong local organizations it would produce if they did!

Source: Stan Burke, Uganda Change Agents Assn.

F. Setting the rules of the workshop

The motivation group is in charge of establishing the rules. They need to run a brief business meeting to decide on the following:

Hours of training, meals, rest, recreation

The facilitators can give some guiding information to help this process. This information could include:

- ✔ Hours needed to cover the topics chosen by the participants
- ✔ Any known restrictions such as hours the generator functions to watch a video, cooks' availability for meal times, etc.
- ✔ Once the participants have this information they can make a schedule of the hours to be kept during the workshop. Display the workshop hours in a prominent place.

Rules of conduct

Participants establish these rules and post them in a prominent place. Guidelines might include the following:

- ✔ Everyone must be listened to and respected;
- ✔ Everyone must arrive on time;
- ✔ The group will decide on consequences for someone late or sleeping.

These six activities A–F will normally take all of the first morning of the workshop to accomplish. After finishing them, the participants can focus on the other content of the workshop.

Making the workshop environment exciting, appropriate, fun, and encouraging; principles for every workshop

Powershift

Shift the power to the participants

Some things we have already mentioned will contribute to this. Others are new ideas:

- ✔ **Work groups** gradually take on more of the responsibilities and authority of the workshop. (Pg. 118)
- ✔ If **questions of time or organization** arise, put them in the hands of the group to decide. For example when someone brings a sick animal during classroom hours, the participants can decide to see it or not. If you cannot visit a farm at the prescribed time or an activity must be canceled or changed, don't make the decision yourself as a facilitator!
- ✔ Everyone **asks permission** to enter and leave the workshop – even the facilitators! Ask the motivation group for permission to leave.
- ✔ **Encourage the participants to question and challenge things.** For example, start this off by catching yourself as a facilitator in a big word. Ask someone, "Do you know what ... means?" If that person can, have him or her define it for everyone. If it is a word unknown to all, ask them, "Why do you let me use words not everyone can understand? Aren't I excluding you by using these words?" Have people discuss that concept. "What can you do about my big words?" Let them decide to ask for clarification and to control the word use.
- ✔ When doing dynamics with the community where there is writing or drawing involved, **put the pen in their hands,** and give them the control.

In a workshop in China, extensionists were learning about the participatory methodology for the first time. Small groups had developed tools for a participatory needs assessment and went to the village to do them together with the people. After the first day, one group said they had learned nothing new from the farmers.

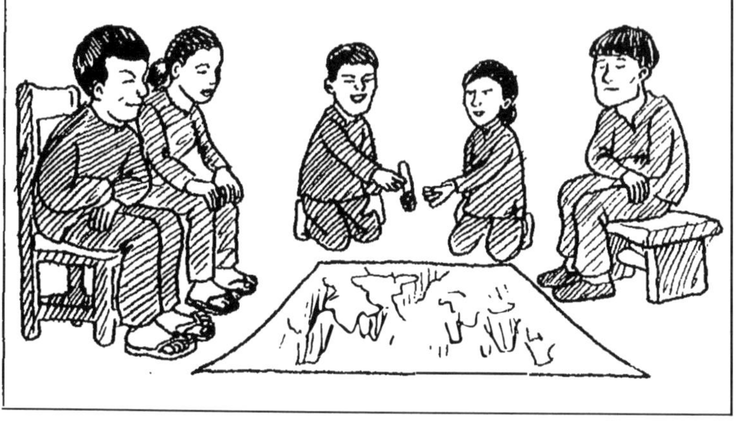

This was curious, as all the other groups had done some powerful learning about the difference between their perceptions as extensionists and the priorities of the people.

On the second day of field work the facilitator went along with this group. Although they were using a "participatory" technique, the extensionist was writing down everything and asking leading questions. The list was the extensionist's list. The facilitator requested that the extensionist give the pen to the farmers and ask each one to put a priority area of need on the list. As the farmers took the pen and wrote, they also explained why they thought the way they did. The list was completely different!

It is very important to give up control. We may think we are being participatory but then we do everything from our own bias as a facilitator. If we put the pen in the hand of the participants, the control goes to them.

✔ If the group is generating a list of items or a final schedule, have one of the participants do the writing on newsprint, if appropriate.

✔ After the first day, at the start of each day of the workshop, there should be a business meeting. The work of each work group is presented and evaluated by all. Have one of the groups, usually the motivation group, run the meeting. The facilitator is a participant. Does it take longer? Yes! But the payoff in the self esteem and ownership of the participants is well worth the time. Everyone will see the leadership of the meetings improve each day.

Choose appropriate tools and *dynamics*

- **Culture** may dictate in many cases what tools work best. Make sure it is culture and not the facilitator's bias preventing the use of a new tool! Perhaps a facilitator feels awkward doing a puppet show, singing, role playing or telling a story. Or perhaps the facilitator cannot see the value of the new tool thinking it not professional enough, too much like playing a game, and not like "real learning." All the more reason to involve the participants in the development of the tool! Once a tool has been tried and evaluated, the people can decide if it is an effective way for them to learn.
- Try to **vary the activities.** Don't use the same type of dynamic such as a role play or brainstorming over and over,. The training team, when they are developing a workshop, can put a list on the wall of all of the types of dynamics they know; then they can think through the list as they decide the most appropriate way to begin. Not every topic needs to begin with a game or role play. Some programs rely very heavily on the technique of putting a question before a small group and then sharing in plenary. **A well formulated question for a problem everyone is aware of can be a powerful tool to open a good discussion.** Remember that practice can also be a good dynamic. Have a practice session of something people commonly do, like tick dipping the animals, and then have a discussion afterwards.
- **Make the topics and the energizers interrelate.** Have one dynamic serve two purposes. For example, if a group is formed for a work activity using a set of pictures of kinds of medicinal plants, the medicinal plants should relate to the overall theme of the workshop. Let the groups explain the use of the plant, where it is found, and how it is prepared. Have your reflection-devotional topics relate to the theme of the day and reinforce it.
- Make sure **the work of the participants is shown in a visual display–**it may be written or pictorial, a chart or a diagram or a list of the results in categories. These should also be distributed to the participants as a part of the workshop report.
- **Use things that are local, inexpensive, and appropriate** for dynamics. Stay away from models, tools, costumes and equipment which must come from outside of the community. For example, use objects the participants find for people to describe what they are thinking or their goal for the future. Have people make maps from things found on the ground. Local facilitators make the drawings for the pictures used, not a professional artist. (See "Making our Own Training Materials" page 287.)

Use the farm, the forest, and the local community as a classroom

There are lots of ways to use the farm, forest, or community or things in the community as a classroom. Go there and look at, talk about, or do something together. Or discuss what people see and how it could be improved.

1. Use an area of the farm, forest or community.
Look at the animals and touch them to talk about genetics and buying a good quality animal. Go to the pasture and walk and sit in it to discuss pasture variety and management. Plan together an appropriate land plan for a piece of land all are looking at together. Sit by the side of a stream or pond to talk about the elements of the stream and what happens if the trees are not maintained around it and the banks not protected from animals. Look together at a hill where erosion is obvious to discuss soil conservation. Plant a tree nursery together on someone's farm. See the story from Kenya on the next page.

2. Have Cross-Farm Visits
Using the farm and the village as a classroom, the farmers and village families can also be teachers. It is very helpful for people to visit a farm where a new, different, or revived old technology is in use. The farmer there can share from personal experience.

Some programs in Central America use cross-farm visits as their only training opportunities. The farmers on their farms show and talk about terracing and its results, fodder trees and their many uses, windbreaks and alleys, and leguminous cover crops.

In Kenya, one program has used "farm competitions." For two days all the participants went to visit each others' farms. A group of farmers were the judges and at each farm the owner explained what they were doing and the others gave their advice. They always discussed together what would be needed to improve each farm and there was a prize for the winning farm. This program found that when farmers judged and gave recommendations they were generally more critical in their judging. They also had more practical advice than the extension staff.
Source: Josephine Wangechi Kirui, Kenya

A story from Kenya

A trainer had been living and working in a community for many weeks. He had seen many children sick and dying from diarrhea and had been trying to convince the people of the importance of capping their spring for clean water. He was all ready to help them get the spring capped. But the people did not listen to the trainer because they did not view the contamination of the spring water as important; after all they had plenty of water.

Finally the trainer had a workshop opportunity, and he took the village people in the workshop to the source of the spring so they could talk about it. It was raining lightly.

Tell me what you see here...
Look, there's trash in the water!
And it looks like a person's feces over there.
The farmer on the hill put fertilizer on his land and the rain is draining it into the spring.
This is what we drink!
I'm not drinking this another day!
Let's do something about this spring

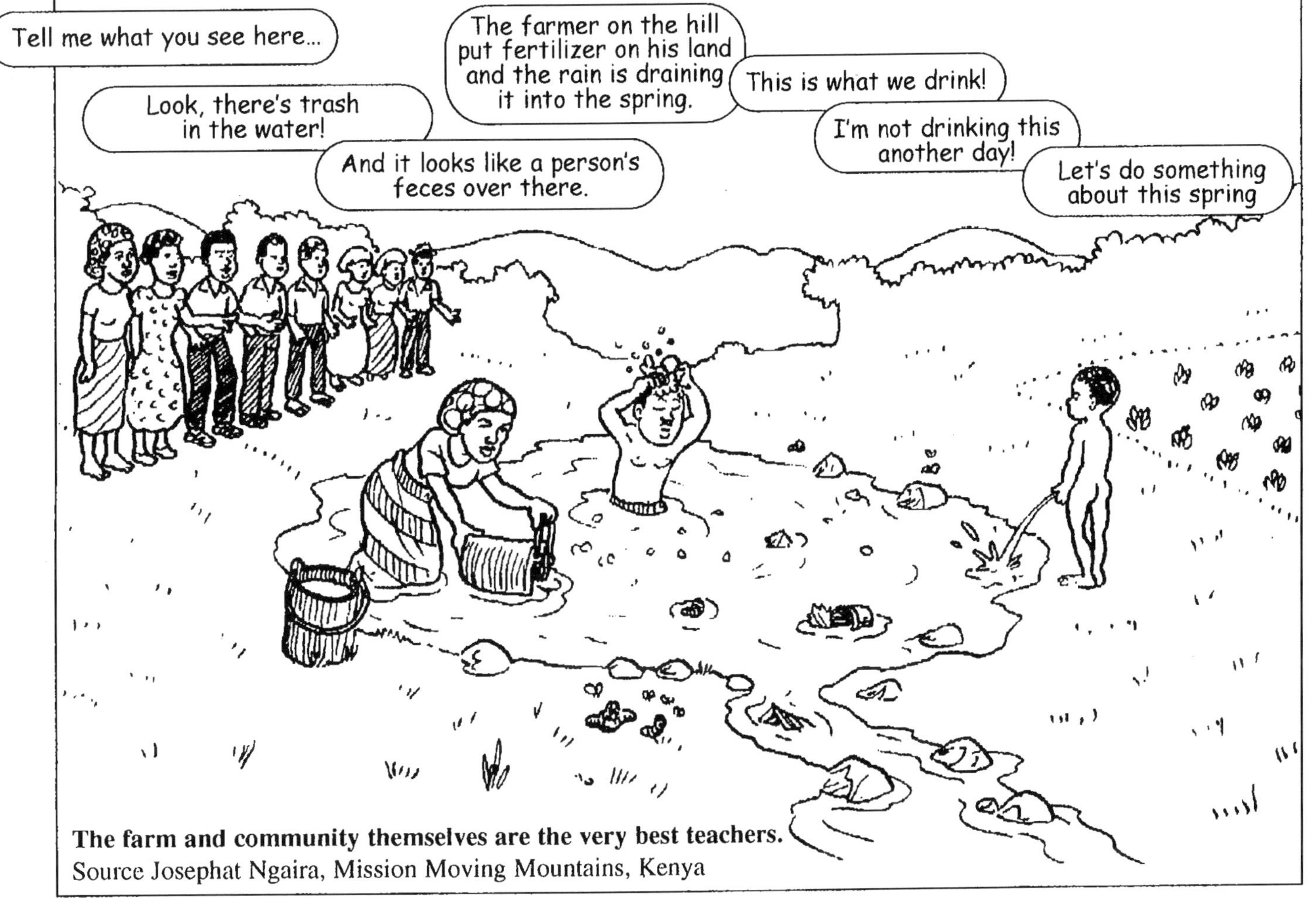

The farm and community themselves are the very best teachers.
Source Josephat Ngaira, Mission Moving Mountains, Kenya

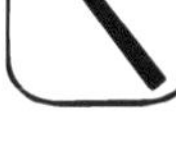

3. Use a simple local object from the farm to discuss a problem and solve it.

An example used to discuss seed storage in Nepal:

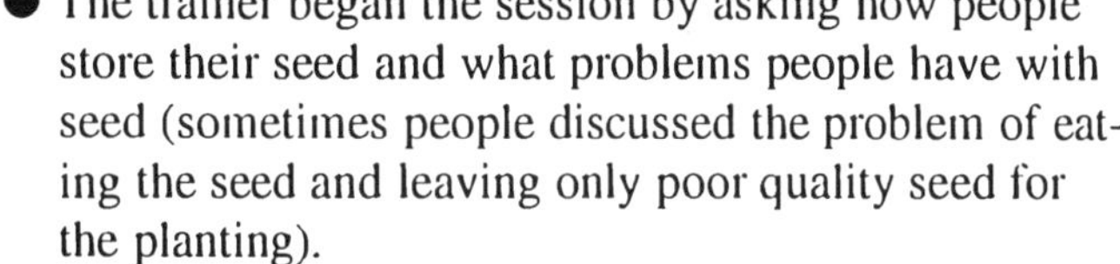

- The trainer began the session by asking how people store their seed and what problems people have with seed (sometimes people discussed the problem of eating the seed and leaving only poor quality seed for the planting).
- The trainer held up a cob of corn which was stored in the traditional way–stacked up off the ground.
- The trainer asked: How many of the kernels are eaten by boors?
- She let each person guess how many to see who could come the closest. There was a prize for the winner.
- One of the participants counted the eaten kernels. With most of the corn stored in this way, most of the kernels are eaten.

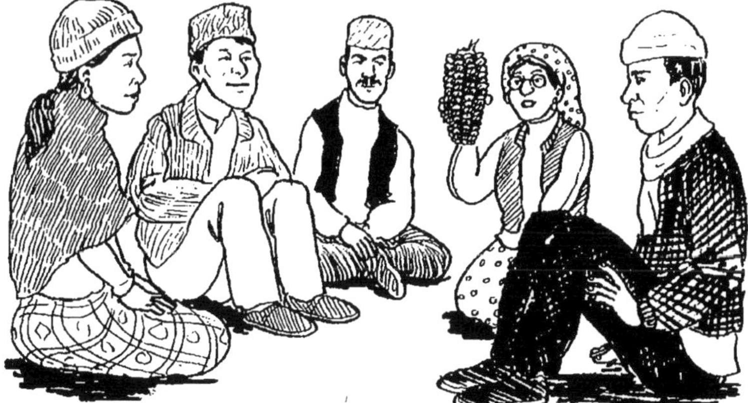

- Everyone was surprised and wanted to know another way of storage. They discussed the use of an herb which grows wild there called sweet flag. They could mix the seed with 20 – 50 grams of dried, ground sweet flag to protect it. The people decided to cultivate the sweet flag to have enough to protect their seed corn.

Include reflection–devotional topics

In the opening section of this book two important ideas were presented for the reader's reflection:

- Many of the issues in agricultural development are social issues.
- A training program must be rooted and grounded in a set of values.

Planning time for people to reflect on and share social issues and spiritual values is an important part of making the workshop appropriate and encouraging. A time of reflection and devotion is commonly scheduled as the warm-up activity for each day of the workshop. The focus of the reflection is a social or spiritual issue related to the other workshop content of the day.

For example, if CLWs will discuss working in their organization during the day, the reflection might focus on the characteristics and values of a person who works with and serves their community. Or this issue might be discussed. "What can we do when discouraged about the organization and its functioning?"

> One of the basic principles of adult learning is :
> **Effective learning will always involve factors of thinking, feeling and doing.**
> All three elements are interconnected and they all change together, not separately.

Here's a simple example of the principle in the previous box involving keeping a schedule of regular vaccination of an animal.

- **What she does:** An owner learns the skills to buy the vaccine and to vaccinate her animal, and she is quite proficient.
- **What she thinks:** She thinks vaccination is important to prevent disease and loss.
- **What she feels:** She must feel the risk involved in the expense and difficulty of organizing the community to vaccinate is less than the risk of the animal getting sick.

Notice that if she **feels** it is too difficult to organize for vaccination, she will not **do** regular vaccination, even though she **thinks** vaccination is important.

When we dialogue about issues in a workshop, we will commonly share what we do and what we think. It is difficult for people to discuss what they feel, especially about serious issues. Because the reflection or devotional time is a time for people to dialogue about what they feel, the reflection topic is related to an important issue from the day's topics.

Many types of dynamics can be used to initiate a reflection. The facilitator needs to ensure that an atmosphere of trust is created. Conclusions from a reflection often help participants to make decisions about other topics in the workshop.

Have fun!

A good sense of humor is a great thing for creating a relaxing atmosphere in which to learn. Jane Vella says, "If there is no laughter, there is little learning." It is important for facilitators to be able to laugh at themselves and with others.

Use humor early in the sessions, not at a time when people are in the midst of a serious discussion. Never let humor belittle a participant or the learning process. Set up some opportunities to laugh and have fun.

Ideas of ways to have fun together:

1. Penalties:

This has the dual purpose of having fun and creating respect for our fellow participants and each other in the workshop. Whenever anyone is late to a session, is caught napping, doesn't ask permission to leave, or loses a game, his or her name gets put on the penalty list. The penalties can be decided by the workshop participants. They choose things like:

- Sing a song
- Dance a dance
- Tell a joke or a story
- Tell a riddle

Also it is helpful for a facilitator to have some ideas of suggestions of fun things for people to do to pay their penalty. Here are some examples:

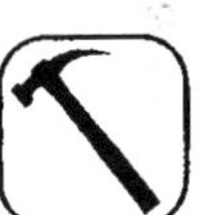

The discourse

The facilitator stands behind the person paying the penalty. Holding a jacket or sweater, the front of which faces the penitent. The facilitator puts her arms through the sleeves of the jacket. She asks the participant to give a speech to his or her fellow learners on some current subject (like wise use of wildlife). As the participant begins to speak, the facilitator begins to do things like scratch the head of the participant, pull up his or her pants, pretend to wipe his or her runny nose, or sweaty brow. It is hilarious.
Source C-CIMCA

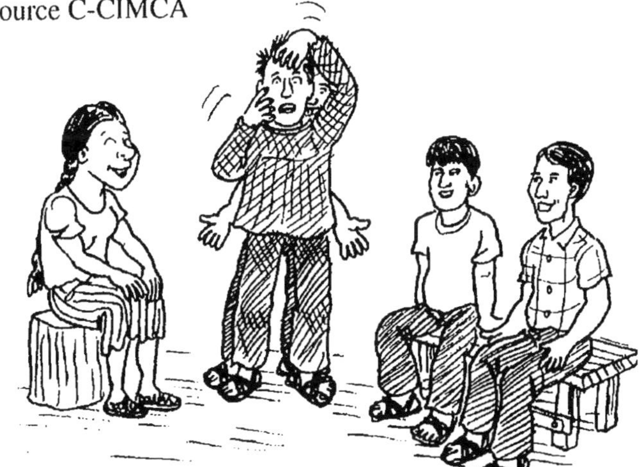

The Kitty
One person goes around the circle of participants meowing and acting like a cat, trying to make the people laugh. The participants have to keep a straight face and pet the kitty on the head. The first to laugh changes places with the kitty.

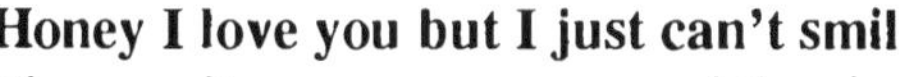

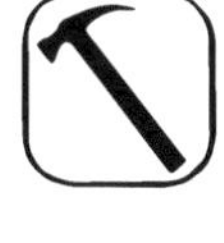

Honey I love you but I just can't smile
The penalty person goes around the circle trying to make each person smile using actions (without speaking). The participants have to say, "Honey I love you but I just can't smile."

How many times a day?
- The penalty person stands in front facing the group, while the facilitator stands behind so the penalty person can't see him or her.
- The facilitator asks: "How many times a day do you do this?"
- The facilitator makes the motions of hand washing
- The penitent, who can't see the motions, makes up an answer.
- The facilitator does different things asking, "How many times a day do you..."

The actions can be: washing the face, sleeping, squating like going to the bathroom, rocking the baby, etc. This is very funny.
Source C-CIMCA

2. In the evening do something fun together.

This builds camaraderie and gives the opportunity to get to know and enjoy one another outside of the training. In different places trainers use different fun things:

- Have a cultural night where people share folk songs and dances from their village.
- Have a night of singing.
- Show videos which can be discussed.
- Provide an atmosphere where people can get together and chat.
- Play sports together.

3. Be willing to laugh at yourself – but not at others.

A natural sense of humor is a great asset for a facilitator. Jokes are normally not recommended. But you can do fun things like the penalty games or like this:
If everyone is sitting in a small group and they need to elect their chairperson tell everyone to raise their finger in the air and on the count of three point to the person they want as leader. This will usually get a laugh.
Source: *HPI Training of Trainers Resource Booklet*

4. Use laughter in tasks and teaching *dynamics* for a great effect. See "Show Me" from "Defining the Situation," page 64 When we all laugh together we are engaged and learning!

Get away from the written word

Don't use written words, especially if women are to be included in areas where literacy is marginal. There are many dynamics which do not require writing skills. For example, games, puzzles, flannel boards, posters, ranking, seasonal calendars, and mapping do not require writing. Many dynamics which are designed for written use can be shifted to picture.

For example:

- In a training needs assessment in Paraguay, everyone was asked to decide what were the two most serious problems with their livestock.
- Then each person found an object to symbolize that problem (such as a dry bone for animals which die because they do not have enough food).
- As each person presented a problem, the object was placed on the ground in the center of the circle of people.
- If it was a new problem it was placed in a new row below the previous problem. If it was a repeat of one already mentioned, it was put alongside the appropriate object.
- In this way the needs were expressed and prioritized by the people in the same exercise.
- The final list of prioritized needs was given to the community with both writing and a picture to represent each need. In this way, everyone understood and participated in defining the needs.

People who are not literate often have fabulous memories. That is where a song or a saying relating to the topic may be very helpful for them to memorize the steps necessary to do something.

In communities with some literate people **an appropriate livestock management manual** which has many pictures and little writing may be used by many in the off hours away from class. Often people have told us they used them to practice their reading as well. Before you print up a lot of manuals though, **make sure you test out both the language and the pictures with the people.** This is called field testing and will make the manual much more appropriate.

Use feedback & encouragement

Three kinds of feedback:

1. The participants need feedback to know how they are doing and to help create the relaxed atmosphere of trust which is most conducive to adult learning. The trainer should remember to give feedback such as "Good idea, thank you" when the participants share their ideas.
2. A part of feedback is **coaching** when a new skill is being learned.

Feedback is very important! There are two places to get more information in this book on feedback: "Listening and Speaking," pg 208, and "Facilitators," pg 50.

We all need to be coached sometimes in the process of training. It may just be affirmation that we are doing it right, or it could be a suggestion of how to do it in a simpler way. People who are having difficulty grasping a technique or ideas or who want a bit more practice will respond to coaching. Talking with and encouraging the participants in an activity, especially the acquisition of a new skill like vaccinating, knot tying, or sheep dipping, encourages them in their learning process. Ask some questions in a small group or one-on-one to help a person think through a complex idea. Make sure your feedback does not judge the person but rather describes the behavior.

3. A third type of feedback is for participants and trainers. This is when we help one another to see how our behavior affects the process of the workshop or the effectiveness of the group. Perhaps one participant talks too much, or another takes over control. It is important that trainers and participants understand how to give feedback in a way which is helpful to others. As Community Livestock Workers practice training others, they will need to receive feedback on their technique.

We learn from our mistakes

We often learn the most from our mistakes. If an atmosphere of trust has been created, it is possible to admit our mistakes and to learn from them. Sometimes adults need to be shocked by their own behavior to realize there is a problem and to reach the level of disequilibrium necessary for them to consider change. If people all fail together and share what happened, they are not isolated in their failure and they want to work together to change the attitudes which caused the failure.

Give people really tough challenges in the workshop so that when they share their knowledge it makes them proud of their knowledge, empowering them in the process.

In almost every workshop we will **schedule one or two "traps"** for people to fall into. They fall into the traps because they are natural actions which contradict what we are saying with our mouths. They also usually generate a lot of laughter. The laughter helps all to look at the contradictions in a relaxed way.

Many examples of traps can be found in this book:

- Show Me ("Defining the Situation" pg. 64)
- Organizations which divide the community ("Learning and Teaching" pg. 24)
- The Budget Plan ("Defining the Situation" pg. 63)
- Deciding for the people – with the banana ("Learning and Teaching" pg. 7)
- Organizing a campaign treasure hunt ("Tools" pg. 285)

Don't be afraid to let people make mistakes!

When the work groups start out at the beginning of a workshop, they won't know their duties very well. Let them do them as they see fit, don't coach them or tell them what to do. When it is time for the morning presentations and evaluations of the work groups, each group will be evaluated by their peers. Encourage people to speak frankly, give good feedback, and really evaluate each group. Challenge the next groups to do better each day.

Often, as a practice session is in progress, mistakes will be made. If it's clear that the mistake won't cause harm to a person or an animal, people should be allowed to make mistakes and to reflect on them. It is in the reflection time that we learn.

As a facilitator, don't be afraid to admit your mistakes as well.

If you admit them, learn from them right away, and take action to correct them, you will be setting a great example for all of the participants. Model a role of self-reflection and of accepting the feedback which is offered.

Is this a question and answer session?

Many feel they have had a participatory training session when they have run a controlled question and answer session. The facilitator asks a question (usually closed) and someone answers, he or she asks another question and someone answers, and so on. When no one answers, the facilitator answers.

Ask yourself as a facilitator, **"Am I causing active discussion and dialogue among the participants or is every participant facing me and answering my questions?"**

"Am I talking more than the participants or am I drawing ideas out of the group?"

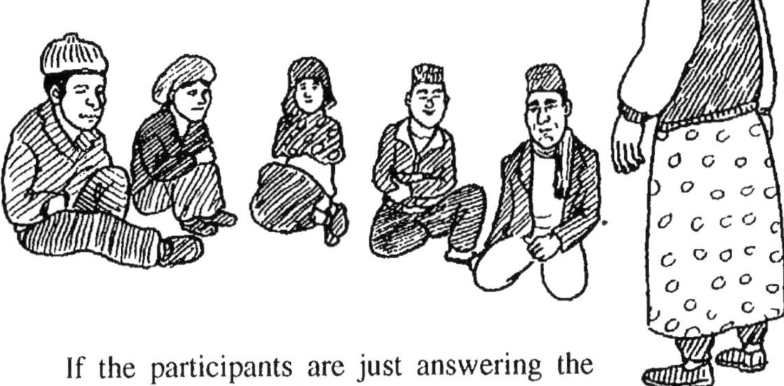

If the participants are just answering the facilitator, there may be several reasons:

☛ **You may not be on an important or generative theme** – If the topic is very important to people, they will want to talk to one another about it to solve the problem. If it is not very important they will answer the questions out of politeness. (See "Listening for important themes" pg. 67.)

☛ **People may not clearly understand the problem** - You can help this situation by an exercise of some sort to illustrate the problem before you begin the dialogue. Have the participants clearly define the problem and its relevance to them. (See "Learning and Teaching" pg. 21.)

☛ **People may feel uncomfortable speaking in a large group** – This can be helped by dividing into small groups first to discuss the problem or question put before everyone. (See "Small groups" pg. 236.)

☛ Culture may dictate that in a training situation people should behave formally and only respond one by one to the questions – **you have not created an open atmosphere of trust** and changed the "culture" of the group. This is very necessary to a participatory approach, to break out of the culture of formal or dominating education. (See "Tips for Good Facilitation" pg. 137 and "Learning and Teaching" pg. 16, and "Women's Participation" pg. 196.)

Some other things you can do to generate dialogue:

- **Be seated;** do not stand and set yourself apart. Be a part of the discussion, not the omnipotent teacher with all the correct answers.
- **Phrase your question as a continuation of the last answer** referring to something the last person said; "What do you think about what Tom said on that thought, Naomi?" That way, people must listen to one another.
- **Refer a question directed at you, the facilitator, back to the one who asked,** or to the group. Resist the temptation to be the expert and to answer all of the questions.

> "Be the guide on the **side** not the sage on the stage."

Ask open questions!

Have some prepared but be ready to think of others on the spot.

Good questions are OPEN: they leave lots of room for participants to contribute their own ideas and experiences from real life. They start dialogue or keep it going. They ask for a deeper analysis. Make sure you do not have a "correct" answer in mind when you ask the question. If you do, the question is probably not a stimulating question.

Example:

Closed question:
Do you have problems with your animals?
Open question:
What are the most serious problems you have with your animals?

Closed questions can be answered with a yes or no or with a short, one-word answer. Or they ask for specific known information given previously, and not from the village reality.

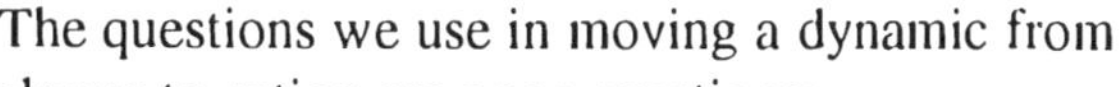

The questions we use in moving a dynamic from dialogue to action are open questions:

- What do you see happening here?
- How do you feel when it happens?
- When it happens in your community, what problems does it cause?
- What are the roots of those problems?
- What can we do about it?

Practice open questions with facilitators and Community Livestock Workers:

Three *dynamics* for open question practice:

1. Listen to the following questions. Which of these questions are open and which are closed? Tell the other people in your group what you feel is the difference between open and closed questions.

Do you like to raise animals?
How can we do this better?
In your experience, what is the best way to control rats?
What is your name?
Which fungicide is best for tomatoes?
How will you use this new way of teaching?

2. Make these closed questions into open questions:

How many kinds of pastures does your goat eat?
Does the hillside show soil erosion?
Are there any questions?
Does your cow have diarrhea?

3. Write three open questions. Each person writes three open questions. Check them with the other people in your small group. In the plenary write some of these questions on large paper and have everyone check them.

Ask everyone, Why do you think we use open questions?

For a sample lesson plan to practice using open questions see: "Write the lesson plan," pg. 106.

Give the opportunity to practice

Much of participatory training is adult learning through discovery. In the process of discovery people are often practicing new skills. For example, many of the communication dynamics (pages 199–208) give the participants the opportunity to practice more effective communication. They also pose a problem to be collectively considered through dialogue.

In livestock and agricultural training, the problem-posing approach is applied to many social situations: Why doesn't the community vaccinate their animals even though they know about the disease problem? The dialogue about this problem may lead to a change of attitude about vaccination of animals. After this, the participants will need the opportunity to try out these new ideas. The best way is to run a training session for the community and organize a vaccination campaign.

"See one, do one, teach one" was the adage when I went to veterinary school. To really learn something;

- First, I see how to give an oral dewormer in a demonstration.
- Then I treat an animal with the medicine.
- But I really know all about it after I have taught someone else how to deworm an animal with the medicine.

Use the practice time in your workshops to give the participants opportunities to see, do and teach. (See "Tools, how to do a practice session," pg. 240.)

Build it together

Talking about chick brooders? Build one together in the classroom. Talking about bee hives? Build several together of different kinds. Discussing corrals? Build one together. Need a head gate? Build one together and use it together to discuss the pros and cons of the way it was built. If you have the option, don't discuss something in class, go to the farm and do it, see it, or build it together. This should not be a demonstration most times. Everyone in the class should get their hands in and do the thing, from the planning stage through the finished item in use.

Closure

There are three levels of closure for every workshop:

1. **Topic Level:** Each topic presented needs a **re-presentation of the ideas** discussed as a summary of what has been accomplished.
2. **Daily**: At the end of each day there should be a **review and feedback activity.** This reviews the materials covered, finds out how everyone is feeling about the workshop, and helps the facilitator know how they are doing and what to change.
3. **End of Workshop: Goal setting, workshop evaluation and a closing ceremony** are scheduled the last day of the workshop. At the end of the workshop it is important to honor the participants in all they have accomplished and in their goals for the future.

1. Re-presentation of the information

The end of every topic discussed in a workshop is the organization of the information and its re-presentation. This is a very important sum-up job of the facilitator.

Here is an example:

A group brainstormed a possible solution to the problem of parasites in their sheep. As they brainstormed, they developed many possible solutions. In the course of the following discussion they talked about different types of dewormers–some traditional and some new–about draining marshes, pasture rotation, separation of animals, and some other ideas. This discussion may have meandered over many ideas. How can the participants keep from being confused and have closure on the topic?

We can reorganize the material into a chart like this:

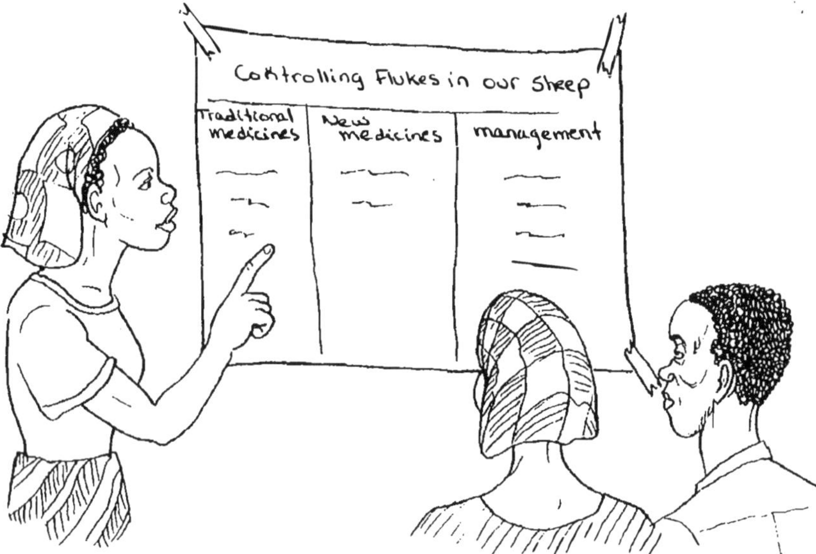

Then the participants can make a plan for the control method they want to begin with. This will bring a sense of closure to the topic. For every topic some similar way of re-presentation of the information discussed is necessary. It can be as simple as a summary which everyone helps to provide. Or small groups can summarize the conclusions in a drama, story, collage, diagram, statue, or song. Or it can be a chart which organizes thoughts into categories. Try it; the more you do it, the more ideas you will have about how to do it better!

2. Daily review, feedback and readjustment

Each day there should be a time for review and reflection. This can be done at the end of the day or at the start of the new day as a part of the warm-up.

A daily review accomplishes a number of things:

- ✔ Everyone revisits the day's material.
- ✔ The facilitator finds out how everyone is feeling–to recognize if there are problems or doubts.
- ✔ People express satisfactions and dissatisfactions with the workshop.
- ✔ The facilitator learns what are the most important topics of the day and what to change in the future.
- ✔ Participants reorganize, draw conclusions, and see connections in the day's material.
- ✔ The facilitator uses the materials to make plans for the next day.

The daily review will bring a sense of closure to the day. Take the time to honor the participant's contributions this day with a thank you. Review the topics scheduled for the next day.

For reviewing topics, please see "Tools," "Games for evaluation and sharing," pg. 268.

The mood meter

This can be used so everyone can gauge the daily mood of the participants and the facilitators: (Note: MAE stands for morning, afternoon, and evening.)

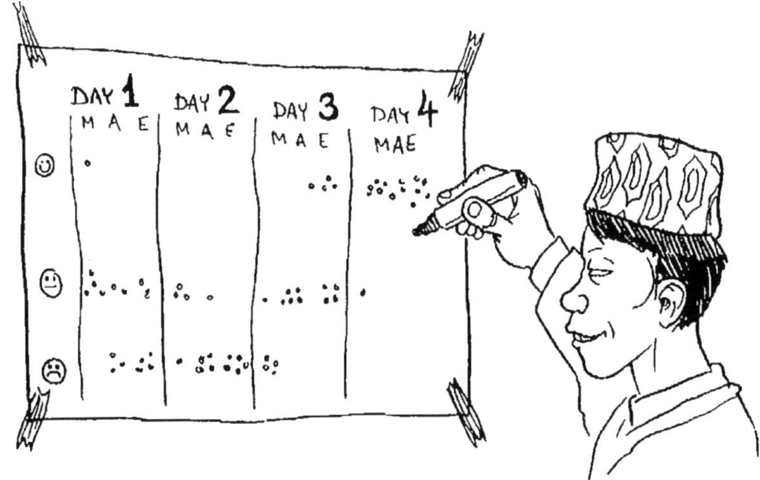

For each session the participants put a sticky dot or a mark for how they are feeling. The mood of the workshop can be gauged by everyone this way. At the end of the workshop draw a graph to show its course.
Source: Heintz Peter Mang

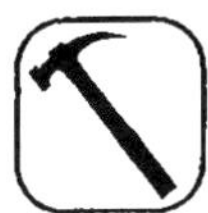

Value feedback

The facilitator needs feedback as to how the workshop is going and how he/she is doing. Here is one way this is done. For other ideas see "Evaluation," "Evaluating a Workshop," pg. 161.

Three questions

These three questions are posed to everyone, or to "walking and talking" groups of two, or to small groups. They discuss them briefly then report back to everyone:

1. What value did you learn today?
2. What thing was most useful today?
3. What would you suggest we change?

3. The last day of the workshop

The last day of the workshop, three important things need to happen:

1. **Goal setting.** This is where each person decides on personal goals for putting the workshop information into practice. See "Follow-up," pg. 149.
2. **Workshop evaluation.** We all take time together to evaluate the workshop. See "Evaluation," pg. 161.
3. **Closing ceremony.** It is important to honor the participants' work during the workshop and the goals they have made for the future. Stress the contribution they are making to their families, their village and themselves. Provide a certificate, or a letter of attendance for them if it is appropriate. This ceremony does not have to be grandiose, but it is a time of closure and passage for the participants.

A closure *dynamic:*

- Draw a large picture of a human body and place it on the floor in the middle of the circle of participants.
- Give each participant three small sheets of paper and a marker or crayons. Have each person write or draw on each paper what they are thinking, feeling, and doing as they leave the workshop.
- Randomly have each person place their papers on the head, heart, and feet of the large drawing on the floor as they tell what they are thinking, doing and feeling

Source: Community Partnership Center, Knoxville, TN

Workshop reports

A workshop report should be given to the participants of a workshop within a reasonable amount of time after the workshop. This report contains the responses, ideas and plans the participants contributed during the workshop. All of the detail of the workshop is not included. Also the techniques and activities are not included. It is a summary report of the conclusions drawn by the participants. Generally, it will be a combination of writing and drawings to make the report as simple and easy to understand as possible.

Here is what one page of a report looked like:

(See the tool in "Defining the Situation," page 63.)

Recommendations:

- The institution that does the assessment must take the community's opinion into consideration.
- The communities must be informed about the specifics of the program or project.
- Institutions must share experiences with one another.

To deeply analyze the theme of the self-assessment the exercise called, "The Game of Investments" was used. The people in each group had the time to consider and invest in the types of projects according to the priorities the groups gave. They chose based on the interests of the institutions and technicians.

This chart gives us the details of the situation:

PROJECTS	ROACHES	MOSQUITOES	FLEAS	FLIES	BEETLES
Irrigation	-	-	-	-	-
Green Houses	-	-	-	-	-
Health Post	-	-	6	3	1
Livestock Improvement	5	4	5	4	5
Environment	2	3	3	3	2
Artisan Products	-	-	3	1	-
Agriculture	5	5	3	5	4
Credit	5	5	3	5	4
Others	4	8	-	-	2

TRAINING	ROACHES	MOSQUITOES	FLEAS	FLIES	BEETLES
Health	3	9	8	3	2
Animal Health	5	5	7	3	4
Nutrition	2	6	-	3	-
Gardening	2	-	2	1	3
Bee Keeping	0	0	0	0	0
Administration	2	0	0	4	4
Others	4	0	0	0	4
Perennial Crops	2	0	6	5	0
Agroforestry	2	6	2	6	3

After adding up the investments according to priorities, we arrived at the conclusion that we alll fell into a trap! We found many justifications for our fall, among them:

- The previous discussion was not very helpful
- The time to think about it was inadequate (in other words, we felt pressured).
- We decided with the mentality of technicians without thinking about our community members.
- The instructions were not clear enough (you only asked us to invest, not think).
- We got confused because we don't have much knowledge of the methodology we are learning.
- We need to use similar methods to describe the reality of the context in which we work.

Tips for good facilitation

☛ **Ask questions which are open and specific.** Open questions will start a dialogue because they do not seek a correct answer. (See "Ask open questions," pg. 132).

★ Make your questions **specific.** If they are vague they won't generate dialogue.

Vague question:
What diseases do your animals have?
Specific question:
What diseases do your cattle get this time of year?

★ **Don't keep repeating the same question over and over** for different people to answer. If people don't respond to the question, rephrase it.

☛ **Enable everyone to participate.** Some shy people will tend to stay silent. Small groups will help everyone participate in this situation. Also, it is helpful to go around the circle and let everyone give an answer to some questions, or give an idea. You can also use someone's name and ask that person a question directly. But please also respect people's need for safety. Allow them the opportunity to begin to participate gradually without forcing them.

☛ **Plan for silence.** Don't be scared of it. Initially if a group has not used a particpatory process there will be more silence. If no one answers the question, don't answer it yourself! Rephrase the question, or give an example. If the topic is a moving one, or one which requires deep thought, plan for a period of silence. Many times when there is silence, the resulting dialogue is profound. In some workshops where everything had to be translated because of mixed language participants, people had more deeply internalized the subject and the results were astounding!

☛ **Keep the discussion on course.** Although some meandering is very productive, some people will always try to take the discussion completely off course in a non-productive way. You can go back to the last question and repeat it, or acknowledge the answer and return to the subject by something like, "That is important, and later we will return to it." Make sure you return to it later! You can make a list of these "tangent" topics on a sheet of paper to help remind yourself to return to them. We sometimes use a drawing of a refrigerator or a bookshelf on large paper where we write the tangent topics. As we discuss them we take them out of the fridge or off the shelf.

☛ **Expect conflict and use it for learning:** Arguments are very good for getting all the points out in a situation and allowing feelings to be expressed. For example, we know people may object strongly to a new way of teaching. Use their objections to open good dialogue about problem-posing education. On the other hand, arguments can also consume session time, cause a block in the discussion and limit the dialogue to two people. A facilitator should be able to deal with arguments which become non-productive.

If it is a strong argument you can:

★ Clarify the points of disagreement;
★ Make sure it is not just miscommunication;
★ Summarize the disagreement and the points;
★ Move on, acknowledging both sides;
★ If the person aggressively challenges you in order to derail the workshop or meeting, ask that person to come up and to tell everyone how to do the thing he or she was challenging you on or to assist you in the training. The arguer will either agree and begin to help and be engaged in the process or will be quiet.

What if the disagreement is between the facilitator and a participant?

When relationships are strained and the air is charged with emotion, an attempt to teach is often perceived as a form of judgement and rejection. –Steven Covey

Don't borrow strength from your position and authority to force people to agree with you. State the problem clearly, make an agreement to disagree and table it. Come back to it later and in a different way.

☛ **Keep the discussion practical.** If someone gives an abstract idea, ask them for an example.

☛ If you have a **very dominant participant:**

★ Give polite feedback about the behavior. It may be best to do this one on one, instead of before the group, so the person is not embarrassed.

★ Limit eye contact with that person since the eye contact gives permission to speak.

★ Give him or her a task to perform.

☛ Keep track of the discussion, **recording comments** on large newsprint (or have a participant do the recording) where it is appropriate to use written tools. Refer back to people's comments, and organize and represent the ideas for further discussion.

☛ In closing the discussion, review the main points which people brought out. Remind people of the purpose. Confirm the decision for action they have taken.

Adapted from Terry Bergdall, 1993

☛ **Celebrate group work.** At the end of a small-group presentation or the end of a group discussion which has been very productive, have applause for the work done or sing a song in appreciation.

☛ **Honor individual contributions.** Assume wisdom lies behind every participant contribution. Ask sensitive questions with respect.

☛ **Honor the group.** Pay attention, even when you are not facilitating (such as during small- group work). Don't casually sit and chat or read a newspaper when participants are planning for their future.

☛ **Demonstrate the power of teamwork.** The facilitators are a team. Even when a person is not leading the discussion he or she should be actively engaged in what is going on and ready to assist in any appropriate way. You can take notes, write group responses on large paper, or ask appropriate questions if the group gets bogged down. At the end of a topic or in the team meeting in the evening, the facilitators can evaluate one another for improvement in the process.

☛ **Don't be a visiting VIP.** The aim is to empower villagers and to encourage their self-confidence and self-reliance. Demonstrate identification with the villagers through similar dress, neat but not fancy, no fancy hairdos, nail polish, etc. Don't expect special treatment. Don't keep participants waiting, or if you do, pay your penalty for being late! Don't eat separately. Mix with the participants in friendly conversation during workshop breaks. Avoid sitting in a chair above those of the participants or sitting in the important-looking chairs.

☛ **Sit in the circle with everyone else,** not apart or behind a desk Don't stand to lead the discussion unless you need to point out something, then sit back down. Have a separate person do the recording so you can be seated with the group.

☛ **Keep the discussion from being chaotic.** Sometimes when the group discusses a generative theme the participants are so highly engaged that they begin to have side conversations in twos and threes. There are many ways to bring the group back to working together and listening to one another. Here are two suggestions:

★ **Have a hum session.** Formulate an open question related to the discussion and ask the participants to discuss it with their neighbor in the circle for two minutes. Once they have discussed the idea, each pair can report their thoughts and the dialogue continues.

★ **Pass the stick or marker or roll of tape.** Help the participants to see that the discussion is disorderly and fragmented and that some good ideas are being lost. Tell the group you will give an object (a stick or a magic marker or a roll of tape, etc) to a person and she will share her idea. When she has finished she can choose someone to pass the object to, or another person can request the object. The only person allowed to speak is the person with the object.

☛ **Listen more than you speak.** Do not interrupt.

Things not to do

☛ If you are doing small group work or brainstorming or in any way asking the participants to develop a list of items; above all else **DO NOT MAKE A CORRECT LIST AND SHOW IT AFTER THEY HAVE DEVELOPED THEIR LIST.**

Why?

- This suggests that the knowledge of the trainer is more important than the knowledge of the participants.
- It devalues the work done by participants.
- It sets up the traditional teacher-student roles we are trying to avoid.
- It does not respect the knowledge of the participants.

What can I do instead?

- Process the trainee's list. Go through the list together and discuss each point, eliminating the ones the group decides are not correct. (Please see "Brainstorming," pg. 238).
- If you want to organize things in a specific order, make a new list together, asking the participants in a plenary session what the correct order would be after all groups have presented their input and it has been discussed in general session.
- Even if you want to have a clean list you can use the participant's list, crossing out the responses the group decides are not correct and making a new list as review for the final product.

You may say, "It's all the same whether I show my finished list which was prewritten or write one in front of the group." But there is a big difference: **One is a product of your work alone and the other is a product of the work of the group; they own it and will put it to use in the future.**

☛ **DON'T USE TWO DRAWINGS OR STORIES OR ROLE PLAYS WHICH SHOW FIRST "THE WRONG WAY" THEN THE "RIGHT WAY"**

Why not?

- A picture or role play or story should always pose a question or a problem; it should never give the answer. The participants will provide the answer.
- You may say, "What if the people don't know the answer?" Most times this is not a problem. The purpose of the picture dynamic is to open the discussion, put everyone in the same place to discuss a common problem. This suggests the people already have experience with the problem, and gives them the opportunity to share their experience in an undirected way.
- The trainer who gives the right and wrong way runs the risk of not analyzing with the people the whole problem. The trainer may view the problem in one way and the people in another way. Putting the "correct" way in front of the people limits the discussion and the creative ideas to solve the problem.

If there is a case where it would be extremely beneficial to demonstrate a correct and incorrect way to do something, for the sake of the discussion, let the people present the right and wrong way. This can be done with a role play or a story.

For more ideas please see "Tools," "Stories and role plays," pg. 243 and "*Dynamics*" pg. 18.

☛ DON'T GIVE THE ANSWER IN YOUR DRAWING OR ROLE PLAY; POSE A QUESTION.

☛ DON'T ASK , "DID YOU UNDERSTAND?"

People will always say, "Yes"

Instead ask, "What have you learned?"

☛ DON'T TAKE OVER FOR THE PARTICIPANTS.

This is especially true in small-group work, or any task which requires a group product like a map or chart.

☛ DON'T MOVE PEOPLE AROUND TO SIT WHERE YOU WANT THEM.

If there is a problem or for some reason people need to be moved around, bring it to the attention of the organization committee. Or suggest a game to move people around randomly such as fruit basket turnover (see "Tools," pg. 275), or say, "All the people with this color garment or with sandals change seats."

Linkage

One of the greatest criticisms of village-based programs who train Community Livestock Workers is their lack of linkage to other programs. There may be government-paid technicians or others from outside institutions who work in the same area who do not even know the people who have been trained to work with livestock in their communities. Sometimes there are government benefits the people never receive, such as free vaccine, because there is no linkage to these programs. This is often also hampered by the distance and poor travel conditions between the village and the government center. Often government workers have been assigned areas too large for them to cover.

Some things which have been done to improve linkages with other programs:

1. **From the planning stage, when the stakeholders are identified, call together representatives of other organizations and the government to participate in the planning phase.** Have these government representatives commit to their participation in the training program, assigning them specific tasks as they relate to their program. Investigate government requirements for Community Livestock Workers. Discover how the participants can be certified and recognized by the government. Make a plan for that certification.
2. **Invite people from the government, the university, or the veterinary laboratory to present a section of a workshop on their program,** say vaccination. While the government worker is at the workshop, have the participants hold a meeting with the worker to raise their questions and to establish how they will work together in the future to accomplish the vaccination program. Or the laboratory worker can come to work with the participants on necropsy technique and good sample taking. Plan a discussion with the lab worker on how they will establish lab services for the communities.

From the Rural Development Center Community Forestry Experience in Nepal:

- Local people know about the services which should be available from the government. But often the local government extensionists do not have the resources to provide full extension work.
- The program works with the community and the government worker to change the attitude and build trust.
  - They give time for participants to develop questions for the local government official. In the course of their training they analyze the community problems and have possible solutions. They ask the government official about these.
  - The government official comes to the workshop, or the people go to the official's office. The government agent knows there will be difficult questions and comes prepared to answer them.
  - The meeting is arranged for later in the workshop, since by the middle or the end of their training the people have the confidence to express their ideas.
  - At the end of the workshop, in the goal-setting phase, they include some goals which could only be accomplished with cooperation between the government agent and the people.

3. **Invite people from a trusted pharmacy to participate in the workshop.** Work with them on their part in the workshop so it is also participative. Combine it with a section in the workshop where people are discussing problems with misuse of medicines, or the problem of adequate and dependable supply of medicines, or the establishment of a cold chain. Give the participants adequate time to prepare for the meeting, and let the pharmacy owner know there will be difficult questions to answer. Hold a meeting with the participants and the pharmacy owners to decide how they can best work together in the future. Encourage everyone to be open and honest.
4. **Establish linkages to other Community Livestock Workers.** One of the common things to emerge from a close-knit group during a workshop is the desire to meet again and share experiences. In many cases this desire is transformed into the formation of a Community Livestock Worker organization. This organization holds meetings for mutual support and idea exchange. They assist one another in maintaining the cold chain or in the purchase of vaccines and medicines. They may link to a livestock producers' organization. As we discuss in workshops, problem-posing education should not be exclusive. As a result, some of these organizations have decided to open to other community workers in their zones. They have included health workers and literacy workers and popular educators. They provide a support network to encourage one another and work together on specific projects they feel will help the larger zone.

Chapter 7

Follow-up and goal setting

by Karen Stoufer

This chapter covers the following topics:

Why have a follow-up program?

What happens after a training workshop is finished? **Is our work as trainers complete?**

The training event is exciting and important. The participants feel they have learned much to apply when they arrive home. Some specific training events will not require any follow-up for the person to immediately apply the new knowledge, skills and attitudes.

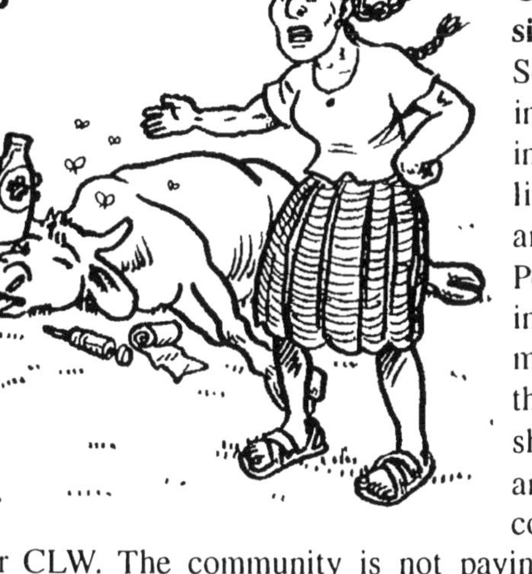

Consider this situation:
Some cases of illness in animals or problems in the community with livestock production are very serious. Perhaps the CLW feels inadequate. The community does not help the CLW when he or she goes to take care of animals. Perhaps the community doubts the skills of their CLW. The community is not paying for medicines and services. These situations can lead to a learning opportunity or to discouragement and abandonment of the CLW position.

The same is true for a basic community training.

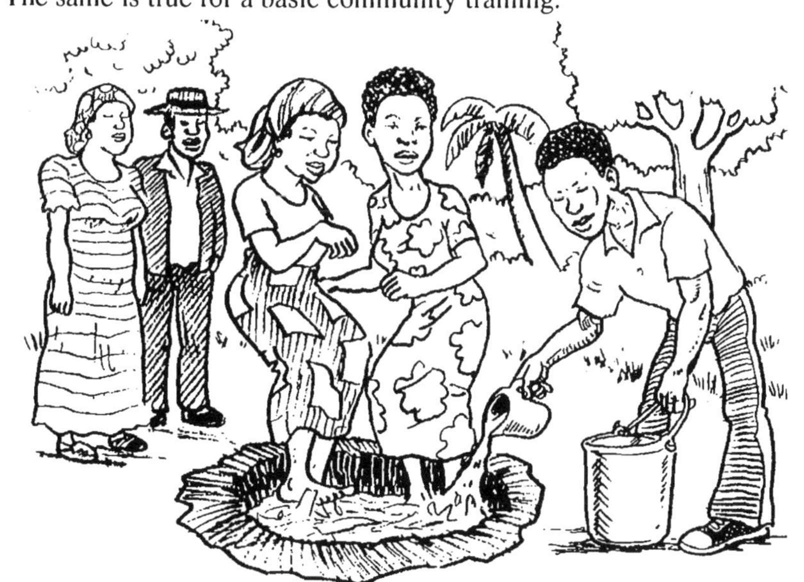

The workshop participant may feel they have learned well how to make silage, as they have participated in making a pitful during the workshop.

But they get home and begin to make the silage and they can't remember how much molasses to add. So the silage is ruined, they are discouraged, and they never make it again!

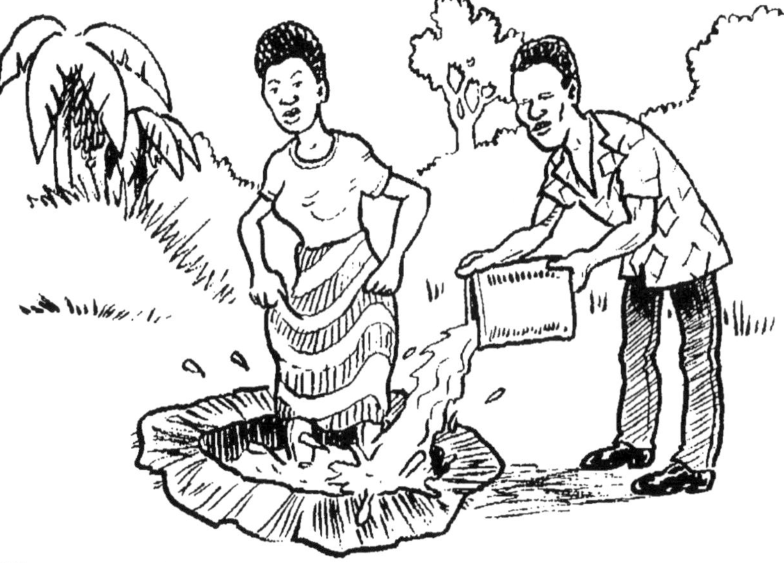

What can we do as facilitators to help insure that workshop participants apply their new knowledge? Or to make sure that they have an opportunity to interact with someone about the problems they have and the new ideas they are using?

Plan an appropriate follow-up program!

Although follow-up is a separate chapter here, it is really a part of the implementation of a training program. The CLWs should be given the opportunity to dialogue about possible problems in their community during the process of the workshops. (See "Reflection/Devotional," pg. 126).

Follow-up is important in any type of agricultural training. The extent of follow-up will depend on the goals and extent of the training.

Follow-up of basic community-level training

In Uganda, Heifer Project has a program which consists of a long series of one-day practical trainings for implementing a zero grazing facility. They provide this follow-up:

1. Extensionists (trainers) visit all participants.
2. Members who have previously implemented the technology provide group support.

In Bolivia following a community training, the participants have these resources:

1. Those who have previously implemented the technology provide group support.
2. The CLW visits participants.
3. A supervisor from the grassroots livestock association visits participants.

Follow-up of Community Livestock Worker training

When training Community Livestock Workers, a coordinated follow-up program must be planned. Make sure you plan the follow-up at the same time as the workshop is planned. The training program from the Rural Development Center (RDC) of the United Mission to Nepal has an impressive record of CLWs who continue to provide services to their communities long after training has finished. (Young, et al 1994) They feel many factors contribute to their record, but one of them is the well planned and implemented follow-up program after training. The rest of this chapter, **written by Dr. Karen Stoufer,** describes their program in detail.

Why do a follow-up visit?

To raise community awareness of the abilities of the CLW.

During the follow-up with an outsider expert, a community meeting is usually called. This meeting is to:

- **Make the community aware of the services** of the CLW and how to use them;
- **Listen to concerns the community has about livestock** and show how the CLW's newly acquired training can help meet those needs;
- **Recognize that the solution to many of their problems is to work together with the CLW.** If the CLW was or ginally selected by this same group to attend the training, it is a good idea to reinforce this bond and the dual accountability of the CLW to serve the community and the community to enable and support the CLW in the work.
- **Discuss payment for services** of the CLW. Some CLWs charge for their service, others only for the medicines. Some work independently, some are part of a community animal health committee. But whatever the system, the community at large needs to understand how it works and why they are being charged. The sustainability of the program is dependent on the CLW being able to continue to work and replace the medicine supply.
- In dispersed communities, the meeting sometimes serves to **introduce the CLW** to people.
- **Set up case visits** among community members' animals during the follow-up time.

These are some of the tools used to conduct the meeting:

- Simple illustrations can show farmers the types of services available, such as preventative dewormings and vaccinations, sick animal examination and diagnosis, general husbandry advice, dystocia management, etc. (See "Tools," pg. 250 and "Learning to make and use pictures" pg. 289.)
- Puppets are great for community meetings. Puppets are especially good in the hands of the people. (See "Tools," pg. 246.)
- Songs are also very good for motivation and awareness, for consciousness raising as well as helping the workers in their work.

As a trainer or facilitator, please don't "show-off" your own knowledge but build on the trust the people have in the CLW and his/her own knowledge and skill.

Raise the standing of the CLW in the community

Much will be accomplished during a well-run community meeting where the CLW's skills are **marketed and respected** by the facilitator, usually seen as an outside "expert." However, in small, remote locations, just the fact that outsiders have gone to some trouble to come visit the CLW, and that they attach importance to the CLWs work, will enhance the respect local people give to the CLW. In some communities, if the facilitator eats in the home of the CLW and stays in the CLW's home overnight, that will also show the respect and importance that can be attached to their animal health work.

Encourage the CLW

This is a time to renew the relationship established during the workshop. It allows the trainer to show personal concern and care for the CLW as a person.

Tips for the good encourager:

✔ Be interested in meeting the CLW's family, seeing their livestock, and discussing general issues of interest to the CLW.

✔ If there have been difficulties, or even mistakes made by the CLW, this is the time to show how the difficulties can be overcome or avoided in the future.

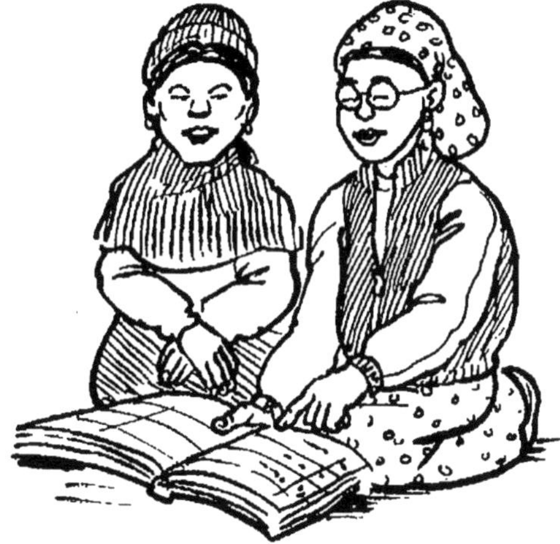

✔ Remind the CLW of his/her successes during the training (perhaps laughingly recall the first time the CLW tried to put the needle on the wrong end of the syringe), and let the CLW realize how much knowledge and skill he/she has and that mistakes and difficulties can be opportunities for learning and improving.

✔ NEVER criticize CLWs or their work in front of any member of the community or family. Corrections should be made in private and done in a supportive, encouraging fashion. If the CLW has forgotten some information, let him or her find it in the manual or in notes. In this way, CLWs will not be dependent on trainers but able to learn on their own.

Refresh and extend the CLW'S knowledge and skills

The RDC training program includes extensive training in the keeping of records for each animal case seen. When CLWs graduate, they are given a medicine box with the medicines they have been taught to use in the workshop.

The follow-up has these goals:

1. Ascertain the level of the CLWs' knowledge through **informal discussion, review of the case records, and examination of the medicine supply.**
2. Introduce new topics if the CLW seems to remember the training workshop content well.
3. Review topics needed by the CLW: use one-on-one coaching.
4. **Observe their practical skills.** Ideally, there will be one or two sick animals in the village to visit and examine. These may be ones that the CLW has already seen and possibly begun to treat, or ones that were mentioned at the community meeting. The facilitator and the CLW should visit the animal together. The facilitator needs to let the CLW lead in the examination and diagnosis and treatment as well as in talking with the owner. The CLW can consult with the facilitator, but the trainer should not take over.

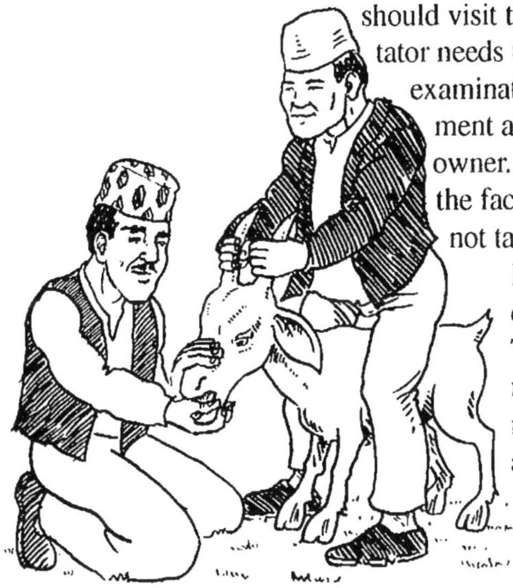

Have the CLW prepare dosages during the follow-up session. The facilitator should bring medicines to practice with rather than using the precious and limited supplies of the CLW. The giving of advice or teaching of farmers is an important skill, and should be reviewed and practiced as well.

Gather feedback on the training workshop

In order to continually improve the training of new CLWs, feedback from the active CLWs in the field is crucial. Follow-up visits may be the only time that these data can be gathered. All CLWs should be asked,

- "What topics or sessions have proven most useful to you in your work?"
- "Which subjects have not been useful at all?"
- "What information/skills have you needed that were not taught during the training?"
- "What advice would you give us to make our next trainings better?"
- "If you attended training again, what topics would you like included?"

Certain topics may not be relevant to the CLW's specific geographical area. Other problems may be seasonal, and if you are visiting the CLW less than 12 months after training, those topics may not have been useful YET. However, in general, if the CLW is not using those skills, no matter how enjoyable he/she may have found the class on that topic, it may not be relevant or appropriate to continue to teach it.

This type of feedback is part of an evaluation. For further information please see Evaluation, pg. 163.

Check the CLW'S medicine supply

The RDC program provides the CLWs with a medicine supply to begin their work. Later, the CLW must replenish the supply from the sale of the medicines in the box. The trainer and the CLW should go through all of the CLW's medicines together. Each medicine should be checked. For each one, the trainer should ask the CLW the following questions:

- "What is the name of this medicine?"
- "What do you use it for?"
- "What is its expiration date?"
- "Is it clearly labeled, in your language, with the name, strength, and expiration date?"
- "Is it kept in a water-proof, rat-proof, and child-proof manner?"
- "Do you have an appropriate amount of stock on hand for particular problems?"

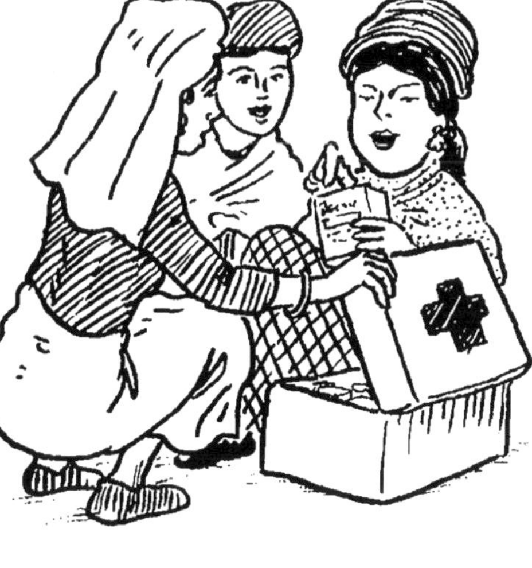

Dealing with restocking:

- Discuss how, when, and from where the medicines are restocked.
- Is the CLW marking up the cost of medicines enough to cover the restocking?
- Are there problems with clients paying?
- Are there problems getting the medicines needed when restocking?
- Do they have any new medicines on hand that were not covered in the training? If so, are they comfortable with their use? It is a good idea to discuss the new medicines in detail.

Consult with the CLW about their own farm

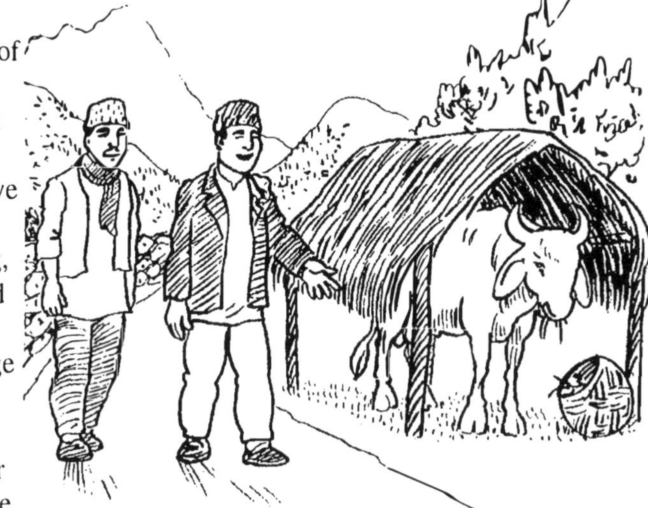

It is more important to admire than to advise here, as part of the encouragement that should be given to a CLW. If husbandry practices have been changed as a result of the training, the facilitator should be sure to recognize this and acknowledge the CLW's efforts. The example the CLW sets for his/her neighbors is far more powerful than all the treatment and teaching he/she will ever do.

Opportunity for the trainer to see local conditions

At the community meeting, the facilitator will have the opportunity to hear about farming practices and specific livestock problems of the area. The facilitator should also walk around in the community and observe conditions. Information which may be useful to the facilitator includes:

- Prevalent livestock diseases
- Cultural practices
- Fodder/feed types and availability
- Evidence of zoonotic diseases
- Socio-economic conditions
- Agricultural/agroforestry practices

Give the CLW an opportunity to ask questions

Many CLWs work in remote situations where veterinary advice is not available. Follow-up visits allow them an opportunity to ask someone they trust, the facilitator, about problems they have had, new ideas or rumors they have heard, topics they never understood well during the training but neglected to ask about then, and specific problems in their locality.

Review record keeping

The kinds of records that CLWs keep depends on how they were taught and the purpose of the records. In general, the minimum amount of record-keeping needed is the best. If the government requires statistical reporting, then this must be done. Otherwise, statistics are of little value to the CLW.

Information on animal cases handled can serve as a tool for continuing education with the CLW. Not only can the facilitator discuss these cases with the CLW, but the CLW can, on his or her own, refer back to them in the future. When a similar case presents in the future, the CLW can review what was done and what the outcome was. It can also serve as a reminder for future treatment such as timing of a second deworming or vaccination campaign.

Financial records are also important to review. Are clients paying? Are they being charged a reasonable amount? Most CLWs tend to charge too little because of the close relationships among people in the village. The facilitator may need to stress that in order to keep serving their neighbors, they must be able to replenish their medicines, etc.

Goal setting: a key

We have previously discussed in this manual the importance of a training program having a vision and goals to work toward. Having an individual set of goals gives workshop participants a sense of accomplishment. They will know they know new things when they do them.

All people who receive training should set their goals for how they will use their new knowledge, skills, and attitudes at the end of the workshop. This can be done in many different ways. Participants should leave the workshop with their goals in hand. If they keep those goals posted in their houses in a prominent place, they will have them in front of them constantly. This helps them to move toward their goals.

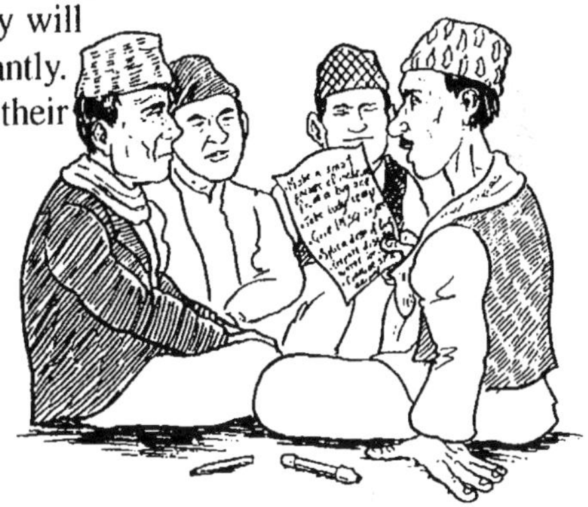

Here is a step-by-step process which is followed in RDC workshops to help participants set their goals. This is used in all RDC workshops, in animal health, kitchen gardening, and community forestry.

A. Make a list by brainstorming, of the course contents, all of the things learned during the workshop. (See "Tools," pg. 238.)

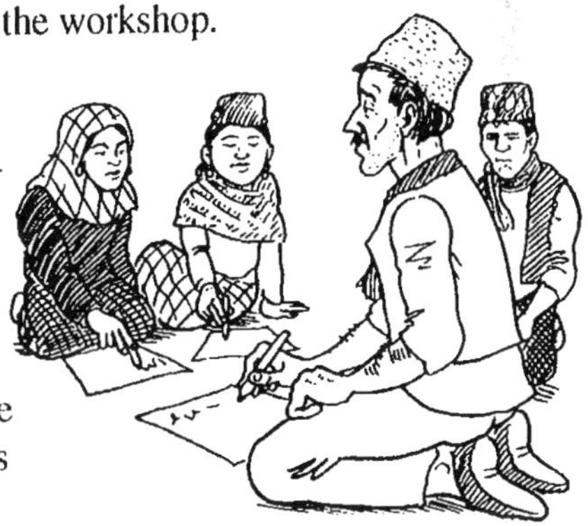

B. From this list **participants set their own goals** for the follow-up visit. The participants set a list of at least three goals, involving their new skills, which are practical for them to apply during the follow-up time period. They also choose things they are eager to try.

Here are some goals from workshop participants:

- Conduct a community meeting and explain the value of preventative worming in livestock.
- Administer preventative liver fluke medicine to 15 water buffalo.
- Assist the community to establish a community tree nursery. (This could be an individual goal, or the community could write their goals jointly.)
- Construct a pit latrine on my own farm.
- Teach three neighbors what I learned about how to plant beans.

For goal setting in community workshops:

- Ask; "What goal would you like to set for yourself?"
- Ask; "How will you do this task?"

The person prepares an action plan.

- They set the goals: with one action plan for each goal.
- They sign the paper and say when it will be done.

C. In addition, in Nepal there are a number of **skills which the CLWs are expected to know,** understand, and be putting into practice. These are checked out in the follow-up visit.

D. Fill out the goal-setting form:

- **Three copies are made:** One for the participant, one for the sending organization, and one for the facilitators.
- **Plan to give people two hours** to complete their goals. Do it in small groups with people from their area.

E. Dialogue with the participants about their goals, first in a small group, then with the whole group of participants.

Sample goal setting form: one page for each goal.

Name of Program: RDC Horticulture Agronomy Training Support Program
Follow-up Form

Name Address:

Objective: Teach at least 5 neighbors the new skill learned

Goal 1:

Action Plan:

Supporting project follow-up comment:

2nd follow-up RDC comment.

Planning follow-up visits

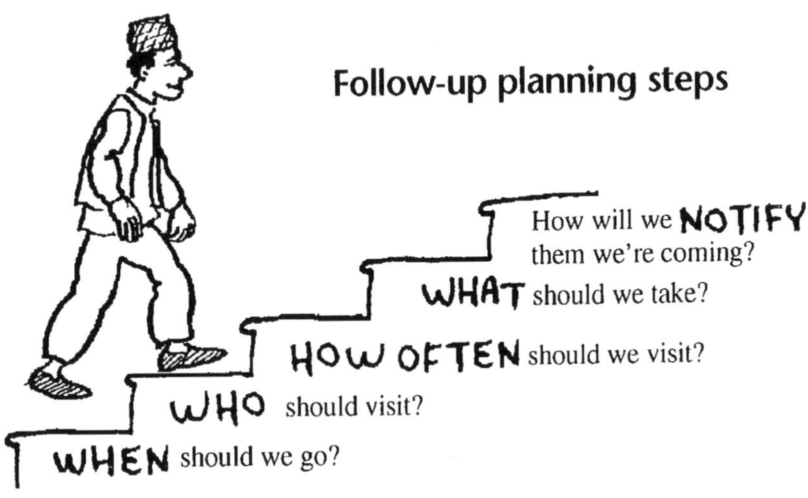

When should we go?

To time the follow-up visit consider these things:

1. **The interval following training.** If the facilitator waits too long to visit, the CLW may become discouraged or cease working. If the facilitator visits too soon, the CLW will not have had time to perform many services, or implement goals, nor sufficient experience to benefit from case discussions with the facilitator.
   The livestock population density of the area the CLW serves and the prevalence of disease will influence how fast the CLW gets that experience. The natural support for and bonding between the CLW and the community also influences this. In the hills of Nepal, each CLW serves an area up to a half day's walk from his/her home and anywhere from 15–70 households. More than three months but less than a year seems an appropriate post-training interval for a follow-up visit in Nepal. During that time the CLW will have had the opportunity to implement the goals from the workshop.
2. **The seasonal work patterns of the community.** The period of seasonal migration for off-farm labor, planting time and harvest time usually are unproductive times for a visit. Everyone is too busy or the household decision-makers are absent.
3. **When the community wants the visit.** Set the time together with the CLW and the community.

Who should visit

Helpful guidelines:

- At least one facilitator that the CLW and/or community already knows should visit.
- In many cultures, women facilitators should be accompanied by at least one other woman, especially when travel involves an overnight stay.

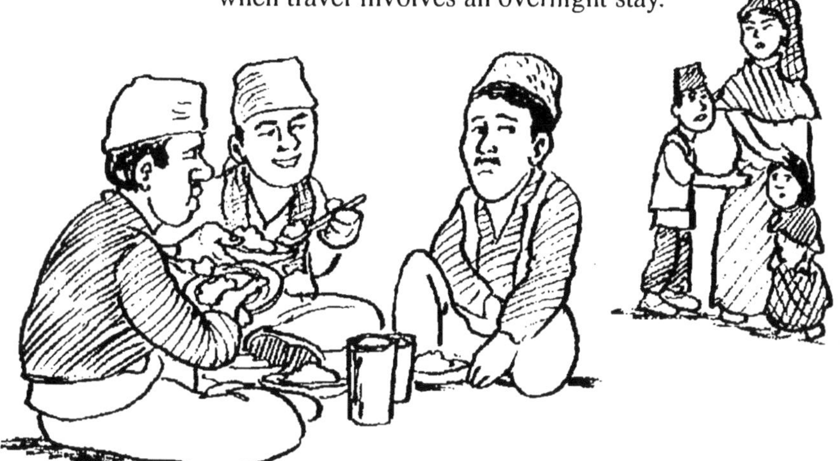

- In food-deficit areas, too many guests can impose a real hardship on hosting families. Even when facilitators pay for their food, it may be that there is no more to be had at any price, and someone will go hungry as a result.
- Too many visitors can draw attention away from the intended focus on the community or CLW or their accomplishments. Go in pairs or threes.

How often should we visit?

A successful training and follow-up will have the following results:

- The community has the awareness, information, and skills to use the CLW's services and incorporate any modifications to existing husbandry practices as they see fit.
- The CLW has the knowledge, skills and confident-yet-serving attitude to encourage, recommend, treat, and model what they have learned.
- When new or additional information or materials are needed, the CLW and the community know where and how to access them on their own.

Options for achieving these results:

A. One visit by technical facilitators, with subsequent visits by locally-based community development workers or project staff to facilitate problem solving as the need arises.

B. One visit by facilitators to communities with well-established unity and communication/support systems.

C. Two visits by facilitators. This would be particularly effective if:

- subsequent refresher or advanced trainings were given between visits.
- certain specific projects are being implemented, such as:
  - a community fodder-tree nursery,
  - vegetable gardens for seed production,
  - breeding program with improved livestock breeds, where progress over time can be a helpful discussion point.

What should we take? General guidelines

Bring appropriate tools.

Don't bring fancy tools or exotic medicines that will never be available to the local community. For example, don't worm every cow in the village with a gun paste-wormer and expect the villagers to then believe that a piece of hand-cut bamboo is just as good!

Don't bring teaching tools such as audio-visuals in foreign languages or tools that require more education to understand than many villagers have.

Some things you might bring on your visit:

- A rectal thermometer (in case the CLW's thermometer breaks),
- Expired medicines to allow the CLW to practice calculating and mixing dosages,
- A photograph of the workshop to talk about what people are doing,
- A few simple training materials such as a poster or flip chart that can be used at a community meeting and then left with the CLW for future reference,
- A copy of the goals the CLW set and, if appropriate, the workshop certificate.

Implementing follow-up

Five main types of activities usually comprise a follow-up visit to a CLW:

1. Home and community visit
2. Community meeting
3. Practical exercises
4. Review of case records
5. Question-asking

For your program the steps may be different. Make a checklist together with all of the trainers of what will be covered in the visit.

Local support system

When Community Livestock Workers have problems or questions, who do they refer to?

Planning ahead with the CLWs about how they will be supported in the future can be a key to long-term success. Take the time to work with them on setting up a local network of livestock workers and other educators. Work with other organizations and institutions in the area with agriculture programs. Help them to establish linkages to existing government people and programs.

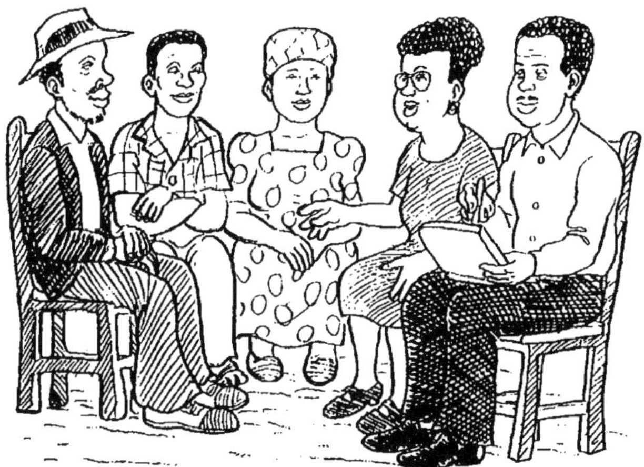

Suggestions for establishing a support system:

The CLWs in the Berlin area in Bolivia set up an organization of CLWs with their own leadership and regular meetings. They did this during the course of their initial training. CLWs used these meetings to discuss problems in doing their jobs in the community and how each of them has solved problems. They also used the time to coordinate vaccination and worming campaigns, to ensure that villages where there are no workers are covered, and to develop their coordination with other organizations and institutions such as the government programs. They have also used the meetings to plan projects and write grants for improvement of their zone, their organization, or their community.

Set up a linkage, credibility, and respect for the CLW by the government technician who covers the area. In this way the CLW has access to vaccines and some support from the government worker. (see "Linkages," in "Implementation," pg. 140).

Some nongovernment organizations (NGOs) have provided for their workers to be available and living in the area to support trained CLWs. If the NGO is to become an institution which will always be available to the area and will integrate into the long term government program, perhaps this is a good policy. However, if the NGO plans to move from the area at some time in the future, there should be a local structure in place to support the CLWs.

Follow-up workshops

Follow-up workshops can be an alternative to home-visit-based follow-up. They could also be used as a supplement to individual follow-up. In this situation, several CLWs from different communities meet together for one to several days with the trainers.

Advantages of follow-up workshops:

1. Exchange of ideas between CLWs. Sharing of difficult and successful cases gives time for teaching of one another and encouragement.
2. Continuing education of CLWs with workshop-style sessions. These sessions can be based on a training needs assessment by the CLWs of their new training needs.
3. Less travel time for facilitators.

Disadvantages of follow-up workshops:

1. The CLWs must leave home and travel. Coordination and communication are difficult.
2. There is no opportunity for meeting with the CLW's communities.
3. There is no opportunity to see the CLWs' actual cases in their communities.

Chapter 8
Evaluation in a participatory program

by Jennifer Shumaker

This chapter covers the following topics:

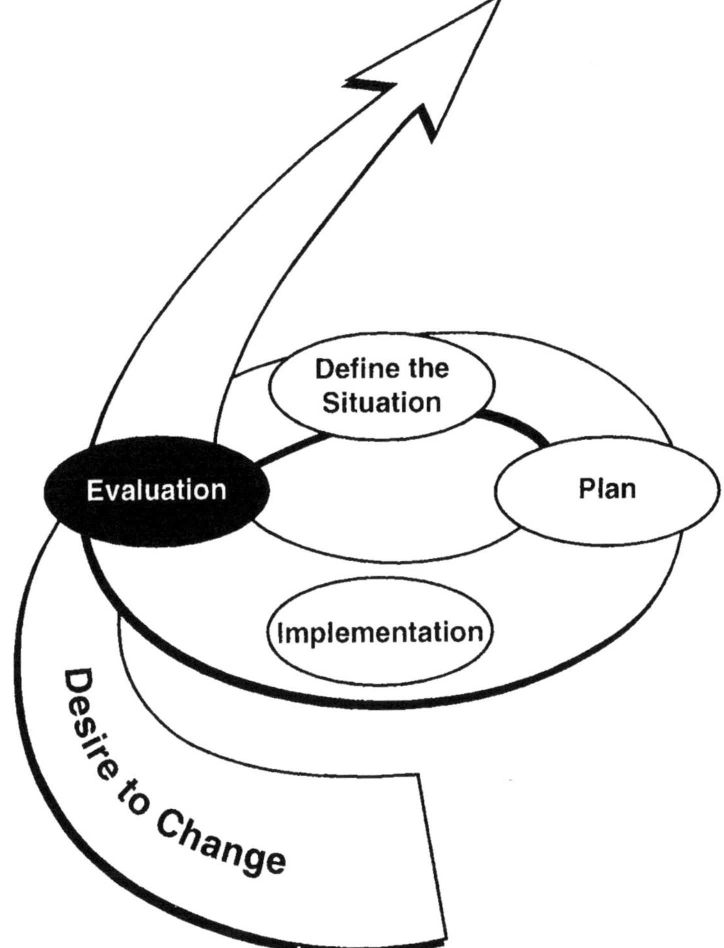

An evaluation is an opportunity for people to **see, feel, and understand that they know something.** We know that we know something **when we do it.**

We know that we have new attitudes:

The farmer in Nepal who begins to plant trees because she wants to save the hillside for her children and travel less distance for firewood knows that she has a new attitude toward soil conservation.

We know new knowledge:

The CLW in Kenya who treats an animal successfully knows that she knows about the disease and its treatment because the animal recovered.

We know new skills:

The community group in Mexico knows that they know the new skills for accounting and marketing their farm products when the cooperative is solvent and makes money for them.

An evaluation is an opportunity for adult learners to **reflect on their learning**. As in the process of dialogue - reflection - and action, taking the time to pause and reflect on the training we have received allows us to see

- How it has affected our lives,
- How it could have been done differently for greater effect,
- What new needs requiring new training have developed from the application of learning.

An evaluation is an opportunity for learning and growth.

Monitoring and evaluation should be ongoing in any participatory training program. This section discusses some aspects of evaluation as it pertains to an agricultural training program. It does not describe a complete evaluation of the program. For more in-depth help in developing a participatory program evaluation, see "References/ Evaluation," pg. 332.

Is there a place for exams?

When examinations are a part of motivating the learning process, encouraging collaboration, and helping learners to meet their needs – yes! If an exam is for judging, causing unhealthy competition, or enforcing a teacher's or program's control – no!

Reasons for exams in a participatory program:

For Community Livestock Workers

- They see clearly **that they know,** and have confidence;
- They increase their **understanding** and **collaboration;**
- They are challenged to do **new thinking** and problem solving.

For communities who send people for training

- They are assured of a **competent CLW;**
- They see that their **needs are being met;**
- They can have **input** for training adjustment.

For trainers

- They can know **how well they are teaching;**
- Everyone can know what subjects are covered well, what needs review, or what changes in approach might be necessary.

Suggestions for effective exams

1. Use an open book

Design the exams so CLWs can use their manuals to look for information and discover solutions to problems. That way the CLW will understand the value of looking something up–not memorizing.

This will help CLWs to do their jobs better. It is always better to look up information–especially drug dosages and symptoms which are confusing–than to try to respond from memory.

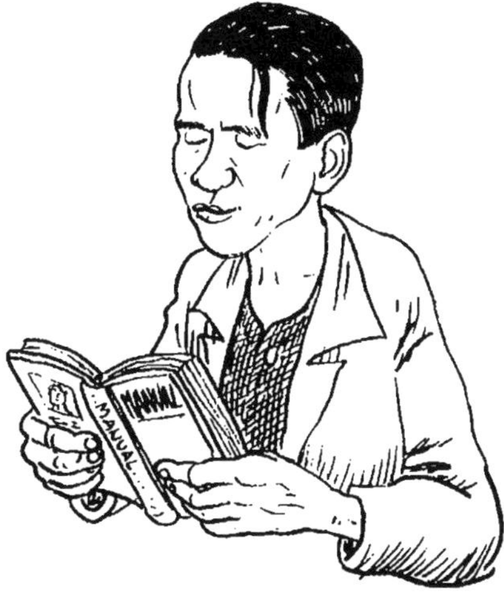

Discussing this will help CLWs to use their manuals when they look at sick animals. If they are affirmed in the use of their manuals, they will not be embarrassed to use them in the community.

2. Use questions which present problems to be solved

Memorizing facts and figures will not help CLWs do their job in the community. Their ability to solve problems will!

Ask questions which present a problem:
A three month old calf is weak and has diarrhea. It sometimes has a soft cough. It eats well and seems normal otherwise:
- What might be its problem?
- What other signs would you look for?
- What questions would you ask its owner.?

Do not ask questions asking for good memory:
- What are the common signs of worms in calves?

The first question gives the learner an opportunity to apply knowledge and use the manual. It helps him or her to think logically and solve a problem. The second question asks for a set of memorized facts.

3. Ask questions needing a brief written or oral answer

There are many types of test questions which can be used.

- **True–false:** These can be guessed right 50% of the time and may encourage guessing.
- **Multiple choice:** These are better for problem solving but may be difficult for marginal readers to understand. It may take much more time for them to answer and they may feel confused.
- **Written answer:** If the question asks for a long answer, it may make the person with less developed writing skills feel defeated.
- **Short answer:** This is an open question, so it requires problem solving. Because it asks for a short answer it is better for people with limited writing skills.

> **Example of a short answer question:**
> Name three things you can recommend to a farmer who wants to improve the quality of the animals in their herd.

4. Use simple language and express the question clearly.

5. Ask questions related to high-priority topics.

6. Use questions which help CLWs think about new things.

7. Be innovative in the way the questions are asked. Try to get away from an individual written exam.

Here are some examples from different programs of ways to ask questions:

A. Participants ask each other:

- At the end of a workshop, the participants **brainstorm a list of the things they have learned** during the course.
- In small groups they put 1-5 stones beside each topic to rate its importance and relevance to them.
- In their small groups they **design a question for each of the three top priority areas.** Their group discusses the answers. These must also be questions which pose a problem.
- When all the questions are ready, the small groups are placed in pairs. Each person from group one has a partner in group two.
- The people from group one ask the questions of the people in group two. Those from group two ask their questions of the people of group one.
- When everyone has had the chance to discuss the questions and answers, they rotate groups. Do not prolong the question asking and answering session beyond one hour.

Facilitators are process observers and resource people for this question-and-answer session.

Alternatively, the final day of a workshop, participant CLWs can be given the time to design possible questions to be used in an exam. At first, it will be difficult for them to design problem-solving questions. But with time they will become very good at it.

B. Model farm mapping for a community level workshop:

(See “Mapping” in “Tools,” pg. 253.)

In small groups, each group draws on the ground how they would like their farm to look five years in the future. They often use plants, sticks, paper, and other things they find to make their land plan in 3-D.

As each group explains their farm, the different aspects of the workshop they have learned and valued become apparent.

C. Asking about treating sick animals with models or animals:

After a series of workshops, the community organization in San Julian wanted to certify their CLWs. So they wanted an evaluation of the CLWs skills. We designed the following problem-solving and diagnosis exam for these CLW’s.

- There were six stations with a model or real animal to treat at each station. Each model animal had a common disease or problem for the CLW to diagnose and decide the proper treatment for. There was a typical medicine box available for them to choose their treatments. Once they treated the model animal correctly, they were given a set of three questions to answer.

These were the models:

1. A very thin horse with parasites. There were dewormers available and they applied them to the model. After deworming the parasites were removed. The parasites were small pieces of paper rolled up with the questions.

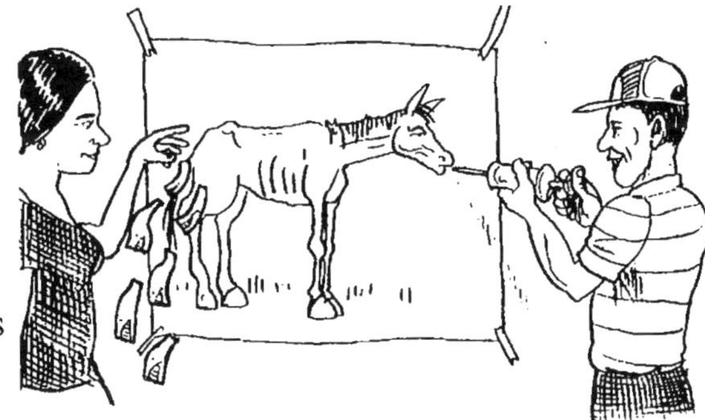

2. A chicken with the symptoms of Newcastle’s disease. The CLWs were told the chicken had diarrhea. They were asked how they could discover the cause. When they did a necropsy of the chicken they found papers with questions inside.

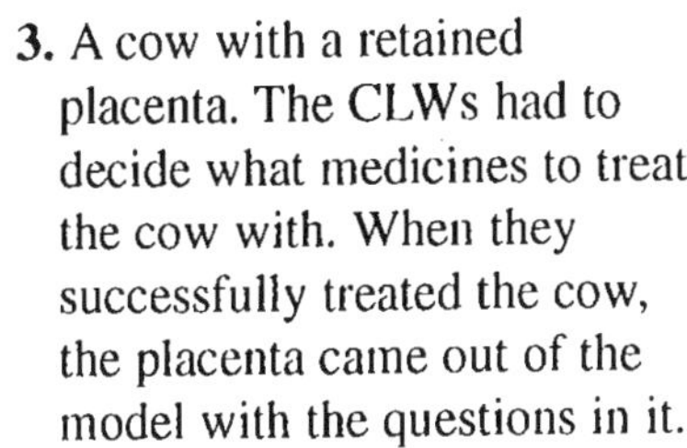

3. A cow with a retained placenta. The CLWs had to decide what medicines to treat the cow with. When they successfully treated the cow, the placenta came out of the model with the questions in it.

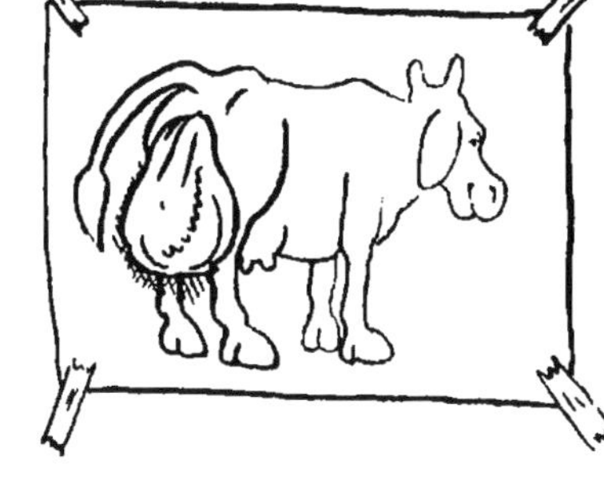

4. A bleeding wound with a stick stuck in it. When the wound was treated properly and the stick removed, the paper with the questions was on the stick.

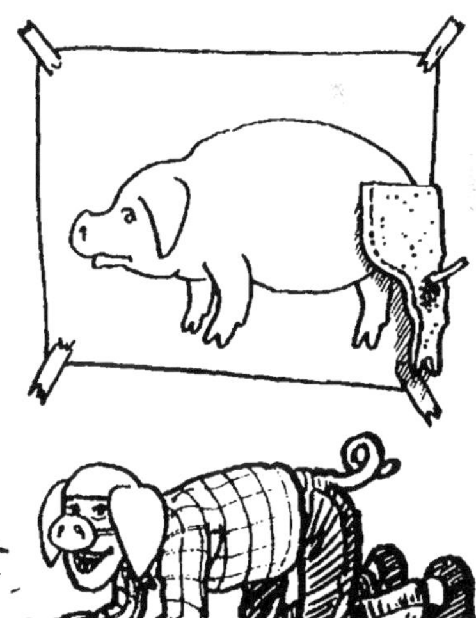

5. A pig which was coughing from pneumonia. When the CLW applied the proper medicine, the pig coughed out the questions.

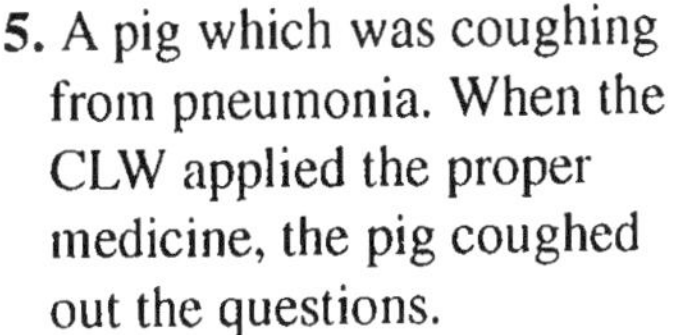

- At each station where there was a model, and a facilitator manned the station, as the "owner" of the animal. The facilitator could give only the information asked for by the learner. In some cases, such as the pig with pneumonia, the facilitator was the model animal.
- All of the CLWs had the same questions to answer and two animal cases to treat. The questions were related to important areas for the CLWs to know. Each question required problem solving about a situation. In this exam situation, the CLWs had the opportunity to show their skills in diagnosis and treatment as well as to think through problem solving. **At the end, all of the stations were visited by everyone and the answers discussed.** Possible differences were discussed as well.

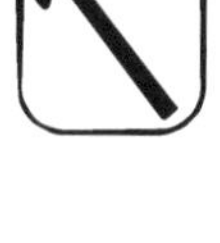

D. Skill testing

Here are some skills which the Rural Development Center in Nepal tests:

- Prepare a dose of powdered medicine for a cow with liver flukes.
- Prepare a single dose of injectable antibiotic from a multidose vial.
- Tube feed medicine to a goat.
- Give an injection to a cow or a goat.
- Take an animal's temperature.
- Pull a calf using a cloth model.

Participants can test one another or facilitators can test participants.

The learner's self evaluation

There are many aspects of training for a CLW which cannot be tested in an exam.

Helping participants to develop the practice of action and reflection will help them to begin to evaluate themselves in many of these areas.

Time given to **dialogue about attitudes** on specific issues during CLW training is very important. The time spent learning to give and receive good feedback will help CLWs in their self-reflection and awareness.

The aspects of training which cannot be tested include:

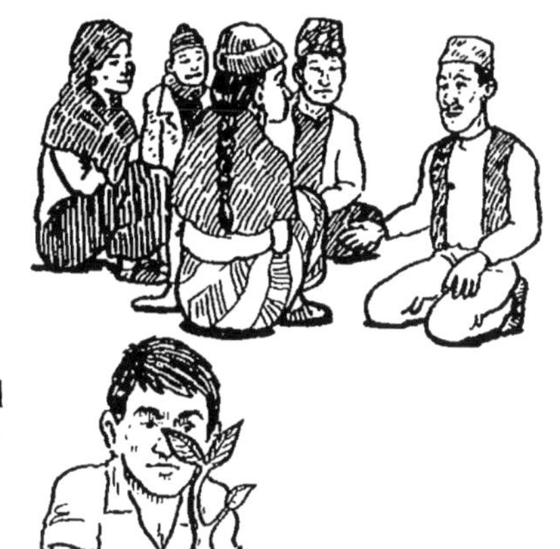

- **Attitudes:** About people in need, soil conservation, working together, serving the community, treating others as equals, and many others.
- **Skills in working with an organization:** What kind of leader is the person? How well can she coordinate a group for planning and doing an activity or year plan? Is he afraid to exercise his new knowledge in his own community?
- **Communication skills:** How well do they consult with others, listen, and give advice? Can they use a participatory method to teach in their community? Do they relate well to all groups in the community –men, women, elderly, and children?

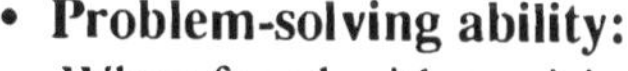

- **Problem-solving ability:** When faced with a crisis situation, how does the CLW respond?

Practice sessions will give facilitators an idea of the CLWs' manual skills and areas where they need special help or more work. Faster students can be asked to work with slower ones so that all perform the skills well.

"Homework assignments" or follow-up visits where facilitators accompany CLWs in their community organizational and training work are valuable times. The facilitator and CLW can discuss together problem areas in communication and organization skills. They can use the practical examples from the work with the CLW's own community.

Evaluating a training workshop

Equally as important as the learners' measuring of their advances in knowledge, skills, and attitudes, is the opportunity to evaluate the content and methods of the workshop.

Why evaluate the workshop?

- To continue the precedent of putting power and control into the hands of the participants. They express how they think and feel about the workshop.
- To know if the content, food and accommodations were appropriate and what to change in the future.
- To know how the facilitator did and what facilitation skills to improve.
- To know if the participants accomplished what they wanted to accomplish in the workshop.
- To insure accountability of facilitators and participants to one another.

Every workshop needs to provide time for this type of evaluation. The results of the evaluation should always be used in the future. Make sure they are recorded in some way, such as on newsprint. When the training team meets at the close of the workshop, they can discuss changing some aspects of future workshops. They should make a plan for implementing that change.

Many methods can be used to evaluate a workshop. Usually the simpler the better!

Here is one tried and true method of workshop evaluation:

A force field analysis

A force field analysis helps us to check out what things are pushing us toward our goals with the workshop or program. It also helps us to know what things are preventing us from arriving at our goal.

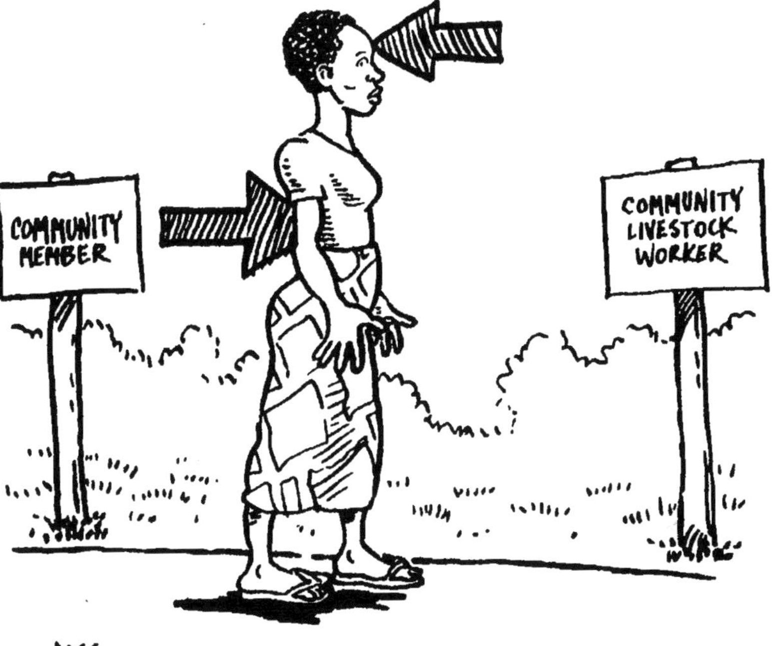

The analysis can be done in small groups. Each group answers these questions:

1. What are the things which have been most helpful or beneficial about this workshop?
2. What are the things which have been least helpful or have caused problems in the workshop?
3. What suggestions do you have for improvement?

Each group presents their results in a plenary session and they are written on newsprint.

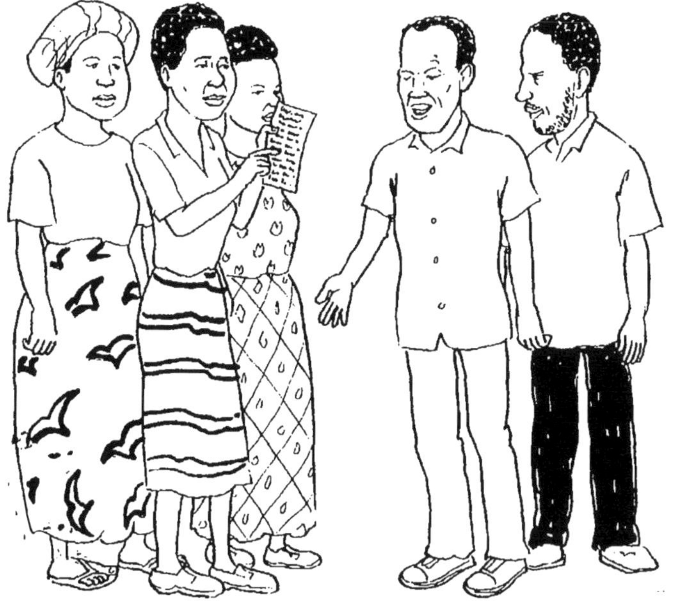

Help people to **get into the habit of not just complaining about a problem but of offering a constructive solution!** This will help them in their own organizations.

In the beginning it may be very difficult for people to offer criticism. They will say, we liked everything! But as time goes on and they see that the facilitator is open to constructive criticism they will share their difficulties openly. The attitude of the facilitator is very important. As CLWs learn about giving and receiving feedback, they will learn to give it well. (See "Feedback," pg. 208.)

This type of force-field analysis is very useful for evaluating each day's work and for the end-of-workshop evaluation. It is best used each day so that participants have an investment in the ongoing changing and improving of the workshop.

The trainer's self-evaluation:

This should be done immediately following a session. When you have a fairly detailed lesson plan you can evaluate your own work better. See if you followed the lesson plan and, if not, why not? It is good for the training team to do this together at the end of a workshop. This way they can adjust and improve for the next training event. Use the objectives for the topic as the road map. Was the objective accomplished by the session? If not, why not? What were the problems in the facilitation of the topic? What suggestions are there for improvement? What were the things done well in the facilitation? What worked well in the topic?

Another way to evaluate the work of the training team is to invite someone, for example another trainer from another program, to visit. She/he can sit quietly through the training and meet with the trainers afterwards, to give opinions and ideas. She/he should remember to praise the things the trainers did well, and share the problem areas she/he saw.

Evaluating a training program

When we join in the process of evaluating a training program we have decided to look at what has been accomplished by the training and if we reached our objectives. The people who participated want to know that they know and are using their new knowledge, attitudes and skills. How can we do the evaluation in a participatory way? There are several good references about evaluating a program in the "Resources" section, pg. 332 to help you. **Jennifer Shumaker,** evaluation specialist for Heifer Project International and coauthor of *Looking Back, Looking Forward*. has contributed the following section on program evaluation.

Who is the evaluation for?

Evaluations will benefit everyone in the program if the recommendations are useful and result in improvements. However, evaluations are not always initiated by the participants in a program.

Most evaluations are done for one of the following three reasons:

1. An **outside funding agency** requires an evaluation to make sure that the resources are being used well. In this case, the evaluation is primarily "for" the outside agency.
2. The **program administration** sees some kind of conflict, and calls for an evaluation to help them make decisions. This type of evaluation is primarily "for" the program management or administration.
3. The **program participants** (ideally!) realize that evaluation is an important part of the whole development cycle, and regular self-evaluations are considered a part of good program management. **Program self-evaluations** are "for" all the participants, and should be done every few years just as exams after tests, or workshop evaluations after each event (See pg. 161). The first few evaluations are generally requested by management. Yet, as they see their participation being taken seriously, the other participants will learn to value this experience. They will also experience improvements over the years that result from self-evaluations.

Program self-evaluations

The following discussion will outline a possible process to use for program self-evaluations. There are many ways to do participatory evaluations. This design is presented for those who are facilitating a self-evaluation for the first time. They may need to follow a prescribed procedure once or twice before changing it for their own situation, just as an experienced cook begins with a recipe and then adapts or completely changes it after trying it.

Participatory self-evaluation is valued by some funding agencies. However, most outside donors still require a professional external evaluator to lead a traditional assessment based on the donor's criteria and methodology. When there are problems or conflict the program can find a trusted and well-respected outsider or team, possibly trained in conflict resolution. The team will usually be better at exploring and resolving conflict than a team of project participants who may already be part of the problem. A basic requirement for an effective self-evaluation is trust between all the people involved.

Program self-evaluations are ideal for situations in which the program administrators, trainers and participants recognize that the program is doing well. They are simply looking for ways to improve. All of the above people can expect the following from being involved in their own self-evaluation:

- increased pride in accomplishments,
- enrichment from sharing experiences and lessons learned,
- motivation to plan and implement improvements.

Who will do the evaluation?

The self-evaluation process involves everyone interested in the program. These people are called the stakeholders. Not all stakeholders will be equally interested in the actual evaluation. For example, administrators of outside funding agencies may not want to take the time to be involved in every step, but they should all be invited to be involved in an appropriate way. At a minimum they should give feedback on the conclusions from a draft report. Certain stakeholders, such as community participants, should have strong involvement in every step.

In most training programs, the stakeholders include:

- the participants in the training,
- the communities who sent them,
- the trainers in the program,
- the managers of the training program.

Others may be added. Depending on the situation, administrators of the outside funding agency, government extension service, or anyone else who has been active in the program can give valuable input. (See Step 1, next page).

The evaluator as facilitator:

In most external evaluations, especially those required by a funding agency, a team of "evaluators" chooses the *terms of reference* (key areas to be evaluated), collects some data, comes to conclusions about the program, and reports their opinions on what needs to be done (recommendations).

In the self-evaluation process we are recommending – one that involves the program stakeholders – the evaluator serves as a facilitator. Facilitators are chosen either from within the program or from the outside because of good facilitation skills. **The facilitator's responsibility is not to do the evaluation, but rather to lead a process in which the key issues, conclusions, and recommendations are decided by a group of program participants.** In other words, the program participants actually "do" the evaluation, and have complete ownership of all the conclusions and recommendations.

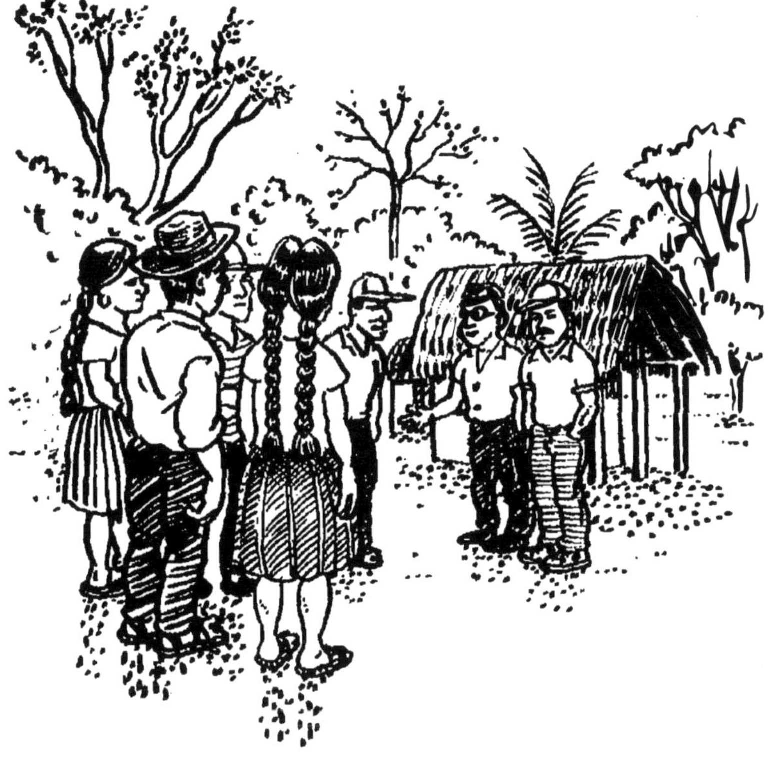

The job of the facilitator is:

- to make sure all the steps of the evaluation are taken as scheduled,
- to facilitate all the meetings,
- to document all the findings, conclusions and follow-up plans,
- to compile the summary report at the end.

How do we do it?

The process of self-evaluation can be separated into the following seven steps.

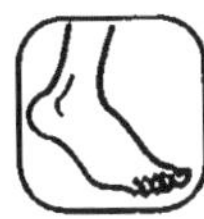

STEP 1: Plan the evaluation.

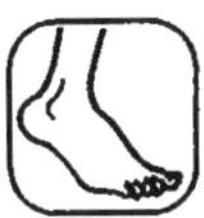

STEP 2: Conduct a design workshop; choose the key issues. Plan how the information will be collected.

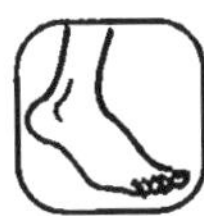

STEP 3: Collect the information: visit the communities and meet with other stakeholders.

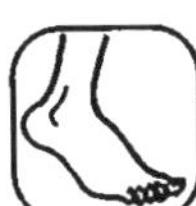

STEP 4: Organize the information from the field visits.

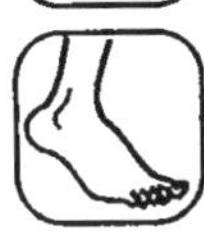

STEP 5: Analyze, follow-up, evaluate; meet to analyze the findings, to make follow-up plans, and evaluate the evaluation.

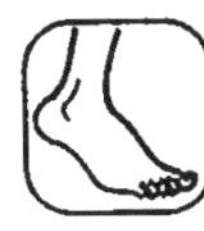

STEP 6: Write a draft report: circulate it to all stakeholders for their feedback before finalizing it.

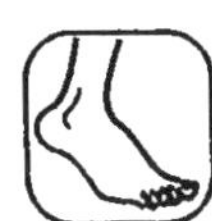

STEP 7: Celebrate the achievements of the program, and share the results of the evaluation.

We will now outline each step in "recipe style." Remember that this process can and should be adapted once you have tried it for yourself.

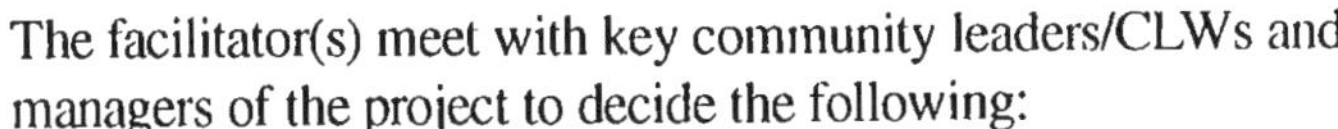

STEP 1: Plan the evaluation.

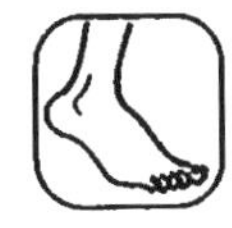

The facilitator(s) meet with key community leaders/CLWs and managers of the project to decide the following:

- **What are the stakeholder groups that should be involved?** (See suggestions on the previous page.)
- From the above list, **who should serve in a "stakeholder group" of 10–30** people (depending on the size of the program)? This team should include respected representatives from as many of the groups of stakeholders as possible, and it will be responsible for the "design" and "analysis" of the evaluation (see Steps 2 and 5). At least half of the people in this large group should be from the communities–including CLWs, farmers, and leaders from each community involved. If the participants in the program are varied, there should be men and women, older and younger, leaders and members of organizations.
- **Who should be part of a smaller evaluation "team" of 3–5 people** trusted in the communities? This team will accompany the facilitator(s) on the field visits, to help interpret the information. A larger group would allow more people to participate, but sometimes a large group causes the community not to share their ideas. For large programs with many communities, several teams could make these visits, each one visiting different communities. In this case, a facilitator should be chosen for each small team.
- **When should all the activities be scheduled and where should they be held?** A tentative schedule of meetings, deadlines and visits (See Steps 2–8) should be made, then checked with the proposed committee and team to make sure the people who should be involved are able to spare the necessary time. Invitations need to be sent at this time. In a large program, it may not be necessary to visit every community. A randomly-selected sample of 5 or 6 communities will usually suffice, especially if every CLW's work has been monitored and supervised regularly.

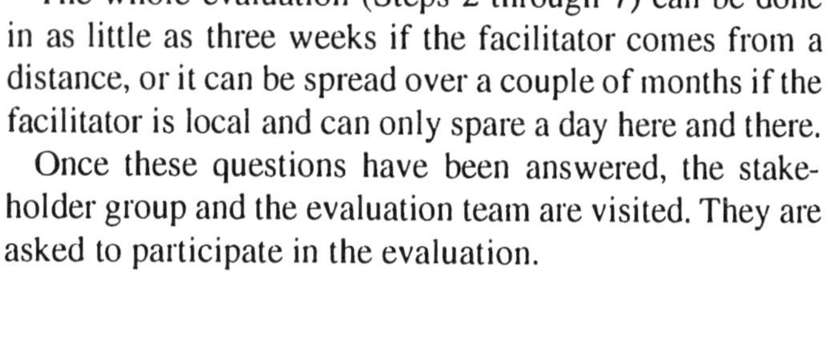

The whole evaluation (Steps 2 through 7) can be done in as little as three weeks if the facilitator comes from a distance, or it can be spread over a couple of months if the facilitator is local and can only spare a day here and there.

Once these questions have been answered, the stakeholder group and the evaluation team are visited. They are asked to participate in the evaluation.

STEP 2: Conduct a design workshop (at least one full day, including evening):

The stakeholder group meets to:

- Choose the key issues,
- Decide how to explore these issues further on the field visits (See Step 3),
- Decide which achievements need to be celebrated.

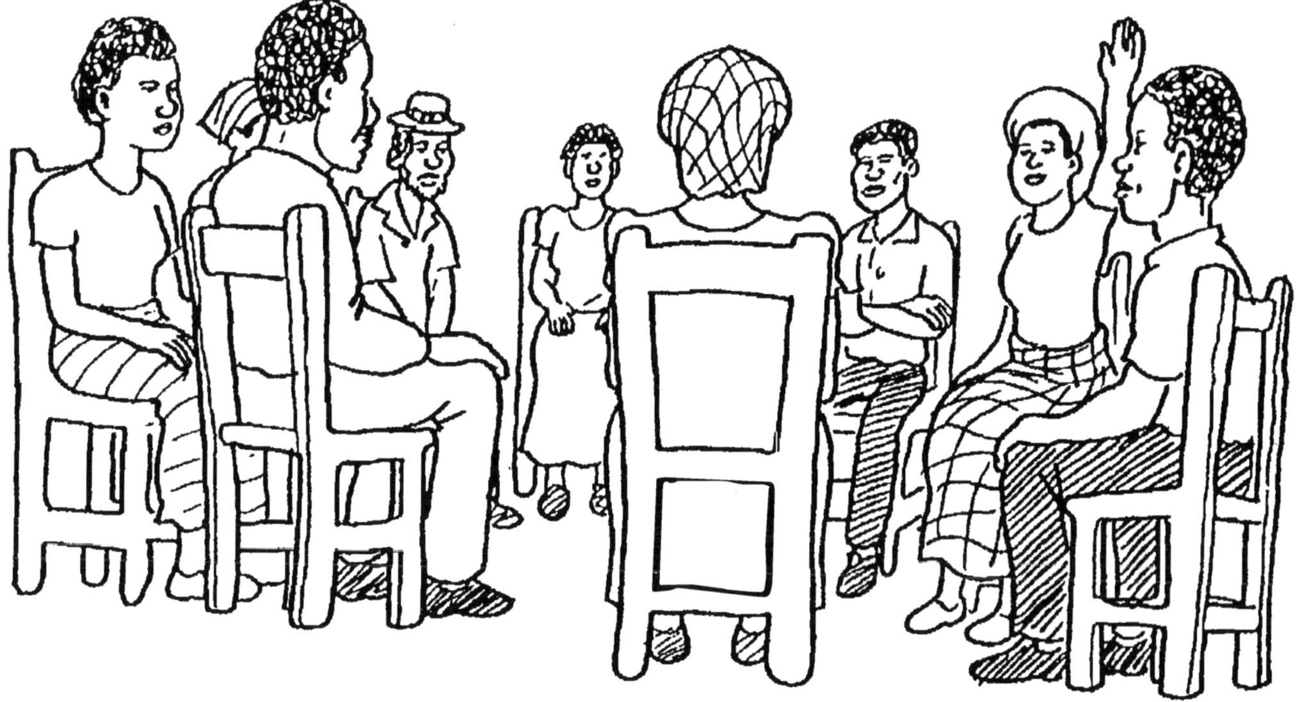

Here is a sample plan for the stakeholder meeting

OBJECTIVE	METHOD	MATERIALS	TIME
Participants know one another	**Welcome** An icebreaker for introductions (See pg. 263.)	Depending on the icebreaker	30 minutes
WHY? **1.** Participants express their reservations **2.** Participants define why it is important to do an evaluation	**1. Buzz groups** (See pg. 242.): *What have been your previous experiences with evaluations?* Participants share their reservations, if any. In plenary discuss how this evaluation can avoid making people feel threatened. Mention that the evaluator is only a facilitator. **2. Buzz groups** *Why do an evaluation?* In the plenary each buzz group shares to reinforce the importance of evaluation in the development cycle. As they share make a list– *"Why do an evaluation?"* If the following goals are not on the list the facilitator can mention them: • Celebration of achievements • Improvements to the program • Participants learn more about themselves by sharing ideas and experiences.	Large paper or newsprint Marker pen	1 hour
Participants hear the evaluation process described	The facilitator outlines the participatory self-evaluation process using the seven steps.	Chart with the steps	15 minutes
	Break		15 minutes

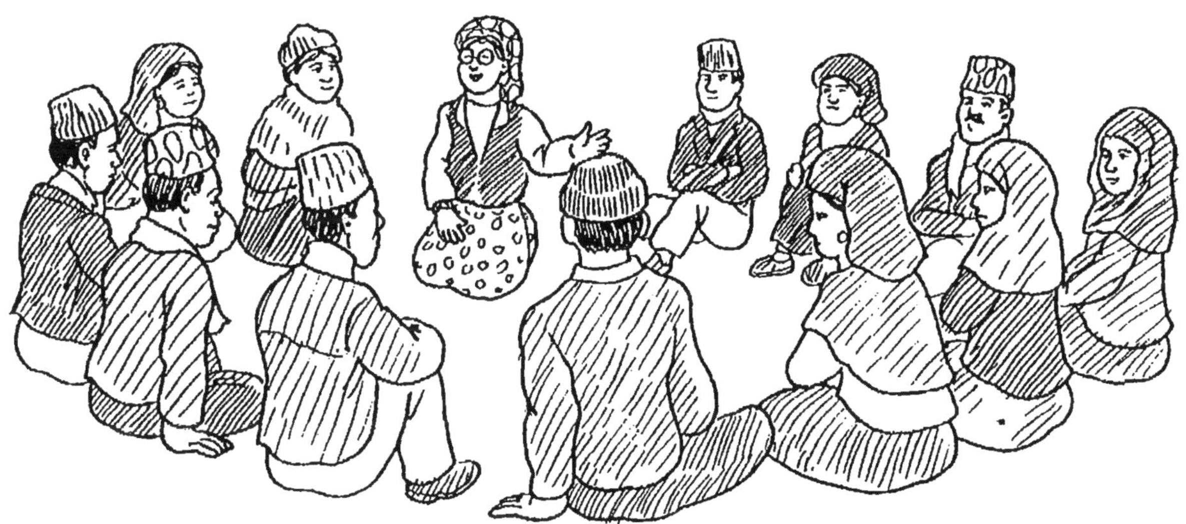

OBJECTIVE	METHOD	MATERIALS	TIME
WHAT? Participants choose the key issues to be considered The achievements to be celebrated. The frustrations/ problems to address for improvement.	**Small Groups** (See pg. 236.) Divide the large group into stakeholder groups. Give each group of stakeholders the same three questions. For example: • What are the strengths of the training program? • What are the weaknesses of the program? • What are some changes that need to be made in the program? Each group writes their ideas on a large piece of paper. In the plenary each group presents their ideas. Silent reflection: Once all the papers are taped to the wall, ask everyone to reflect silently on which ar the most important issues. List the most important issues: Ask people to call out the most important issues and write them on large paper with the title, "Key Issues." These may be other issues of obvious importance to everyone. Some key issues chosen by various training programs: • What participants feel about the training, • change in knowledge, skills, and attitudes as a result of the training, • level of achievement of the goals and objectives of the program, • relevance of the current goals and objectives of the program, • relationship between the CLWs and the communities, • impact of the training on agricultural production, • cost/benefit analysis (cost analysis with qualitative analysis of benefits). Prioritize the list: This evaluation should be limited to three or four Key Issues. Everyone can write on a small piece of paper the three issues most important to them. During lunch two participants can calculate which three or four issues received the most votes. People should understand that other issues will be addressed eventually. On a separate paper write a summary list of the accomplishments and strengths of the program for the final evaluation.	Large paper for each group Marking pens Small pieces of paper	1 hour & 45 minutes
	Lunch		1 hour & 30 minutes

OBJECTIVE	METHOD	MATERIALS	TIME
WHAT? The committee determines what they need to know about each issue.	**Small Groups** (See pg. 236.). Divide the large group into stakeholder groups. Give each group one key issue. Ask the group: "How will we know if we are doing well in this area?" In the plenary each group reports. Together everyone approves the answer for each issue and makes additions or corrections. For example: For this issue, "How would we know if the relationship between the community and the CLW is good?" The list might look like this: • The number of times the community uses the CLW increases over time; • Most people will praise the CLW when interviewed; • The CLW and the community will agree on the role of the CLW; • The CLW will be active in the community; • Participatory methods will be used in meetings and training sessions facilitated by the CLW. This list is called *indicators.* They indicate the truth about the key issue. If there is a need to clarify what indicators are or how to set them, the facilitator can give professional advice.		1 hour
	BREAK		30 minutes

Indicators: With groups who have not had much experience in evaluation, the wording of the list may not satisfy an evaluation specialist as being "true indicators." "True indicators" should be measurable. But for the purpose of a self-evaluation, the participants know the culture and the program so well that intuition and *qualitative* information usually mean more than numbers and other *quantitative* data. So it is not necessary to know the jargon and to have the exact wording. The main goal of the evaluation is to reach sound conclusions and decide on how to implement positive changes. The process and details are not as important as they might be for a professional evaluator preparing a report for a funding agency.

Quantitative indicators: These are indicators which can be measured by numbers , for example, the number of times the CLW was called, or the number of animals treated by the CLW.

Qualitative indicators: These are the indicators of the feelings and thoughts of the people. They are measured by how people were or are affected by something: for example, the CLW was so excited about her work she asked for more information and further training, or the CLW now does his work with much greater confidence, etc.

OBJECTIVE	METHOD	MATERIALS	TIME
HOW to collect the information Participants design the tools or techniques that will be used to explore the key issues or collect information.	**Small Groups** Each small group should have people from each stakeholder group. Assign one key issue to each group. Each group plans what the people who visit the communities will do to help people discuss the issue.(See Step 3 for ideas.) Sometimes more than one tool is needed for a single indicator. Sometimes one tool will serve for several indicators. Be simple and brief.If a simple technique/exercise will provide useful information, don't use a complicated one. A mixture of tools used in the past is: • Examination of project records, • Observations of selected farms, • Semi-structured interviews with individuals and small groups (See pg. 261.) A community group meeting using role plays/ranking exercises/or other participatory tools.	The materials the participants need to complete their plans	1 hour
Each group shares their tools and plan.	In a plenary session, each group shares one of their more complicated tools. They receive feedback on the tools and the plan from the larger group.		1 hour

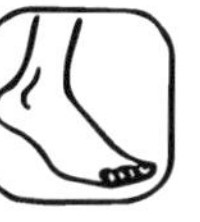

STEP 3: Collect the information

At the start of each visit, the team will give the community/small group/farmer:

1. A complete explanation for the visit,
2. A summary of the key issues that will be explored,
3. Assurance that you are not evaluating the farmers – you are asking the farmers to help evaluate the program.

Community members all need to feel like a part of the evaluation. Some of this preparation will already have been done, since community leaders, farmers, and/or CLWs should have attended the design meeting. But it is always better to give too much information about why you are in the village than too little. You cannot assume that everyone knows what is happening.

Each community visit should include a mixture of activities, such as walking on selected farms, semi-structured interviews with individuals, small group discussions, large group meetings/interviews, and examination of records.

Some sample dynamics for use with group meetings

The following have been used successfully in an evaluation. They are focused on specific key issues as defined by the evaluation team. They are here only as an example, not to use directly.

1. Ranking of workshop topics to determine the most important and the most used (See "Ranking and sorting," pg. 255). In small groups the people considered which were the most important and most used topics of the training workshops they had attended in the past. Each topic was written on a card. The group sorted the cards into three categories: Used often, used little, not used. This dynamic generated a good reflection with the community on their priorities before the workshop and what they have used most from the workshop.

2. Debate – Popular Education vs. Traditional Education, which is best?
This will start an excellent discussion. First brainstorm about what is meant by "popular education" and what is meant by "traditional education." This brainstorm also demonstrates people's ability to be analytical about the methodologies. The size of the debate team is important. If it is a large group (more than 15) each team should have about five people. If it is a smaller group, divide everyone into two teams. Flip a coin to decide who debates on which side. Write down all of the responses given during the debate. See page 9.

3. Walk together through the land of the participants, looking at their animals. Do a semi-structured interview (pg. 69). and record the answers. The semi-structured interview facilitates a flow of conversation rather than following a formal question and answer format.

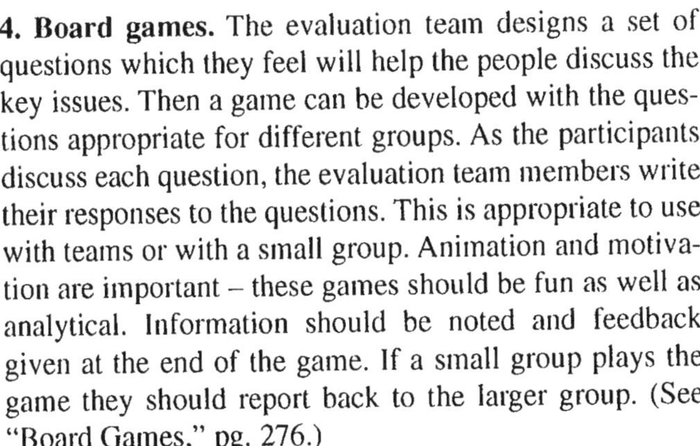

4. Board games. The evaluation team designs a set of questions which they feel will help the people discuss the key issues. Then a game can be developed with the questions appropriate for different groups. As the participants discuss each question, the evaluation team members write their responses to the questions. This is appropriate to use with teams or with a small group. Animation and motivation are important – these games should be fun as well as analytical. Information should be noted and feedback given at the end of the game. If a small group plays the game they should report back to the larger group. (See "Board Games," pg. 276.)

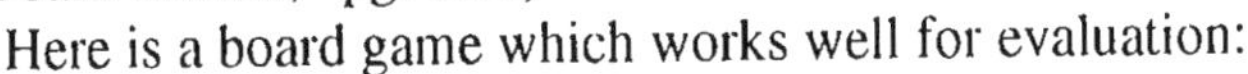

Here is a board game which works well for evaluation:

• **The road to our vision** (can be modified, for example "The road to better production," or "The road to women's participation," or "The road to soil conservation," depending on the key issue being explored). See "The road to our vision," pg. 276.

5. Role plays. These can be used for the community to demonstrate how members felt a situation was before training and how they feel it is after training. For example, in one evaluation, the people wanted to know how training in organization strengthening had affected the community organization. In a community meeting, the whole community was divided into two groups to create two different role plays. Half the community demonstrated how a community meeting was conducted years ago (before training) and half the community role-played a community meeting now (after training). See "Role Plays," pg 244.

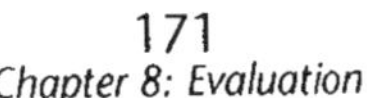

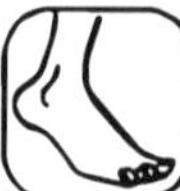

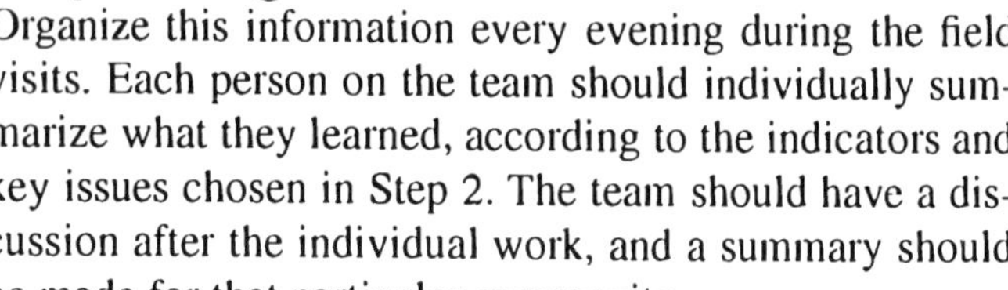

Step 4: Organize the information

Organize this information every evening during the field visits. Each person on the team should individually summarize what they learned, according to the indicators and key issues chosen in Step 2. The team should have a discussion after the individual work, and a summary should be made for that particular community.

For example, we can use the key issue, "Relationship between the CLWs and the communities." A community might do a role play called; "Participatory methodology used during the parasite training sessions conducted by the CLW." Each member of the visitation team lists observations made during the role play and during the community discussion after the role play.

A list of all the team members' observations might look like this:

- The CLW was very knowledgeable and confident.
- Young people participated as well as older people.
- The participants weren't talking enough.
- The trainees didn't seem to be very excited during the role play.
- The CLW talked very loudly, and didn't give the people enough time to answer.
- All the parts were there, but it all seemed too mechanical.
- The trainer seemed impatient.
- No live animals were used in the role play, even though the instructions made it clear that this was an option.
- No women spoke up or were called on for opinions.

Note: We are using a more negative example because this will lead to more interesting analysis and conclusions. It is important to give equal attention to positive experiences. In some cases there will be nothing negative to analyze.

Here is an example of a list from another village, where there were only positive relationships:

For the indicator: "The CLW will be active in the village"

- The CLW lives in the village and shares the same language and culture as the villagers.
- The CLW participates in all the village meetings and festivals.
- The villagers show much respect and affection for the CLW.
- The villagers ask the CLW's opinion on many issues unrelated to livestock.
- The villagers often give small gifts to the CLW in return for his generosity.

The team should also look at the other indicators and list their own observations: the number of times the CLW is called to treat the farmers' animals; the attitude of the farmers towards the CLW, etc.

The group can arrange these into a summary table, making sure all are in agreement. The summary might look like the one on the following page:

Table 1

KEY ISSUE: Relationship between CLWs and community:	COMMUNITY: XXXX	CLW: yyy
INDICATOR	**SOURCE OF INFORMATION**	**FINDINGS**
Number of times CLW is called on	CLW records Project records	Increased by 14% over the past two years – is called repeatedly for problems
Farmer attitudes toward CLW	Individual interviews Group meeting	CLW has been helpful and is always ready to treat the animals, but isn't patient enough to show farmers how to take care of problems themselves.
Roles of CLW defined by CLW and Community	Interview with CLW and Group meeting of farmers	CLW sees his role as treatment of animals; farmers see his role more as trainer, to teach them preventive techniques.
CLWs involvement in community activities	Community records CLW interview Group meeting	CLW only comes to the community to treat animals. He no longer lives in the village.
Methodology for parasite training sessions	Role play in village XXXX	CLW has excellent technical knowledge to treat the animals CLW impatient and dominating Participants not fully engaged Women not encouraged to participate Live animals not used Mechanically correct, but lifeless (This list is a summary of the comments from the previous list)

Team meeting to compile information

When the summary has been done for each site visited, the team(s) should meet again for a day to compile a general summary of findings on large sheets of paper, to be shared with the whole committee in the analysis meeting. The same table (above) can be used as a format for the general summary. The summary should be as detailed as needed for good analysis, but need not include every detail. If the findings are different for different CLWs, however, more detail will be needed.

For example, if all the CLWs in the area have summaries resembling the one above, the problem may lie in the training of the CLWs. However, if most of them have very different summaries, and the one above is the exception, the problem could be in the personality and approach of the individual CLW, and the solution will be very different.

Sometimes the team cannot resist doing analysis during these team meetings, and coming to conclusions and recommendations. When this happens, the team needs to recognize that this is not the final product. These recommendations should not be presented to the committee at the time that the findings are presented. The team must remember that they are part of the larger stakeholder group, and they have the chance to give their input into the analysis meeting just like everyone else. This only becomes a problem if the team develops a sense of ownership in their own conclusions and dominates the committee.

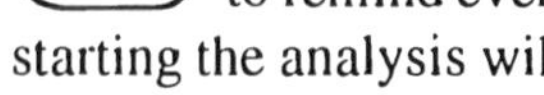

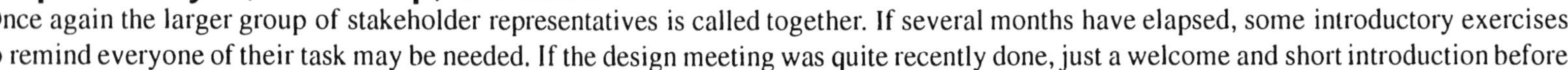

Step 5: Analyze, follow-up, evaluate

Once again the larger group of stakeholder representatives is called together. If several months have elapsed, some introductory exercises to remind everyone of their task may be needed. If the design meeting was quite recently done, just a welcome and short introduction before starting the analysis will be sufficient.

The following is an example of a lesson plan when there was only 13 days between the analysis and the design meetings, so there was little need for review.

Plan for the analysis, follow-up and evaluation meeting:

OBJECTIVE	METHOD	MATERIALS	TIME
Participants are reminded of the reason for this meeting.	**Welcome** A brief presentation and review of the 7 steps of a self evaluation process. Point out where this meeting fits into the whole process.	Chart of the seven steps	15 minutes
Participants make a list of their hopes and fears for this evaluation	**Brainstorm:** (See pg. 238.) In plenary the participants share first what their hopes are, then their fears for this evaluation based on what has happened thus far. The facilitator or a participant writes a list titled "Hopes" and another list titled, "Fears." Keep this list for the evaluation of the evaluation. If there are severe problems arising from the process of the evaluation,divide into small groups to suggest solutions to the problems. Each small group deals with a different problem.	Large paper Marking pens	30 minutes
Participants make a list of the weaknesses and strengths of the program	**Identifying the weaknesses and strengths**** Presentation of findings: Working with one key issue at a time, ask the team(s) to present their findings. Tape all the findings on the wall. Divide into small groups: Each small group makes a list of the weaknesses which have been found and another list of the strengths which have been found for the first key issue. Each small group presents their list. Make a summary list of the weaknesses on another large sheet. List on a different paper any new strengths that have been observed, or particular people/activities that should be celebrated and recognized at the celebration meeting. Move on to the next issue until the accomplishments and weaknesses for each key issue have been listed.	Findings from each group in chart form. Large paper Markers	1 hour
	BREAK		15 minutes

**In this session, you will find that interpretation plays a major role. A key part of the day will be sorting out which problems are simply the result (effect) of deeper problems (causes) that must be identified if good solutions are to be found. Sometimes an indicator will give confusing results that need to be interpreted. For example, we had decided that if the number of times the CLW was called increased, this would indicate a good relationship between the CLW and the community. However, when combined with the other indicators, we found that the CLW was probably creating dependency on himself for problems that could be solved by the farmers themselves. This resulted in a large number of calls. This is an example of why more than one indicator is needed before a good interpretation can be done.

OBJECTIVE	METHOD	MATERIALS	TIME
Participants analyze the weaknesses and create a list of the causes of the weaknesses for each key issue in the program	**1.** Remove the original lists of findings, and put all the new lists of weaknesses on the wall in full view. **2.** For each weakness, discuss whether this is an effect (caused by a deeper cause), or if this is the real cause that should be addressed. For example, in the case of the CLW yy in community XXXX, we should discuss whether the weakness is the actual CLW (in which case the CLW might need to be replaced) or if the attitude of the CLW was just an effect of a deeper cause;for example, poor training of the CLW's in general (in which case the solution would be for more training. **3.** To help interpret the findings in this way, you should look at other data or observations. In the case of the CLW yy, we can look at the situation for other CLWs who have received the same training to see if they are experiencing the same weaknesses. **4.** If the weakness is already stated in terms of the real cause, and not just the effect of a deeper cause, leave it on the list. If the weakness turns out to be an effect of a deeper cause, add the deeper cause to the list. **5.** Several weaknesses may have the same basic cause. Identifying these "causes" is the equivalent of "conclusions" of a traditional evaluation. **6.** After leading the discussion on several issues, find out if the group feels comfortable enough to continue this process in smaller groups, to speed up the process. If not, continue facilitating this session until every weakness has been analyzed in this way. **7.** You should now be left with a new list of real "causes" that should be addressed. ***	Lists of weaknesses Large paper Markers	Variable
	LUNCH		1 hour 30 minutes

***A smaller group of committee members can take this revised list of causes/weaknesses and categorize it during the lunch, or the whole group can do it if they still have energy! There are usually some weaknesses that are repetitions of others, and several small "problems" can sometimes be combined into a single cause. Usually the list of separate issues becomes shorter, with some sub-categories under larger issues.

OBJECTIVE	METHOD	MATERIALS	TIME
Participants write follow-up plans	**Follow-up plans** Small groups: **1.** Divide the weaknesses and causes for the key issues among the groups. **2.** Each group will decide what needs to be done about each of the weaknesses and causes they have been given. **3.** Each group makes a follow-up plan for each weakness or cause category. At this step it is important to have the decision-makers in the meeting, so that real follow-up plans can be made. If a group has no decision-makers their plans will be considered tentative, but should be taken seriously by the decision-maker when he/she receives it. The follow-up plan should look like a strategic action plan, with the objective, the responsible person/s, the deadline, and the resources needed (for example, see table 2, on the following page). If there are many issues to be dealt with (and there often are on the first evaluation), there may not be time to complete a follow-up plan for each issue. In this case, the small groups should simply develop an objective, and leave the actual plan to another meeting or to the manager of the program. This objective becomes the "recommendation" of a traditional evaluation, and since it was developed by the participants, it is likely to be useful and relevant.	Lists of categories of weaknesses and causes Large paper Markers	Variable
Participants evaluate the evaluation process	The last hour of the meeting should be devoted to evaluating the evaluation process. This evaluation will be the same as the evaluation after a workshop (See page 00), and is designed to identify changes that would improve the next self-evaluation.		1 hour

Table 2 A sample follow-up plan for an evaluation

WEAKNESS and/or CAUSE	OBJECTIVE	TASKS	PERSON(S) RESPONSIBLE	DEADLINE	RESOURCES NEEDED
Most CLWs in community XXX are not effectively involving women in the village in training sessions, the cause is inadequate training in gender awareness.	A training session on gender issues will be offered to all existing CLWs. Those CLWs from community XXX will be required to attend	Trainers A and B will be asked to conduct this session. If they cannot do it, C and D will be asked.	Mrs. T will make these contacts. Mr. P will organize the sessions.	Contact will be made by April 10, alternatives contacted by April 20 if needed. Training Session will be held in mid-June (dates to be finalized depending on the trainers)	$500 for transport, lodging, and trainer fees
One of the CLWs is not relating well to the community. Cause seems to be the wrong choice of CLW	CLW will be presented with the findings and asked what can be done. If he is willing to make changes; he will be given a probation period; if not, he will be relieved of his responsibilities, and the community will be advised about what qualities to look for in their new choice of CLW	Approach the CLW with these findings, and supervise the probation period or relieve the the CLW of all responsibilities.	Mr. P will contact the CLW, supervise the probation period, and/or relieve the CLW of his responsibilities.	CLW will be approached within the next two weeks, and the probation period will last 6 months. If a new CLW should be chosen, this should be done before the next scheduled training session begins.	No additional resources needed.

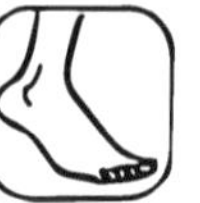

Step 6: Write a draft report

The facilitator/leader can either write the report, or can assign parts of the report to different team members. The draft report should be written within two weeks of the analysis meeting. Since most of the people who need to understand the report will have been involved all the way through, there is no need to include lengthy written descriptions of findings.

One way to organize a report:

Section 1 PURPOSE: One paragraph which describes the purpose of the evaluation (from the design meeting). At the end it directs the reader to the appendix which should include all the information on dates of activities, the communities visited, and people on the team and committees. This appendix can simply be the notes from the design meeting.

Section 2 STRENGTHS: The strengths that have been identified and celebrated, including any individuals who should be recognized for exceptional contributions to the program.

Section 3 FINDINGS and SUGGESTED SOLUTIONS, FOLLOW-UP PLANS: The findings, conclusions and recommendations should be organized according to the key issues identified in the design meeting.

For example:

Key issue 1:
Findings: One paragraph summarizing the findings
Suggested solution/follow-up plan:
This is where the report should be careful to list all the decisions made in the analysis meeting. If action plans were made with the decision-maker's participation, this should be noted. If the decision-makers were not involved, the action plan should be called "suggested" or "tentative."

Key issue 2:
Etc.
Etc.

The report doesn't need to be a long masterpiece. The main purpose of the report is to have a historical record of findings and decisions made, so that the next self-evaluation can build on this one. In some cases, the findings are useful or interesting enough that someone may want to write up an article for wider distribution. In our experience, evaluation reports are never widely read. However, much attention is given to the importance of sharing evaluation results. Short, concise articles about specific issues that arose and how they were solved might be very useful to the wider community development and training audience.

The draft of the report should be read by the whole committee to make sure the decisions and findings are recorded as accurately as possible before the report is finalized.

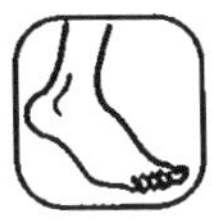

Step 7: Celebrate the achievement of the program and present the evaluation results

If the program is small and the communities are close enough for one large meeting, this can be a program-wide celebration. If the communities are spread out, there can be several celebrations. The leaders on the committee who have been sent by their communities can lead these celebrations.

There are several important reasons to hold these celebration meetings:

- to recognize the people who have made exceptional contributions (we have often written award letters for these people),
- to share the results of the evaluation,
- to celebrate in some appropriate way the accomplishments and strengths of the program (by a skit/play/entertainment, a special meal, or whatever is culturally significant).

It is during this meeting that people realize how evaluations are beneficial for the program. If the results are never shared, and the strengths never recognized, the communities might see evaluations as merely a required exercise that is designed to judge and criticize the program.

Ideally, the final report will be distributed in this meeting. But often the report takes time to finalize, and the celebration should happen soon after the field visits. As long as the draft report feedback has shown there are no problems with the way the decisions are recorded, the celebrations can be held before the final report is distributed. The focus of the celebration is on accomplishments, and these are seldom disputed in the draft report.

Section 3

Issues In Agricultural Training

Each of these issues will affect the quality of your training program in agriculture. Gender balance and family participation are necessary for successful training. If people don't communicate well, they won't participate. If we are training in an area where there are traditional practices, they should incorporated into any agricultural training program.

Chapter 9

Valuing the role and participation of women

This chapter covers the following topics:

If you are involved in a livestock project or training, whether in a city neighborhood with small animals or in a rural village, look around and see who is participating in the program. Is it mostly men or mostly women? If livestock provide the financial base for most families in the community, and your program has mostly men or mostly women, is it fully participatory? It may actually be excluding one or the other.

Livestock production affects the family nutrition, health, well being, and wealth. Since the whole family is so greatly affected, both men and women should be considered in the program. If the training program is appropriate and immediately applicable, it will include women's and men's training needs.

The invisibility factor

Why do agricultural training programs and projects which do not reach the whole family or which focus only on men get started? Many individuals in a community do not value their own work. In particular, village men and women tend not to value the work of women. As a reflection of this problem, sometimes development programs do not consider the roles of both men and women in agriculture in their planning. Some call this the **invisibility of women's work.**

Consider this true story of how **action is used for analysis:**

In the highlands of Bolivia there was a farmers' cooperative which allowed only the men to be members. They had some problems as an organization, and often found themselves less effective than they wanted to be. They asked for organization development help from an outsider institution.

When this institution began working in the village they asked why the women did not come to the cooperative meetings. The men replied that the women did not work with the crops or in the co-op and were therefore not allowed to be members of the cooperative. In addition, they would not allow the women to have training or credit.

So the institution planned a two-day training session for the women and through a mother's food program obligated all the women to attend the training. During the time the workshop took place, all could see that most of the crop and co-op activities of the village stopped. The women analyzed this situation.

At the next meeting of the co-op, the facilitators asked the men what they thought of the women's training. The men answered emphatically that the training was bad because it had stopped them from their work. Why? asked the institution. The men said they had to cook and wash and take the animals to pasture and see the children were all fed and off to school, and it didn't leave any time for the crops. Some had been in the midst of planting, and they talked about how they had to stop planting because normally the man plows and the woman plants. So the facilitator discussed with the men how the women played a vital role in the production of crops, even though they were not always in the fields. They also discussed the women's roles in the fields in the planting and harvesting and in feeding any hired workers. They even discussed how many of them consult with their wives about the crops they plant and make decisions together with their wives.

The story in the box can be used without its ending to allow the people to analyze the situation and draw their own conclusions of how women participate. The dialogue can be rich as people see the direct application to their village organization.

Source: C-CIMCA

Because many communities do not value the work and role of women, they also prevent them from full participation in community life.

My husband would not let me go to the meeting. I have to clean and take care of the children. Besides, I'm tired from working so hard.
I think the women should participate and vote in these meetings.
What does my wife know of important things? She doesn't work. All she does is spread gossip!

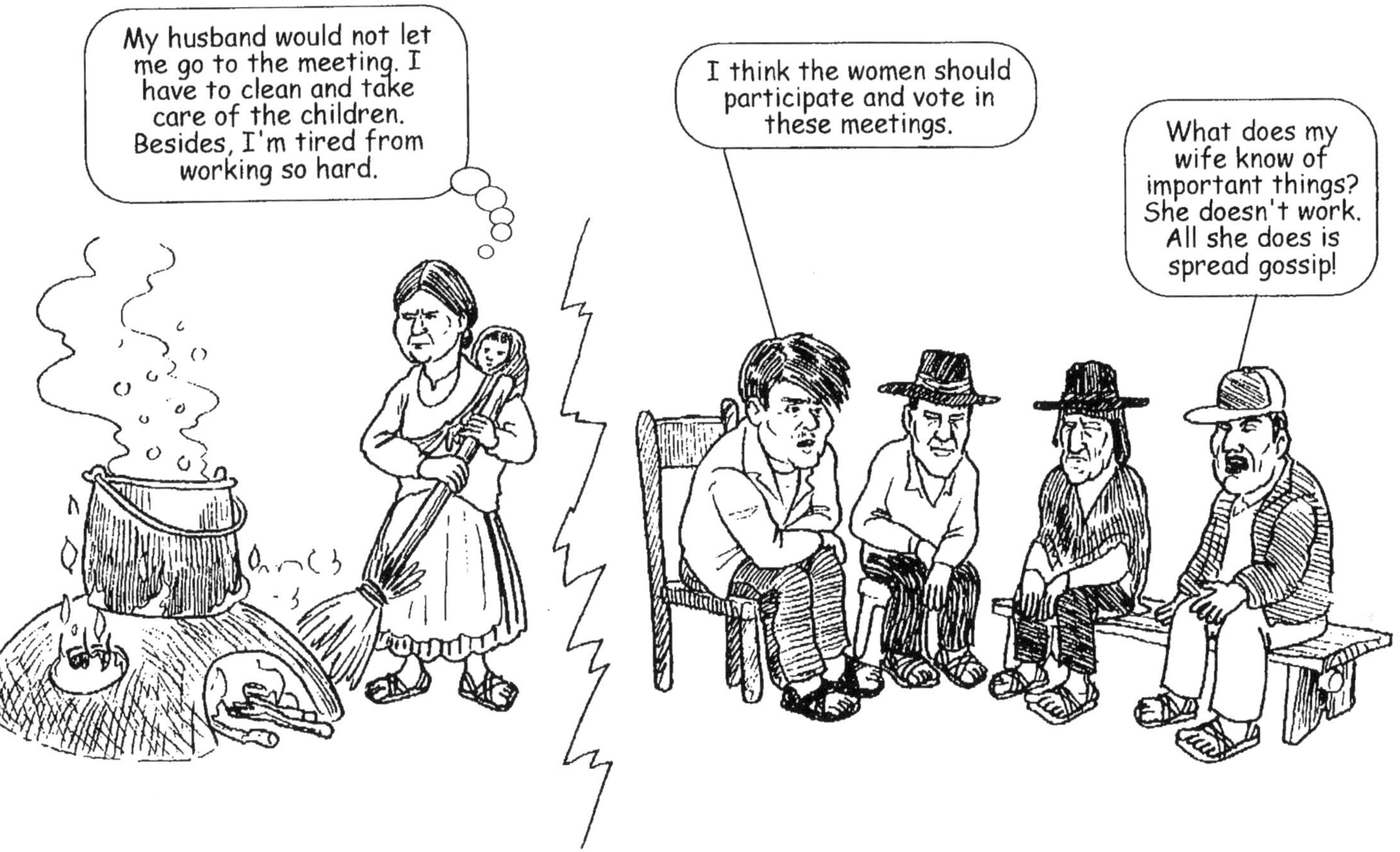

You can ask your group of participants and trainers if this happens in their communities. What is the truth in this situation? What is the myth?

This view of women's roles only hurts the community as they lose half of the available resources the community has for the wise solution of its problems. It is like a bicycle with two tires. No one notices that both are important until one of the tires has a flat.

In many areas people are realizing how this situation damages their community and the families in the community. They are acting to make changes which fully involve the women of the community. They are building stronger families who work well together for their own future.

Lets look together at how one group analyzed people's roles in livestock care:

- They brainstormed together a list of all the jobs involved in caring for the family cow.
- Then they made this chart for ranking by drawing a picture on the ground:

- Everyone decided who spends the most time at each job. For instance, if the pasturing (be it herding or cutting fodder) is done by women, children, and grandparents, they put more rocks for the person who does the job more often and fewer for the ones who do it less often.
- Once the people ranked the jobs, they began to discuss them. They looked at the amount of work done by each family member.
- From the analysis of this chart they all began to **recognize and to value the work everyone does.** But they especially saw how much the women work in livestock management.
- The people used this information to define their livestock project and to decide who should attend the training. They based their decisions about who should receive training in caring for cattle on who would use the training most. Can you see from their chart who should receive the most training? If our training program in livestock production or agriculture is to be immediately applicable and relevant, we will consider the woman's role and her training needs as well as the man's. We will also look for ways to strengthen the family and the way they work together.

For more information on ranking see "Tools" page 255.

So, how can we erase the invisibility factor? How can we be sure our program trains the people who really need it?

What about gender analysis?

One way is to create an awareness of this invisibility factor. Once people are aware, they can make decisions about the training. Creating awareness is called gender analysis. There are many ways to do gender analysis and many good resources on it. (See "Resources" pg. 335.)

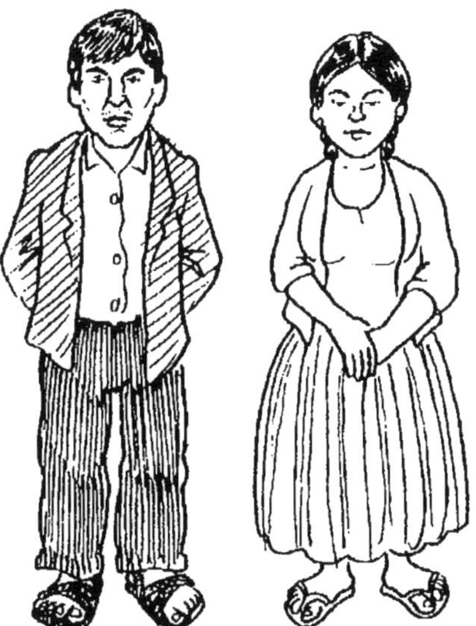

Sex refers to whether a person is physically a man or a woman. This is unchangeable and universal. It is defined by biology.

Here are some brief definitions:

Gender refers to the roles or characteristics society has given people, such as who washes the clothes and who drives the car in a family, or who is supposed to be meek and who is supposed to be strong. This is changeable and not universal. It is socially or culturally defined.

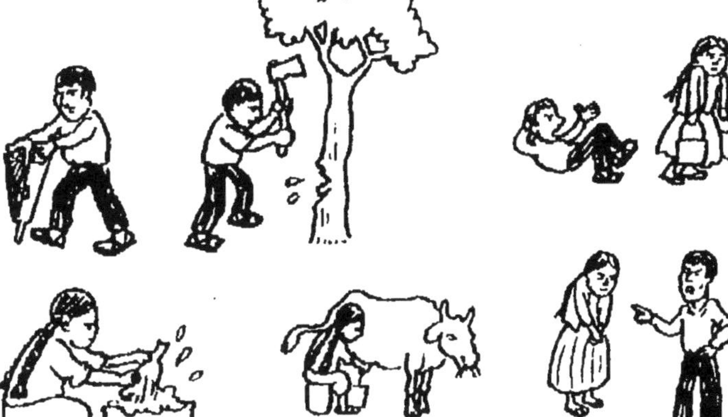

Gender analysis is a process of self or collective awareness and reflection on the roles or characteristics a culture or society has given to men and women.

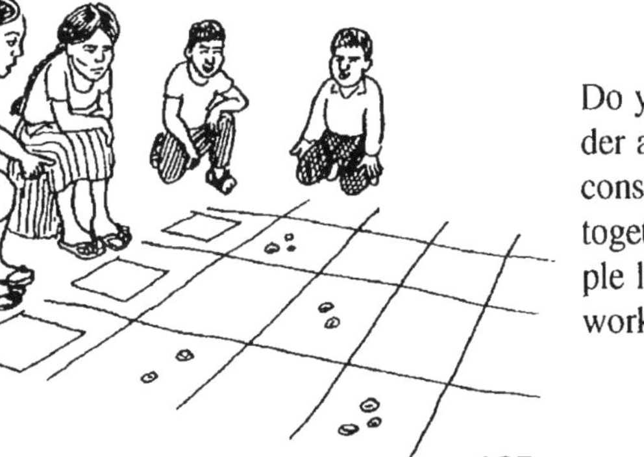

Do you see that word *process* in the definition of gender analysis? Remember the **process of awareness** or conscientization (see pg. 22)? It requires working together on a deep analysis of the actual situation people live in. It is not something that happens once in a workshop and is finished. It is a much longer process.

Why is gender analysis so important in agricultural training?

☛ So that within families, people will **appreciate the work of one another.** In this way they become more mutually supportive and stronger as a family unit. Animals receive better care, and production increases.

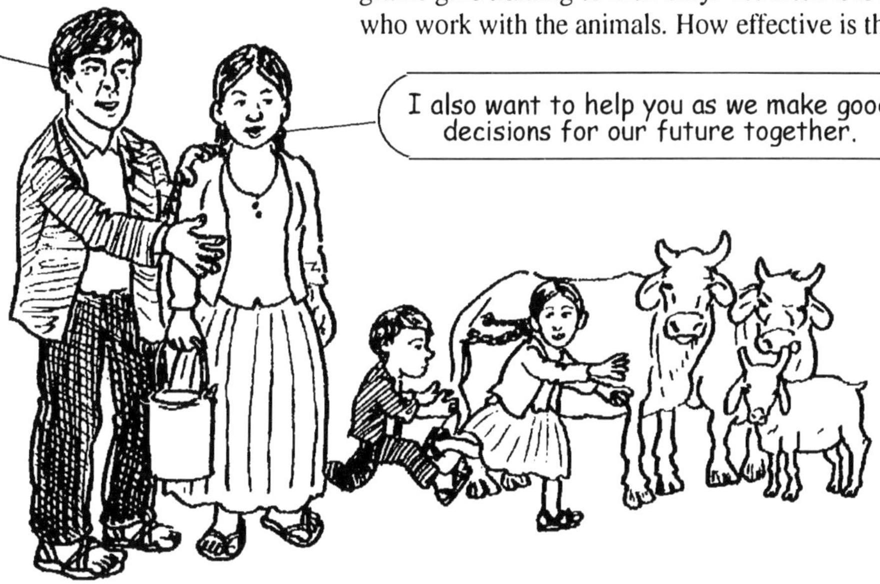

☛ So that people, especially women, will have a greater appreciation for the contribution they make to the family's work and production. Both women and their husbands begin to value the women's role. This **builds women's self esteem** and helps them to be proactive participants in their family's and community's development.

☛ So that the community doesn't lose half of the value of its people's ideas and work. Women are 50% of the population, 50% of the problem and 50% of the solution. When the women participate, **the community organization is brought to far greater effectiveness.** The organization's livestock-related activities, such as marketing animal products, community irrigation, soil erosion protection, livestock loans, etc. will be more successful.

☛ So that **appropriate training** is given to people for whom it will have an immediate use. Many livestock programs give training to men only. Yet often it is the women who work with the animals. How effective is this?

☛ So that livestock **projects do not place a greater work burden on women** who are already overloaded with work, without concrete benefits for them. The project can help the woman to decrease her current work as the benefits of the project increase her access and control of resources.

A true story:

In the lowlands of Bolivia a women's group decided they would like to begin moderate scale egg production in their community. An outside institution agreed to help them.

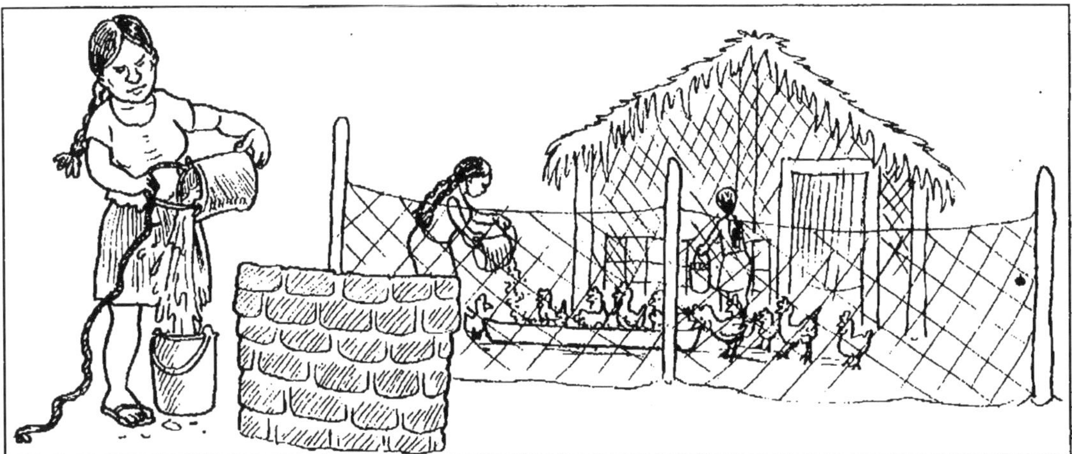

The women took technical training on chicken and egg production and marketing. They took out a loan and built their facilities to house 1000 chickens, including a well and a grain mill. They entered production with excellent management. The chickens did very well and began to produce many eggs. The women investigated the market and developed dependable customers. Although it was much work for the women, they began to see the economic benefits which they controlled, and they valued the work they were doing.

When the husbands saw the women's enterprise was beginning to earn money, they became suddenly interested. The men took over the management of the books and began making "loans" to themselves. Then as the women saw less and less benefit, they lost interest, so the men also took over production. They hired someone to do the work and made short-cuts. Eventually the business went broke from mismanagement.

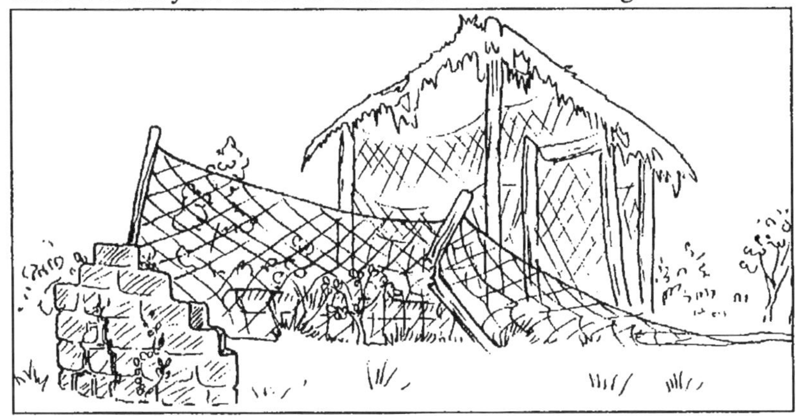

- What happened here?
- Have you seen it happen before in some other form?
- What could this outsider organization and the community have done differently?

The outsider institution in this case went to work with a women's group. No one gave much value to the women's possibilities and the outsider institution did not try to involve the men from the beginning. There was no dialogue about the roles and responsibilities in this project, who would own the resources, or the potential effect on the women, the men, and their families.

What is analyzed in gender analysis?

Many aspects of women's and men's lives are considered in the process of gender analysis. For livestock projects and training, some of the most important are:

People's roles in the family, on the farm, in society:

- What are the specifically livestock-related roles?
- Who cares for the animals and plants the pasture?
- How do the other household and family roles support this livestock work?
- What is a woman's life like from birth to death, and how does that differ from a man's life?
- Are these roles important?
- Who participates in the local organization, and how do they participate?

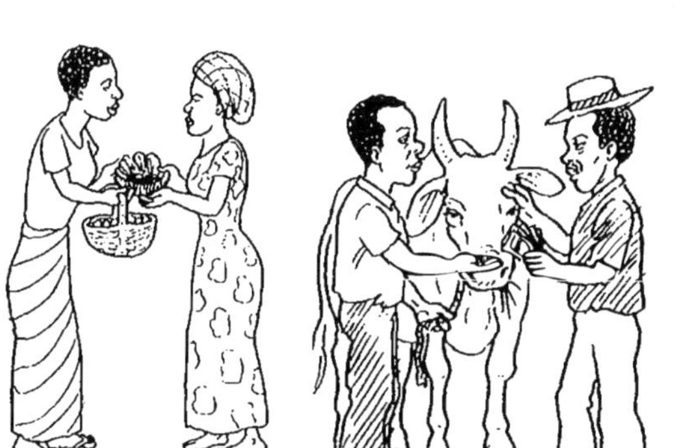

People's access to resources:

- Who is able to get milk and eggs, posts for fencing, animal loans, money for the care of sick family members, land to raise animals on or plant an agroforestry system?
- Who sells the animals and their products?
- Who benefits from the work of the local organization?

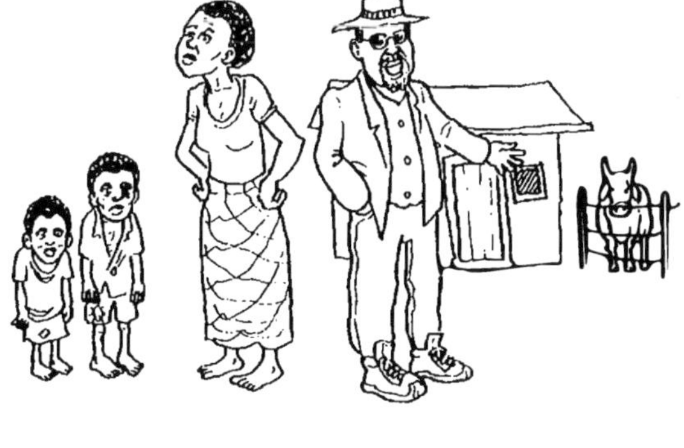

People's control over resources:

- If a man or woman can get the money for the things he or she needs, how does he or she get it?
- Who controls the money?
- Who owns the house, the land, the animals?
- Who can inherit the land or animals?
- Who do the children belong to and how many children are there?
- When crops, animals, and their products are sold, who controls the money and what is it used for?

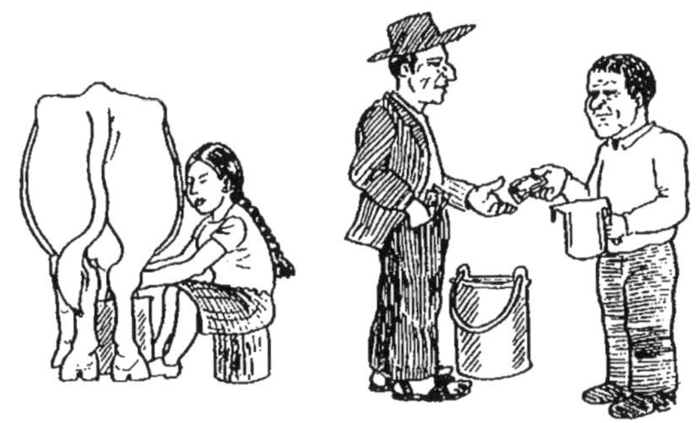

Every livestock program, project or training should be analyzed by the community for these three aspects:

1. The benefits to women and men:

- What will be the actual outcome of the program or project?
- What will women have at the end? Animals, milk, eggs, money, pasture?
- What will men have at the end?
- Who will control these resources, the men or the women?

2. The incentives for women's participation:

- Why should the women participate?
- What will be the benefits to them, tangible and intangible?
- What will be the benefits to their children?
- Will they own livestock themselves or just be responsible to pay the debt?
- Will they have money from extra milk sales that they control or only more work as they care for the cow?

The only people who can analyze these things are the insiders involved in the program themselves. Outsiders cannot analyze this for the people; they will never have enough information. Outsiders can only help to facilitate the process.

3. The constraints to women's participation:

- What might happen to the women as a result of the project as the women see it?

More work without benefits, a loan to repay without the husband's help, lack of childcare during training with the result that children may become ill, danger from travel on bad transportation, possible assault?

Tools used in gender analysis

In previous chapters several examples of dynamics to initiate discussion about roles and resources have been mentioned. Here are a few more. What others have you used successfully?

Some dynamics to look at people's roles:

1. What is the work we do?

- Divide into small groups separated by sex.
- Depending on how many groups there are, ask each group to draw pictures illustrating the work they do:

Women's groups:

- What work do women do in and around the house?
- What work do women do with the livestock?
- What work do women do in the fields?
- Add another task if it is appropriate to your area.

Men's groups:

- What work do men do in and around the house?
- What work do men do with the livestock?
- What work do men do in the fields?
- Add another task if it is appropriate to your area.

● Each group makes simple drawings of the tasks they complete in each area. Have a large drawing of a woman and a large drawing of a man ready up front.

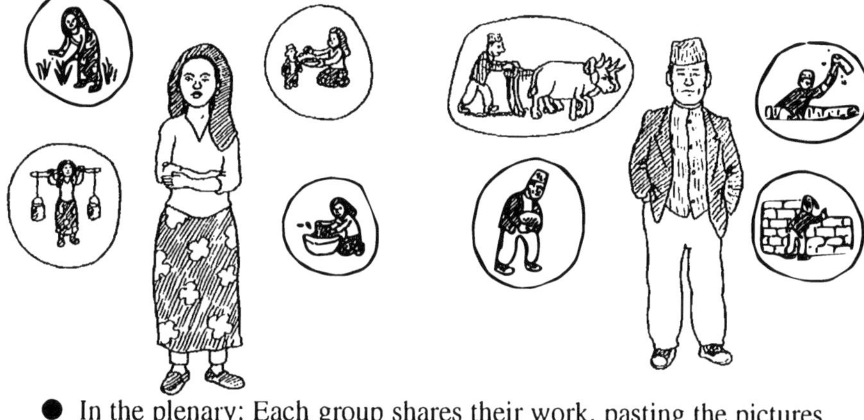

● In the plenary: Each group shares their work, pasting the pictures around the woman and the man.

● Analyze together the resulting drawings with special emphasis on the work of the women and how it contributes to the family production. Does her work have value? Why doesn't she get paid for her work?

● Now, cover over the woman's picture. Ask, "How would the family and the farm produce if the woman were not there?" Do the same with the man's picture. Ask, "What could we each do to appreciate the work of the women and the men in our families?"

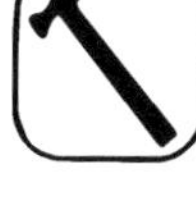

2. A woman's life from birth to death

● Divide into groups of 4–5 men or women. If you have outsiders and village people together in the workshop, put the outsiders into their own group.

● The group task is to answer these questions:

What is a woman's life like –

When she is born?	As a child?
As a young woman?	Before marriage?
As a mature woman?	In her old age?

● Have each small group answer this and then present it to the whole. If a comfortable situation has been created, the reality of the women will come out here. Depending on the confidence level of the women, the facilitator may need to encourage the women's groups. From this dynamic the men's different view will be plain.

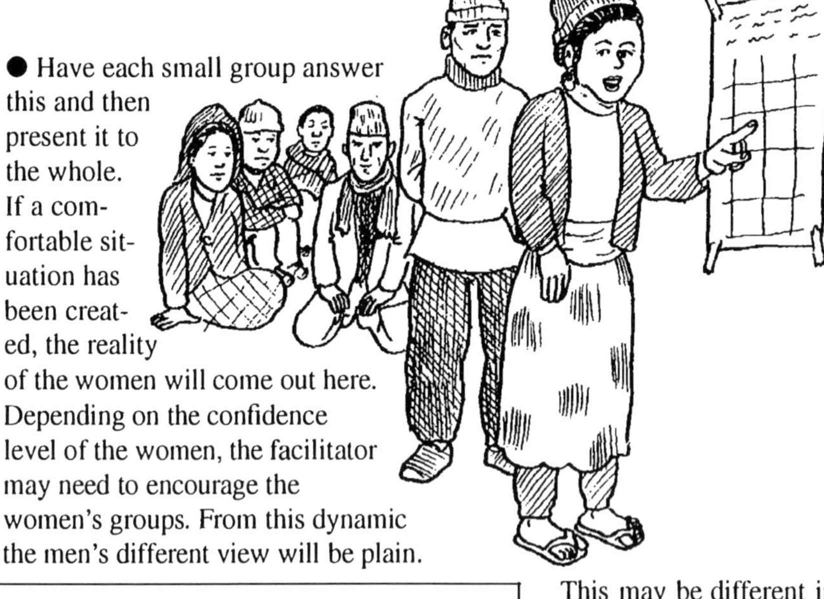

Here are some things people have shared in different communities:

- **From birth** the girl child is not treasured as the boy. The boy baby is given the choicest foods.
- **As a child** the boys will often be off playing soccer or other sport while the girl carries her younger siblings and works to cook and wash and herd the animals.
- **As a young woman** she is not permitted to continue studying but must marry early or work hard at home.
- **As a mature woman** she works very hard from dawn to late in the night. Most often her work is not valued or paid for. She is beaten and abused by her husband.
- **In her old age** she is not respected or listened to. She is not permitted to speak in village meetings or give counsel from her wisdom. The men say she speaks only gossip.

This may be different in your area, but, as an outsider, be prepared to be taken by surprise by the reality. Facilitators can use the difference between the men's and women's perceptions to draw out an effective dialogue and a decision to change. This dynamic has the greatest impact in a family or an organization when men and women are present together in training.

Another way to do this: Have each group pose as silent statues to represent each aspect of the woman's life. The other participants analyze the statues.

Source: Bing Flores

3. Action for analysis

In the highland Bolivian story (pg. 184), the outsider institution used the claims of the men and a training workshop to initiate an analysis in the community. Can you think of an action in your community which would help people to see women's and men's roles in a new light? The aim is always to appreciate one another's work. Men are not the only ones who often do not appreciate or value the work of women. Many very hard working women will say, "I don't work on the farm," or "I don't work for a living." Yet the activities they do are integral to the success of the farm production.

4. Ranking and sorting

Ranking and sorting such as in this section on page 186. (See "Tools" pg. 255 to learn how to do it.)

5. An analysis of a story

One of the previous stories (of the co-op who wouldn't allow women pg. 184 or the women's chicken group pg. 189) can open the discussion about women's and men's roles in livestock production. Or better yet would be an actual situation from your community or a nearby area which most people know about. Tell the story or have a group spend 30 minutes to discuss and plan a role play of a story from the participant's area. Analyze it together. What should the women's and men's roles be? How can the organization or family work more effectively together? How can the community put the other 50% to work in accomplishing its vision for the future?

6. Drawings from Uganda

This series of drawings were used in Uganda for an analysis of roles. The groups organized the jobs people did according to men, women, or men and women. One group arranged them like this:

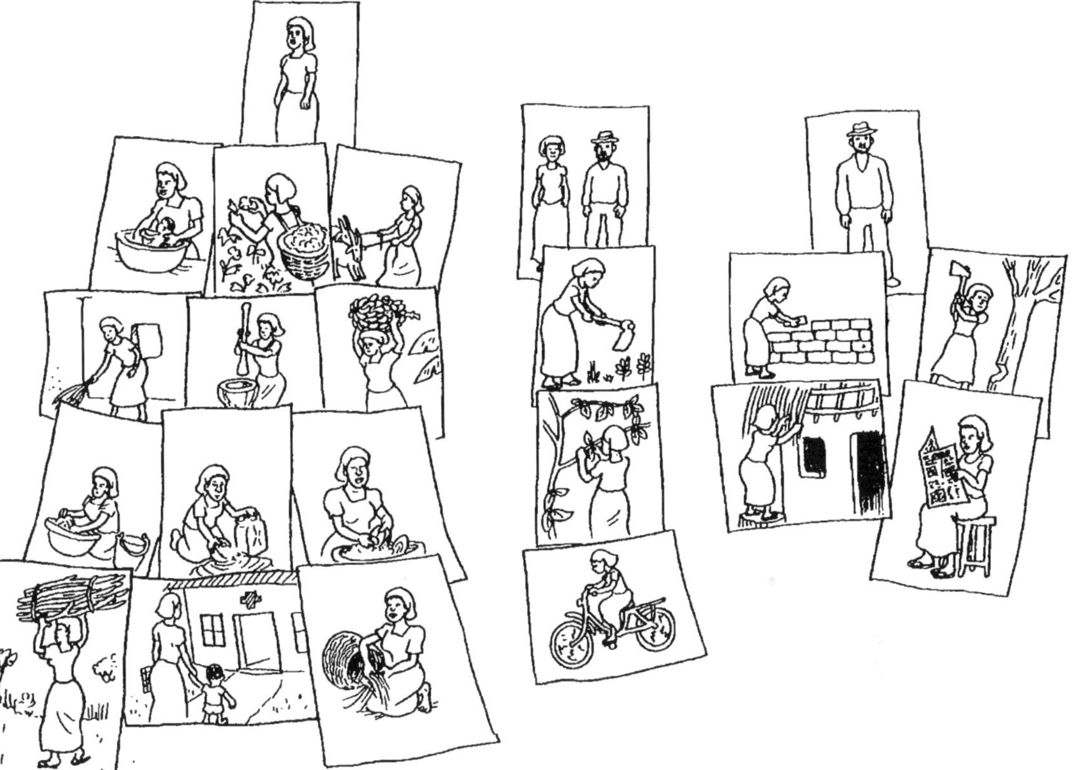

Then they all analyzed if this is the way things should be or if they work the best this way. They were later given time to adjust and change the pictures to show how they would like it to be. Then they discussed how they could make these changes.

Remember, the way you draw the pictures may affect the decisions made by the group. In the Uganda version the women were performing all the tasks in the pictures, even those typically done by men.

Source: A. Beinempaka

Some *dynamics* to look at ownership and resources:

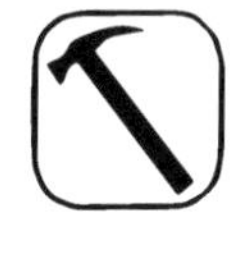
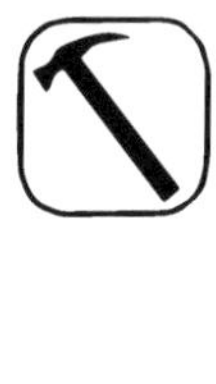

1. Who owns what?

This is similar to the exercise with roles above. It uses drawings of resources in the village (for example, house, furniture, animals, trees, crops, fields, etc.) This set of drawings was organized by a group in a workshop according to how people view ownership of resources in their community.

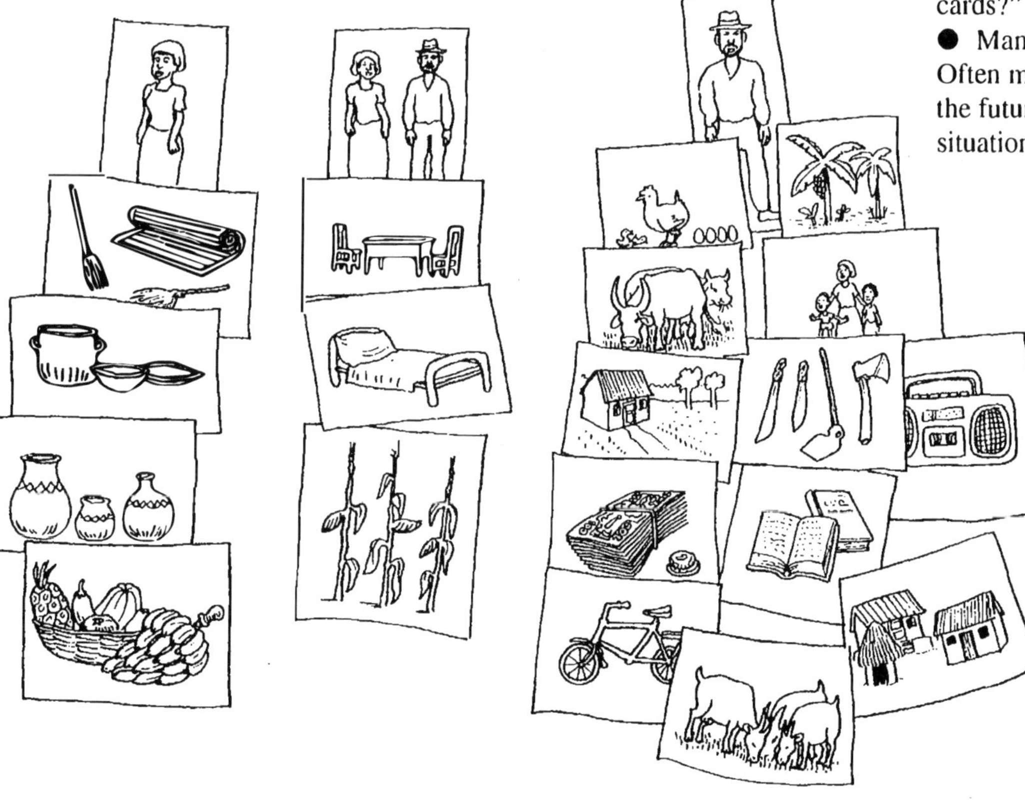

- Each group works with their cards in columns and assigns resources to men, women, or men and women together, according to who owns them. It is important that the group says who "owns" the object, not who "uses" it.
- In the plenary each group presents their opinions about how and why they organized their cards in this way.
- They analyze the current situation asking, "Is it good?" They look at the distribution of roles and women's and men's work as well. They can look at who is doing the work and who is getting paid for it. The next step is to ask the groups, "How would you prefer to arrange these cards?"
- Many myths and taboos come out in the analysis.

Often men and women will make a decision to change in the future. They can discuss how they could change this situation.

2. Flannel board

This is a similar way to look at the control of resources. The people have the opportunity to arrange the resources by ownership first as they are, and then as they should be. See "Flannel Boards," pg. 248.

3. Open-ended stories

An open ended story such as the egg-production story from this chapter (page 189) is very helpful to begin this type of analysis. See pg. 243

4. Resource Map

The community in small groups of all men or all women draw a map of how they perceive the resources in their community. They include what the resources are and who controls each resource. See mapping in "Tools" pg. 253.

Women's participation in agricultural training

I hope you have noticed that throughout this manual there have been suggestions for how to encourage the full participation of women in a training program. These ideas are not confined to a single chapter. This is because a participatory training program must consider women, not as an isolated group, but as important participants in every step of the program. When programs isolate women and offer them "women's" classes in an effort to do something with the women, they are further marginalized within their communities. When programs work completely separately with women in livestock programs, how can this lead to the valuing of the women's role in the home, on the farm, and in the community?

Constraints

Obviously there are many constraints to women's participation, or the issue would not arise. Some of these are:

- Language
- Literacy
- Low self esteem
- Prohibitions against participation in community meetings
- Invisibility of women's work
- Women's work load

Cultural norms are usually given as a major constraint in many societies. In Nepal, where the caste system and religious culture traditionally dictate that women do not speak in front of men, one large training program has these thoughts:

Training with only men or only women:

PROS

- Women express their opinions better.
- Women are relieved of the fear of contradicting men.
- Allows women's training in ethnic groups where women are not permitted to speak in front of men.
- Allows extra training for women not used to technical areas.

CONS

- Either men or women are excluded from the process.
- Most training needs both sexes involved.
- Women do not learn to express themselves in the village.
- No definition of problems and solutions together in the community.
- Tends to reinforce separation and the devaluing of women's roles.

Sometimes this program in Nepal will use mixed workshops, and sometimes they will give the same workshops to separate men's and women's groups.

Practical ways to encourage women's participation In training programs:

- Gender analysis in a community will often be the first step to encouraging women's participation. But sometimes there is great difficulty getting to the point where women will participate in gender analysis.

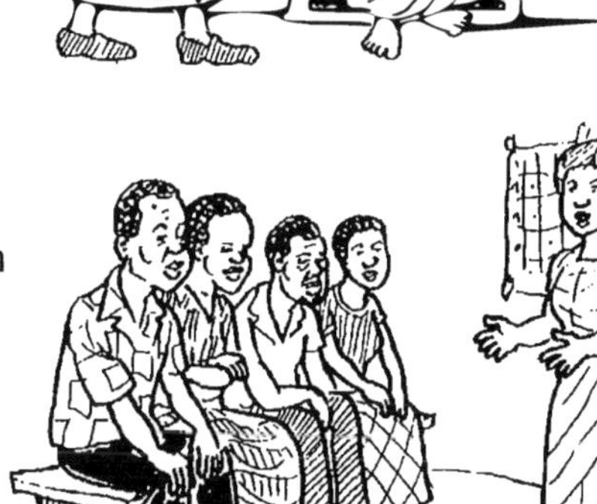

- For the first workshop visit–their homes, talk with them, and invite them personally.
- Meet with the community and let them know the training is for women as well.
- Have women facilitators and staff.
- Have village women as facilitators.

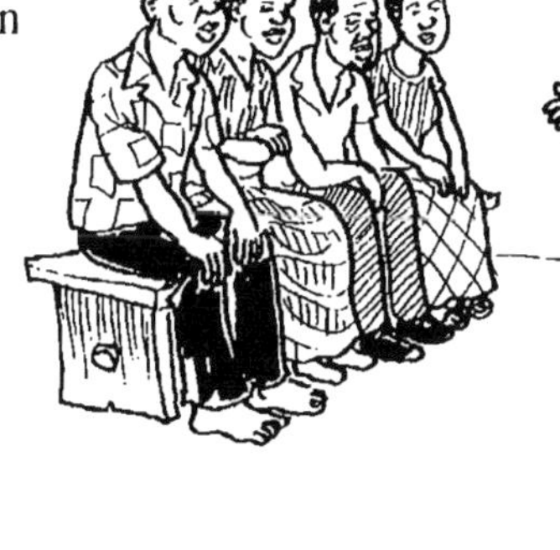

- Use modeling by women facilitators.
- Ensure male staff members show respect to the women on the staff.
- Establish a rapport between the women and facilitators
- Encourage the women to speak.
- Ask for those who have not yet participated to give an opinion.
- Wait patiently for the woman to speak. Many times it takes awhile for them to speak for the first time.
- Encourage one of the women participants who begin to model within the group.
- In sociodramas and pictures make sure women are portrayed in decision-making positions, not only men. If participants design a role play where only men have positions that involve decision-making, you can ask them why.
- Put the women in their own small groups, especially at the beginning of a workshop. This helps the men to see that the women have valid points. The women gain self confidence and self esteem as their ideas and opinions are valued in front of the men.
- Provide child care for the babies of nursing women. If they bring a caretaker, the training program can pay for food and lodging for the caretaker.
- Keep the workshops short. Women come more often if the workshop is not longer than 7-8 days because they have much work to do and it is hard for them to be away from their work and families longer.
- Hold the workshop close to home. Women want village-based training closer to home (not center-based training). Men don't want the women to travel far and be away, and women feel insecure away from home.
- Have several women in the workshop (not just one).
- Provide separate sleeping facilities for the women participants.
- Use the language closest to the first language of the people.

In Kenya, a training workshop was held within a culture who believes the mother-in-law should never look at or speak to the son-in-law. The mother-in-law was the one who had been chosen for the workshop, but the son-in-law also came. How would you have handled this situation?

The facilitators understood that the mother-in-law had been chosen to attend. When the group sat in a circle for training, the facilitators asked the son-in-law to sit behind the mother-in-law outside of the circle. They supported the woman's attending the course and encouraged her to share her ideas. In this way, both participated in the course and the woman's self esteem was raised.

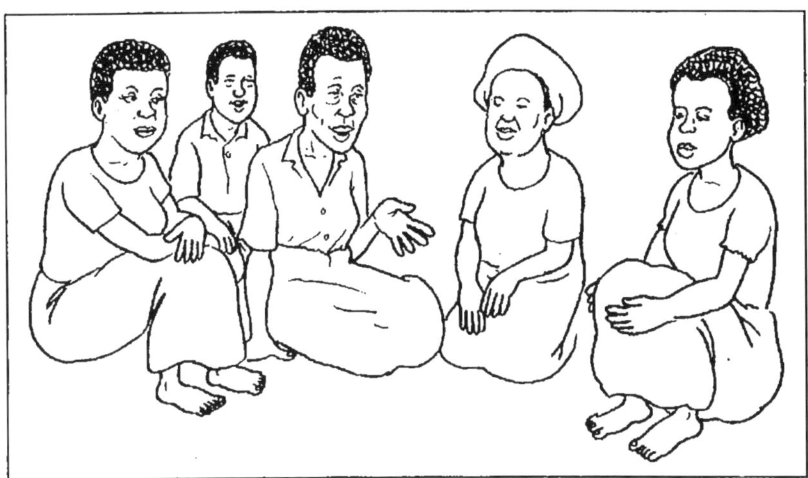

Source: B.J. Lindquist

Chapter 10

Healthy communication and healthy groups

This chapter covers the following topics:

Every idea in this chapter is useful for:

✔ **Facilitators of Participatory Training and CLWs:** to improve their training and relational skills.

✔ **Grassroots Organizations** working in agricultural or livestock production and marketing: to strengthen their work together, help them continue their programs, and make their organization more effective.

✔ **Outsider Organizations** who have participatory training and development programs: to improve the effectiveness and sustainability of their work.

Why is it so important for an agricultural program to train people in effective communication?

Most participatory development initiatives depend on people working together to solve a common problem or to achieve a common vision or goal. Good communication and good group skills are essential for an organization to have success in their work. If, in agricultural development, we want a participatory training program to be effective, we cannot ignore how people relate to one another, how they communicate, and how they work in groups. **When group work is successful, it builds self and group esteem.** Participatory training goes hand in hand with good communication and good group functioning. It builds people's abilities to solve problems without outside intervention. **This leads to long term sustainability** after an outsider group has left an area.

Understanding about good communication is a powerful tool for facilitators and CLWs. When facilitators know how they personally respond and interact in a group, they can evaluate and improve their relational and facilitation skills. This will make them much more effective communicators. Many of the tools in this chapter will help facilitators and CLWs to analyze their approach to communication and group work. They, in turn, can facilitate an analysis by workshop participants or in their grassroots organizations.

There are many good books and manuals available for working on communication, group work and organization strengthening. This book will not try to share everything in these areas. This chapter will share some ideas about important topics to cover and some dynamics which have been helpful in initiating dialogue within the framework of an agriculture training program. For more information see "References," pg. 333.

If you will be using these tools to help an organization to develop, you need to remember: always **start with a participatory assessment** of the situation. The facilitator, together with the members of the local organization, should formulate a plan for assessing the strengths, weaknesses, and vision of the organization. Based on this assessment, the appropriate activities for strengthening the organization can be planned.

Healthy communication

Listening, speaking, understanding, and improving

Did I understand you and did you understand me?

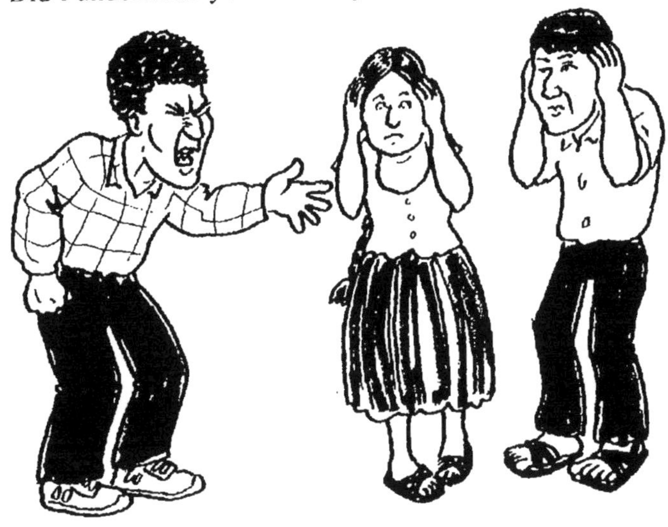

Start working together on good communication skills from the first day of the first workshop. As a facilitator, practice what you are learning about communication, and always model good communication. All Community Livestock Workers need training in good communication to be successful in their jobs!

Listening skills

Many times communication misfires because we stop listening or they stop listening, or we or they never were listening in the first place! The best thing we can do is improve our own listening skills and model really good ones. Give all participants the opportunity to do this.

Some helpful listening skills:

- **Listen actively.** Make eye contact. Affirm what you are hearing with a nod or an uh-huh.
- **Don't tune out** or turn off what the other person is saying.
- **Don't interrupt.** It shows you are not listening, but rather thinking about what you want to say!
- Try to **understand rather than to be understood.**
- **Rephrase** what the other person said in your own words. Then ask if that was what was meant. This insures you really understood. *"What I think I heard you say was..."*

> He who answers before listening, that is his folly and his shame.
>
> Proverbs 18:13

For good information on listening and communication see Hope and Timmel, *Training for Transformation* "References," pg. 330.

Two *dynamics* to help you practice and discuss good listening:

1. This is what I heard you say:

● Make two lines of the participants facing each other so everyone has a partner. Sit in lines, with some space between each person.

● Have a set of pre-written, conflictive statements ready on small pieces of paper. These conflicts should be real ones which generate discussion normally in your group.

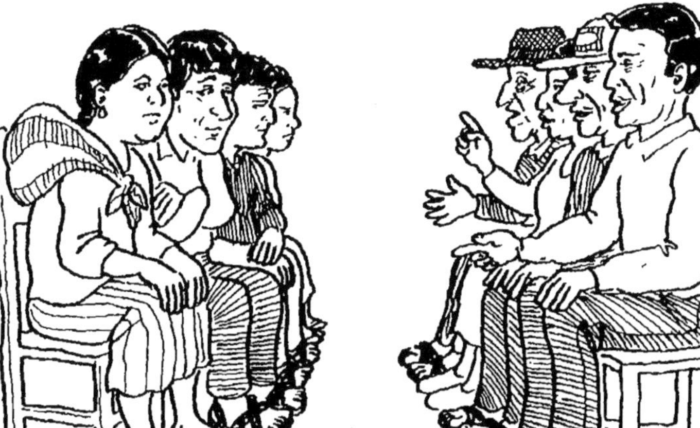

Examples of conflictive statements:

- Women should never be allowed to go to community meetings.
- Men should be the only participants in livestock training.
- It is the man's responsibility to beat his wife.
- All traditional medicines are better than purchased medicines.
- It is better to use the land to produce as much as possible and then move on.
- It is the president's right to take resources from the organization; that is how he is paid for his work.

Use statements which relate to topics which are being discussed in the workshop.

● Each pair has a conflictive statement. Each pair will have a dialogue about the statement. All pairs are talking at the same time. All the people on the right are in favor, all those on the left are opposed. The people on the right have five minutes to defend the statement. The people on the left must practice listening attentively, repeating and rephrasing what the person says. At the end of five minutes, change so the people on the left can refute the statement. Those on the right must practice good listening.

● **When both sides have spoken, ask people:**

- How did it feel when you were listening to these ideas?
- Did you want to respond instead of listen?
- Did it help you to understand the other person to listen to them?
- How did you feel about each other?
- Did you get mad at the other person?
- Did good listening help you to focus on the topic instead of your feelings about the other person?

> My dear friends, take note of this: Everyone should be quick to listen, slow to speak and slow to become angry. James 1:19

● After this discussion, have everyone on the left move down one chair so they have a new partner. The person on the end moves to the other end. Pass all of the topics one person to the right. Now everyone has a new pair and a new topic. Repeat the discussion. Switch in the same way one more time.

● Finish this dynamic with further reflection and dialogue about good listening. The participants should make a list of what they feel are the important aspects of good listening.

2. The telephone:

This simple child's game is very powerful with a dialogue.

● With the participants seated in a circle, the facilitator whispers a message to the person on his or her right. The message could be something like: On the 15th of September, the women's livestock production group will hold its fifth annual livestock fair. Please bring your animals. Everyone is invited.

● Each person whispers the message to the person on his or her right. No questions for clarification are allowed. When the last person receives the message, he or she says the message out loud. Then ask the tenth person what she heard. Then ask the fifth person what he heard. Then read the original message. Do not try to pin the blame on anyone.

● **Ask the four open questions:**

- What did you see and feel happening here?
- Does this happen in our organization?
- When this happens, what problems does it cause?
- What can we do about it?

● Make a list with participants of all of the things they can do to listen well and clarify the message. They may decide to resolve to be better communicators!

Speaking: make the message clear

Just as listening well is essential to good communication, so giving a clear message helps to ensure understanding.

The community of San Martin had a meeting to organize a vaccination campaign. Most people understood they would vaccinate now and pay later. They arrived with their animals and no money. The Community Livestock Worker had paid for the vaccine. After vaccinating, at the next meeting, many people did not pay for the vaccination, or they wanted to pay for the vaccine but not the work. The CLW was discouraged and quit her job because she could not collect and has lost money.

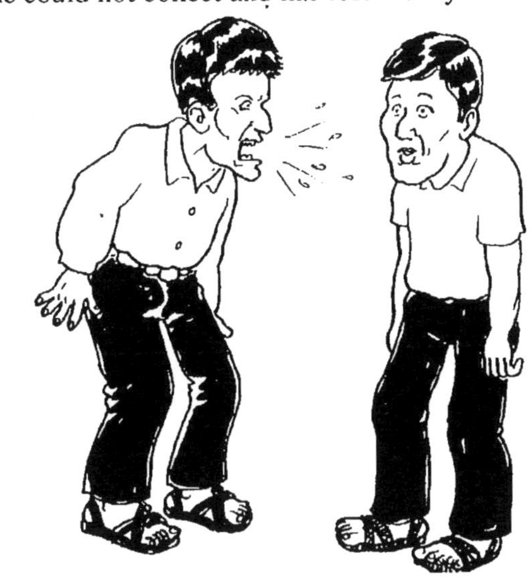

Many times when we think we have communicated something very well, the listeners have not heard the same thing! Maybe they received a partial message, or something totally different from what we were trying to say. This can cause terrible misunderstanding and fights in an organization if it was an important message.

Some tips on giving a clear message:

- Ask the person or group you are talking to to **repeat the message** you have given them in their own words. If it is not correct, clarify.
- **Think ahead about what you want to say** and plan a way of saying it that will be clear.
- **Speak in summary form.** When there is too much information the message is not clear. Say what is essential.

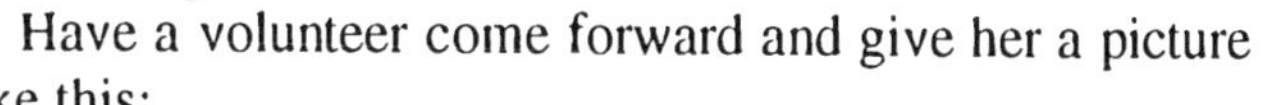

Four *dynamics* about clear communication:

1. Everyone draw this.

● Have a volunteer come forward and give her a picture like this:

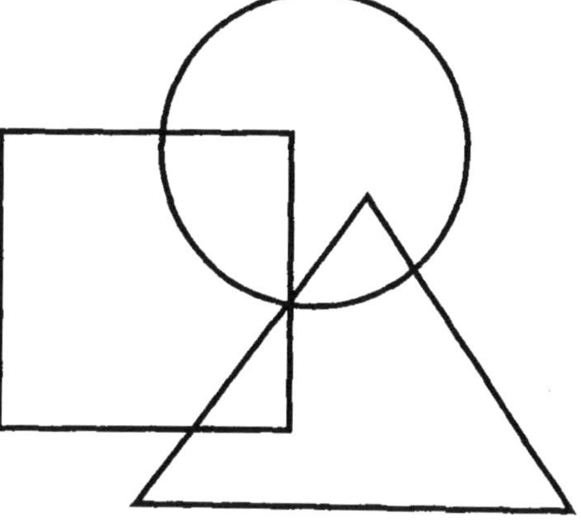

● Make sure the people in the class cannot see the picture through the back of the paper (you can use double thickness paper or thin cardboard). Ask the volunteer to get all the participants to draw this picture on their own paper by telling them what to draw without showing them the picture.

● After one volunteer tries, have another one try, then a third. They will each try to tell everyone how to draw it. After each volunteer, have everyone show their pictures and ask if that is the correct picture. None will be the same. After all three have tried, ask if anyone knows another way to get someone to draw this picture without seeing it.

● If they have not been able to reproduce the picture, you can **tell everyone how to draw the picture as you mime drawing it with your finger.**

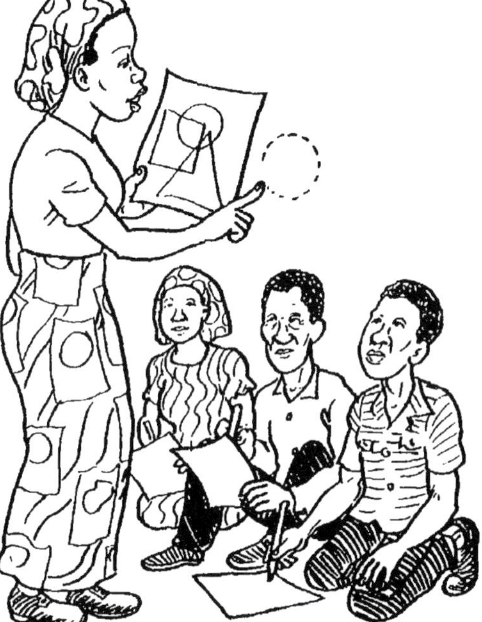

● The results will be remarkably like the original. Finally show everyone the original.

● Ask the four open questions:

- What did you see happening here? Was the message clear?
- Does this happen in our organization?
- When the message is not clear, what problems does it cause?
- What can we do to overcome these problems?
- What can we do when we give a message to insure that the listener has heard correctly? As listeners, how can we be sure we have heard correctly?

● Develop a list from this discussion of what can be done to encourage and ensure good communication.

2. Can you repeat this?

● Have everyone take out a paper and pencil. Show them a drawing which is fairly complicated but clear, for five to ten seconds. The picture can be about legal paper size or a bit bigger. Make it a line drawing, not one which is colored in. You might use the shield of your country or city or an emblem which is often seen but probably not too well known.

● Take the picture away. Now ask everyone to draw what they saw.

● Have people show their pictures to the whole group. Then compare their pictures to the original.

● How did everyone do?

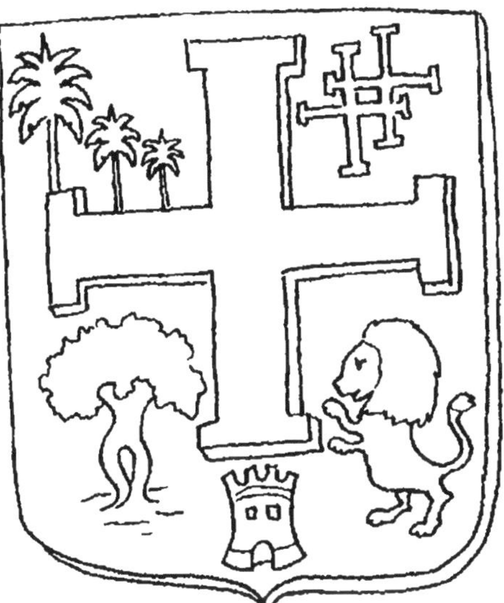

● What did you see happening here? People may get upset that they did not have enough time to see the picture. Have them analyze what was happening in depth. The picture is the same as a spoken message. We hear it often just once, or very rapidly. Afterwards we think, now what did that person say?

● When this happens, what problems does it cause? If the spoken message was important, when we repeat it to someone else, it is different just as our pictures are different. Maybe the next person acts on our message inappropriately, or perhaps it starts gossip.

● What can we do to overcome this problem?

3. A role play.

(How to use this role play? See "Tools," pg. 244.)

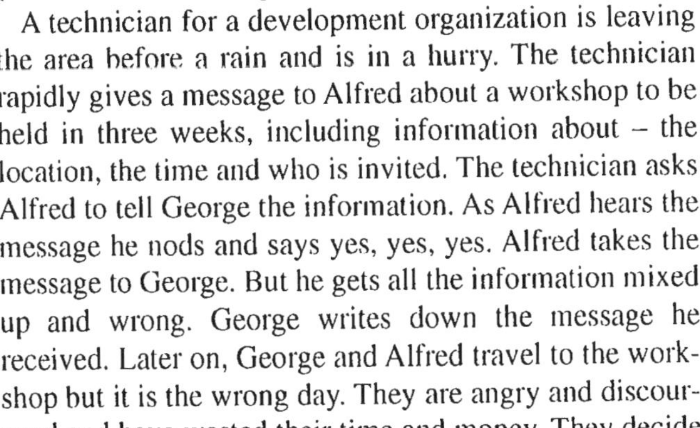

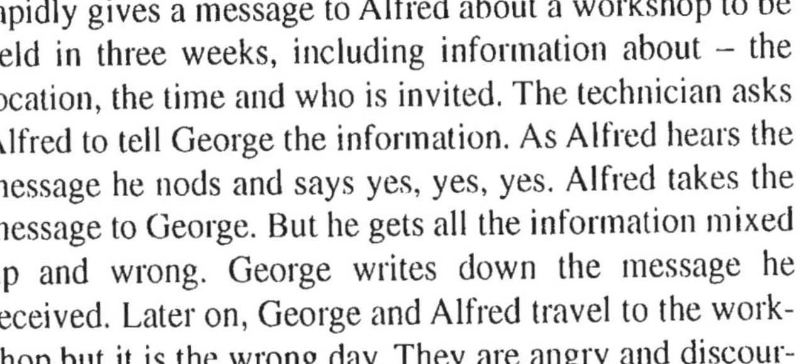

A technician for a development organization is leaving the area before a rain and is in a hurry. The technician rapidly gives a message to Alfred about a workshop to be held in three weeks, including information about – the location, the time and who is invited. The technician asks Alfred to tell George the information. As Alfred hears the message he nods and says yes, yes, yes. Alfred takes the message to George. But he gets all the information mixed up and wrong. George writes down the message he received. Later on, George and Alfred travel to the workshop but it is the wrong day. They are angry and discouraged and have wasted their time and money. They decide never to work with this program again.

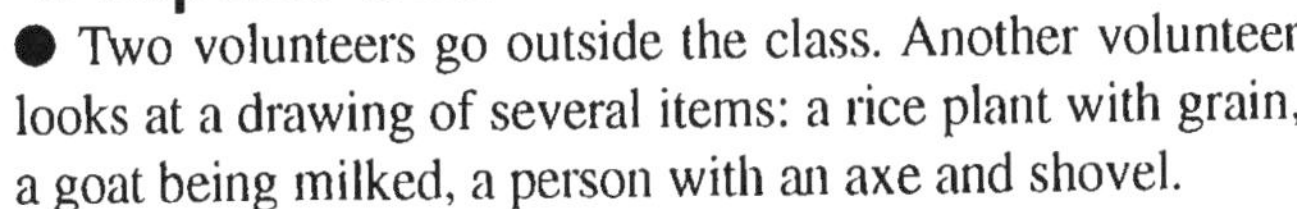

4. Explain this.

● Two volunteers go outside the class. Another volunteer looks at a drawing of several items: a rice plant with grain, a goat being milked, a person with an axe and shovel.

● Put the drawing away. Ask a volunteer from outside to come in. The person who saw the drawing explains it to the one who has come inside. Then the second person comes in from outside. The first from outside explains the drawing to the second. Then the second person explains the drawing to everyone. Now, show everyone the drawing.

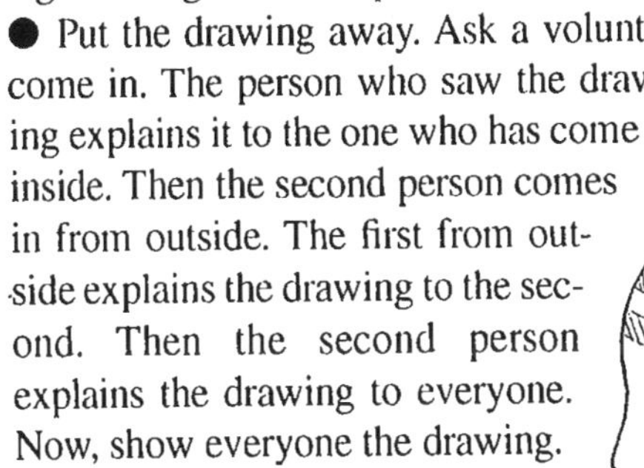

● Use the four open questions to initiate a dialogue about this situation.

● Write down the suggestions everyone has to make the communication clearer.

Understanding: how we perceive the message

SEEK TO UNDERSTAND FIRST then to be UNDERSTOOD!

> A fool finds no pleasure in understanding
> but delights in airing his own opinions.
> Proverbs 18:2

When you and I look at the same picture or situation, we may see two entirely different things. This difference in perception can cause a total break in communication. We think we are talking about the same thing, but we're not! It is important for me to understand how you perceive a situation if we want true open communication.

Two *dynamics* about perceptions, to use when there are misunderstandings:

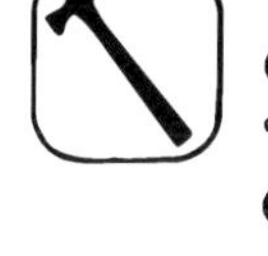

1. What's this?

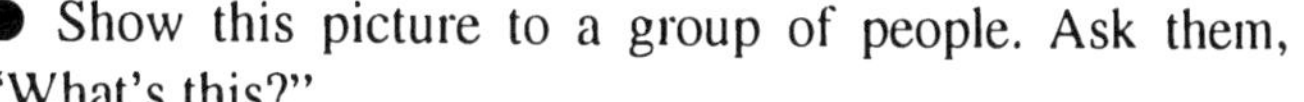

- Show this picture to a group of people. Ask them, "What's this?"
- Everyone will agree it is a rabbit.
- You can say, "But I think it is a duck!"
- Discuss that with everyone, perhaps they will try to dissuade you. Have a disagreement about it.
- **Turn the picture on its side and show everyone the duck.**
  - Who was right? You can agree that both were right.
  - What did you see happening here? See how easy it is for different people to see the same message differently. And both can be right.
  - What problems does this cause when it happens in our organization?
  - What can we do to overcome this problem?
- People will realize they are not always right. They can also make a decision to try to understand the other person's point of view first, before trying to convince them of their own.

Source: International Institute of Rural Reconstruction, Philippines

2. Make this, please.

- Divide into groups of 4–5 people.
- One group will be the observer group. Each observer will observe a different group at work. The others will do the dynamic.
- Give each small group a bag of things found, such as: sticks, plastic, paper, string, rubber bands, etc. Make sure each bag includes paper and a pen or marker. Make sure each bag's contents are the same.
- The instructions are, **"Make a stable."** The first group to finish wins a prize.
- Some groups will try to construct a 3-D stable from the contents. Others may draw one. If no group is drawing one, give the hint to someone so they will. If a group draws a stable first, they win. This should be done with lots of laughter and fun. Make sure the prize is something that could be shared with everyone, if the winning group so decides (like a bag of candy or a box of crackers).
- What did you see happening here? Ask the observer group and open the discussion to all.
- Ask a group who was building and lost, "How did you feel when you lost?" This will initiate a lively dialogue because the groups who were building will think it unfair to accept the drawing if you said make a stable. But as they reflect, they will see that the directions were not very clear.
- What problems does this cause when it happens in our organization?
- What can we do about it?
- How can we seek to understand the other person's point of view?

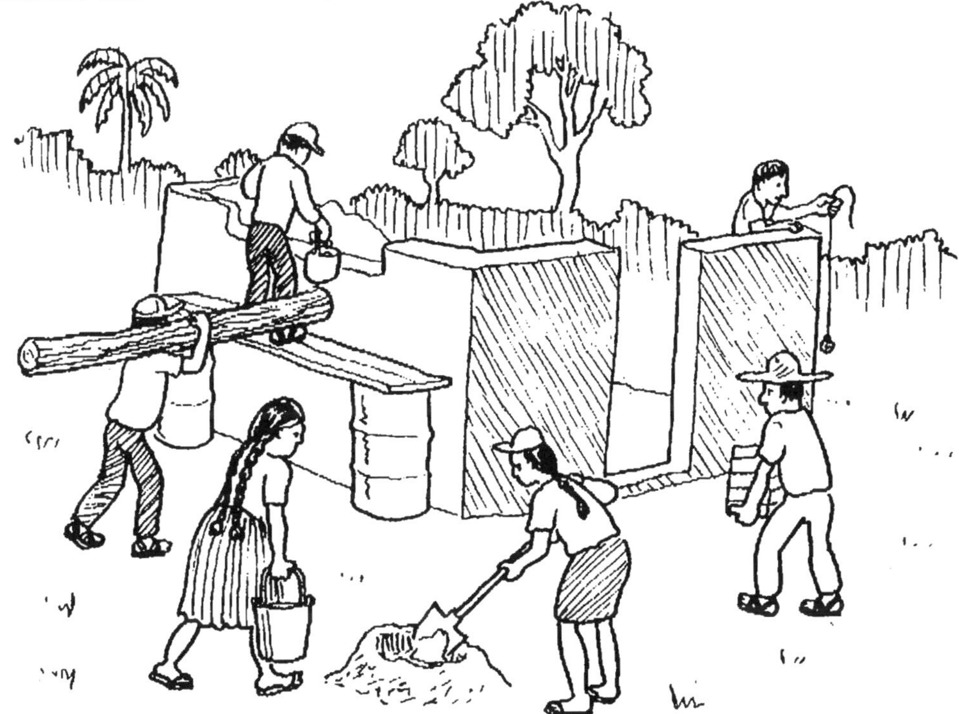

Improving the way we talk to one another: giving and receiving feedback

Many times, because the things we talk about in workshops or in organizing together are so important to people, they cause heated debates. Sometimes people talk about their feelings. They may try to blame someone in the workshop. Or they may tell what they think about the other person in a way that causes pain. This is usually destructive in the workshop as well as in organizational communication. Many times we wait until something is really bothering us and then we blow up at the other person, lashing out from our emotions.

Look at these examples:

You never do anything to help me with OUR sheep! I have to do all the work.
How will our organization ever get better if you never help?!

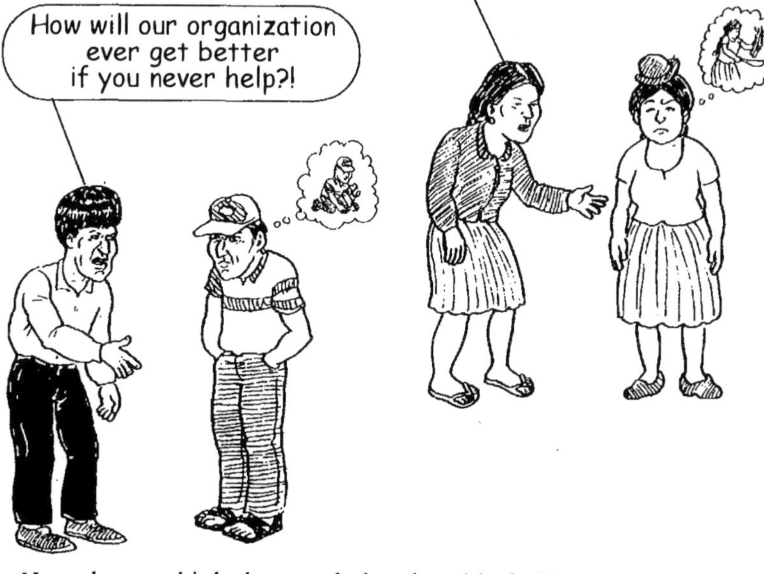

How do you think the people hearing this feel? How would you respond? Why do you think the people spoke this way?

Have the participants think this through and respond.

Inappropriate feedback

- In small groups **have each group role play a situation of inappropriate feedback.**
- Below are some examples of role plays given to groups. Make them appropriate to your area, or create different ones from the organization's experience:

1. John and his officers from the livestock association, are getting ready for their annual assembly. The officers are just getting ready to go into the meeting when the president lashes out at two of them saying, "You two are no help at all! You never come to meetings and you are not ready with your parts of the meeting. I can see I'll have to do it all myself, as usual!"
2. The women's livestock group is having a regular meeting. They are discussing the use of the group ram. Ann yells at Patricia, "You are so selfish! You have the group ram. But you never let us breed our sheep to him. I can tell you just want all his lambs for yourself." The other woman responds, "This group is worthless! I'm quitting," and she storms out.
3. The local church group is having a communal work day to help each other establish terraces on their land for better pasture production. They are working along, but Pedro arrives late. Joaquín says to him, "I'm sick and tired of you not coming on time to anything. We have been working for hours. The next time you come late, you're out of the group."

- We know how it feels to be on the receiving end of negative feedback like this. Usually you don't even want to listen to the person. Your emotions are highly charged and the situation is not constructive. But feedback can be very helpful to us in our relationships, in the organization, or in our family or our work.

So how can feedback be given and received without such negative consequences?

Have the group discuss this question together and develop a list from their answers. Some of the things they may include:

✔Don't heap blame on people or fling their offense at them. Don't judge them. Just **describe the situation.** If we say it judgmentally, the person will automatically want to defend himself.

✔**Describe how the situation makes you feel.** For example, say, "When I can't take my sheep to be bred, I worry that I will fall behind in my production and I will not have the lambs to pay for school fees."

✔**Be specific** and state precisely what the situation is. If you are too general it is hard for the receiver to understand.

✔**Consider the other person.** If we give feedback thinking only of ourselves, it will not help but hurt the other person. Make sure he or she can do something about the behavior before you say anything. (Maybe someone is late because of a serious problem in the household).

✔**Don't wait until you are mad!** Give feedback early on so the behavior can change and so resentment does not build up.

✔Remember about good communication! **Say clearly what you want to say. Make sure the other person understands.** Check back to see that the message was clear.

If all we ever hear is positive feedback, how will we know our behavior causes problems and change it?

Receiving negative feedback is important for everyone's growth. But feedback, even well spoken, is sometimes hard to hear. It is also very hard to give to someone else. Many people don't want to interfere, or they don't want to harm their relationship. That's why we so often wait until we are mad, or until there is a big problem. How can we receive it well and encourage others to give it?

Tips for receiving feedback

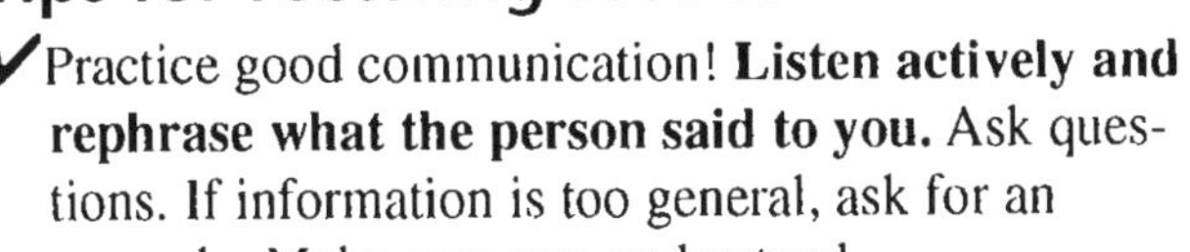

✔Practice good communication! **Listen actively and rephrase what the person said to you.** Ask questions. If information is too general, ask for an example. Make sure you understand.

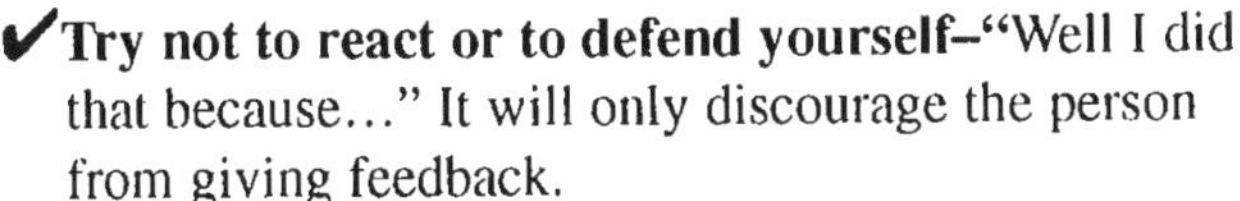

✔**Try not to react or to defend yourself**–"Well I did that because…" It will only discourage the person from giving feedback.

✔**Don't be hurt by the feedback and clam up!** Remember it is one person's opinion and people see things differently. You can check it with others and work on it if you decide to.

Now have the groups return to their role plays. Have them change the role play so that feedback is given correctly.

As a trainer you should plan to always model healthy feedback. If you show you are open and accepting of criticism and correction, people will see its value.

Healthy groups

As facilitators and CLWs we work toward change in the way participants and community members think, feel, and act. We do not want the changes to be temporary. For the changes to be permanent, both the people and their social environment must change. This is why the work of organizations and groups in development is so important. The organizations provide the social environment where change can take place. Discussion and agreement in the organization provide a place for an individual to be encouraged and to develop commitment to change which is not present when one person alone is changing.

Many farmers recognize the importance of organizations and seek to form cooperatives and associations. They expect their organizations to help them get credit, market their products, and perform other services like negotiating with the government and other institutions. But often the organizations fail, for many reasons, and the farmers dreams are not realized. Here is a story of an organization which was successful and which helped its members to realize their dreams.

In the town of San Pedro in the hills of Guatemala, a group of people looked around at their village and their land. Erosion and deforestation due to overgrazing and hillside farming had destroyed their land and dried up their water supply. They could not produce enough crops or animals to feed their families. There were no services for health care or schooling near by. The situation was so desperate their children had all moved to the city. This same group of people went to a series of workshops and decided to make big changes in their farm and village management.

To help them implement those changes, they formed a cooperative. Through the co-op they organized to build terraces and plant trees, they began making compost, they received small loans, they brought more technical help, and they protected and capped springs. When one member had difficulties, the others would work together to help that member out. One of the hardest things they did was to switch their animals from an extensive pasturing system to complete confinement in stables. As a group they decided the confinement was necessary to stop the overgrazing and erosion. As organized members of a co-op, everyone helped to enforce the new law of complete confinement.

Today the area is transformed. Forests of pine trees provide timber for houses. Land is extremely productive. The animals are raised in complete confinement. The co-op, through its members, built a school, health clinic, church, and store for the community. Many of the children of the original group have returned to the community with their children. There is a sense of hope for the future. All of this took place during a 30-year war in Guatemala which severely affected the villagers lives time and again.

What do the people attribute their success to?

They believe their success is due to their hard work and perseverance but their organization also gets much of the credit. The members of the co-op were learning many new farming techniques during the years they were changing their community. Through the organization, they encouraged one another in their decisions to change. When one lagged behind, the others reminded him of his commitment, and he continued on. The organization is not perfect; it has had many problems. But it has also served its members well.

The members of the San Pedro co-op learned about how a group can function well together. They applied much of what they learned in their organization.

The following four sections in this chapter give tools and ideas for working together well in groups. The San Pedro co-op applied many similar skills to the development of their strong organization.

The power of small groups

Successful organizations have usually figured out the power of small groups in thinking things through and getting things done. These are often called committees or work groups. In our agricultural workshops we also work with small groups because good learning, sharing of information and ideas, and dialogue takes place in a small group. So, in the course of our workshops we can help the grassroots organization by giving them tools and knowledge for good group work.

The two jobs of a group: group function and task

What is the work of a group? To accomplish the job or task they have been given, right?

Look at the group pictured on the right:

We must develop a plan of natural pesticide use for our crops.
Let's get out paper and draw what we think would work.
Did you hear about the robbery yesterday?
No, what happened?

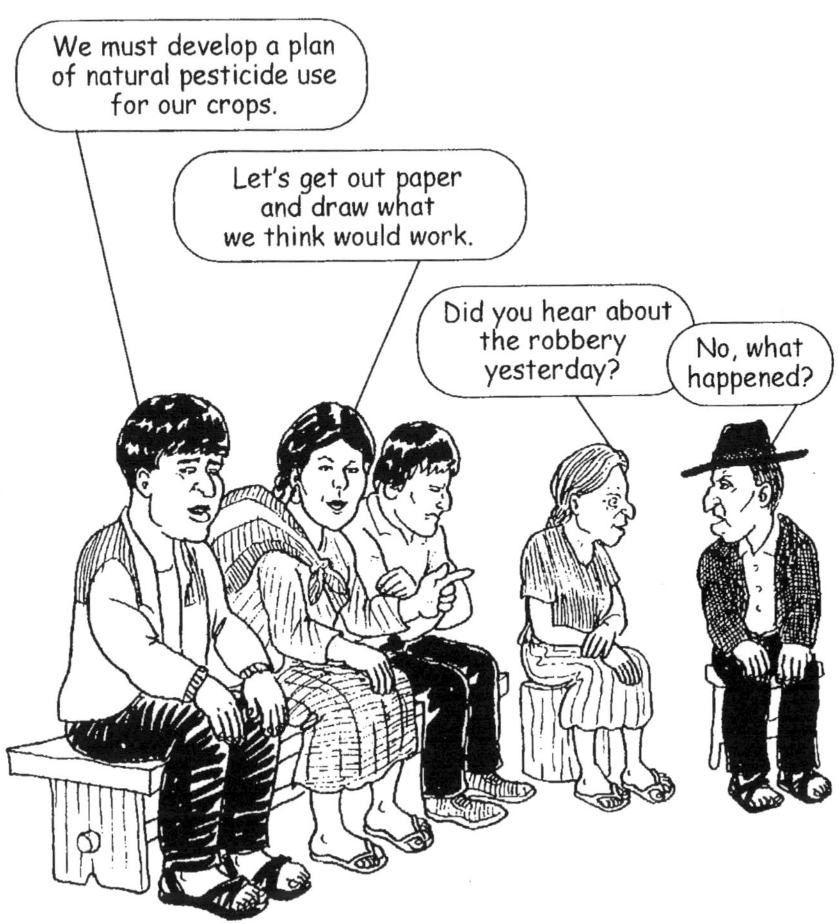

The task of this group is to develop a plan for natural pesticide use in their community. They will need to use their planning, organizing, implementing, follow-up, and evaluation skills to accomplish this task. How well do you think that task will be accomplished by this group? What problems do you see the group having? What could they do differently?

Every group which works well together has another job, besides their task. In this case the task is a pesticide plan. But the other job is to function well as a group. If this group ignores (as they are doing) how the group works together, they will not be able to accomplish their task well.

Two *dynamics* to discuss the two jobs of the group:

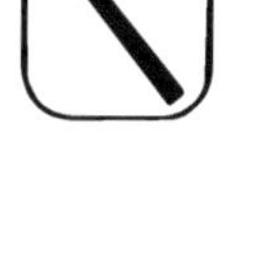

1. The horse

● Picture a horse as it is used for pulling or riding. It needs both its front legs and its back legs functioning perfectly to be able to work. The two jobs of the group are like the front legs and the back legs of a horse. You can point to a horse or show a picture and ask how it would work with only its hind legs working. Would it be as useful? Would you be able to carry the cargo you need to carry? Or could you get where you needed to go?

● The group, like the horse, needs both front legs and back legs working to move forward and get the job done.

● In small groups have people define what is involved in doing the two jobs of the group.

- Why is paying attention to the two jobs of the group important for a good organization?
- Why is it important for participatory training?

● Throughout the workshops the two jobs of the group must be done well in all small-group work. Reflecting on this will help participants to have well functioning groups.

Modified from Vella, 1995.

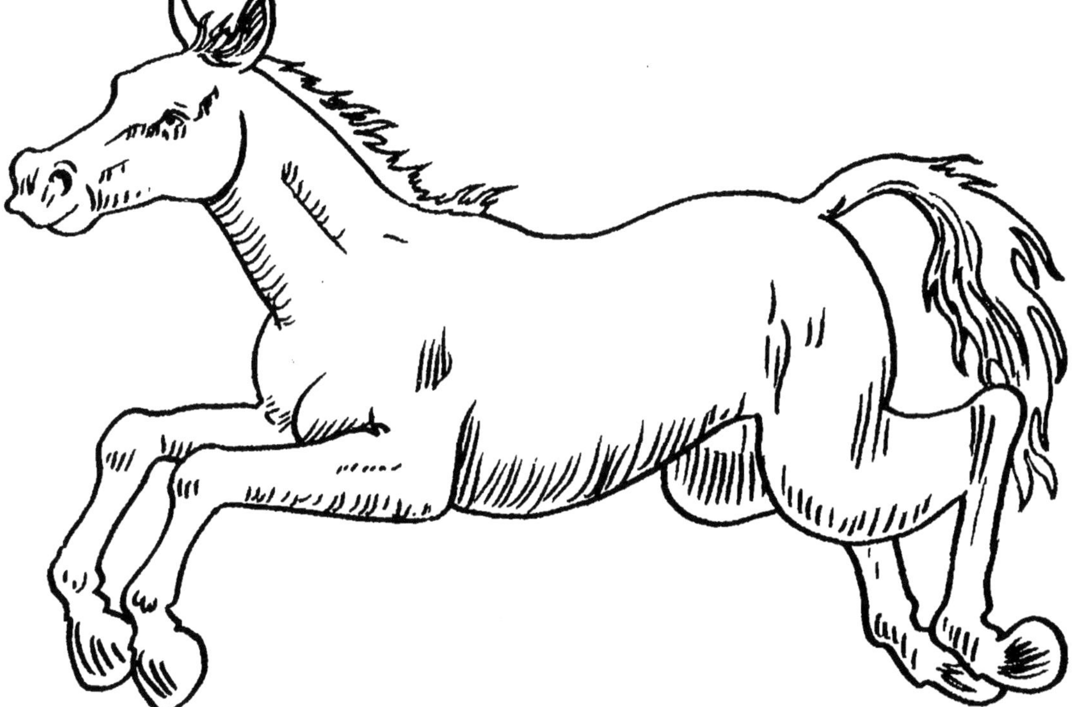

FRONT LEGS
JOB 1

Good group function

- Use good communication skills (question, clarify, listen)
- Make sure everyone participates
- Get everyone engaged in the group
- Help people know how they work in a group
- Use humor appropriately
- Work within a time frame

BACK LEGS
JOB 2

Getting the task done

- State the task clearly
- Stay focused on the task
- Plan effectively
- Keep notes
- Draw conclusions
- Evaluate
- Make decisions effectively

2. Work without talking

- Divide into small groups. One group will be the observer group.
- The other groups will each receive a bag with various objects in them. These objects can include plastic bags or bottles, string, sticks, stones, colored paper, markers, tape, and whatever else you can find. The contents do not have to be the same in each bag.
- Tell each group to build something useful from the contents of the bag. Tell everyone, NO ONE IN THE GROUP IS ALLOWED TO TALK WHILE THEY WORK. This will probably take 30–45 minutes. The observer group is charged with observing how the groups are functioning.
- When everyone is finished, everyone walks around together to all the groups, and each group shows their work. Everyone votes on the best object made.

- **Ask:**
  - How did you feel when you could not talk?
  - How did your groups work together? Ask the observer group to share what they observed.
  - How important is talking to good communication?
  - Was it possible for a group to work well together without talking?
  - What happened in the groups that did not work well together?
- At this stage you can use the image of the horse to talk about the two jobs of the group. Do the participants have anything to add to the lists above in the jobs? Facilitate a dialogue about the importance of the two jobs.

How do we relate in a group?

If every person in the group understands how they relate to others, the group will function better. Each of us approaches the work of the group in a different way. Some of us engage and participate well. Those who are participating may speak as soon as they have an idea, or sit and think before sharing an idea. Others sit back and listen without participating or they may distract people. Still others try to take over the whole process and boss people around.

Each participant should be given the opportunity to reflect on how he or she participates in a group. Through the process of reflection, the participant can decide if he or she is an engaged, active participant in one of many ways. Or the participant can decide if his or her way of working in the group is distracting the group from completing their tasks.

On the following page is a *dynamic* which will help trainers, CLWs and all participants in organizations to analyze themselves. It also provides a good opportunity for healthy feedback.

The animal in you

What we want to accomplish:

- Each person analyzes how he or she participates in a group.
- Everyone defines the importance of honest feedback.
- Each person receives honest feedback about his or her participation in groups.

What you will need:

- A picture of the animal participants in a group.
- A large picture is placed on the wall where everyone can see it:

Each animal has distinct characteristics.

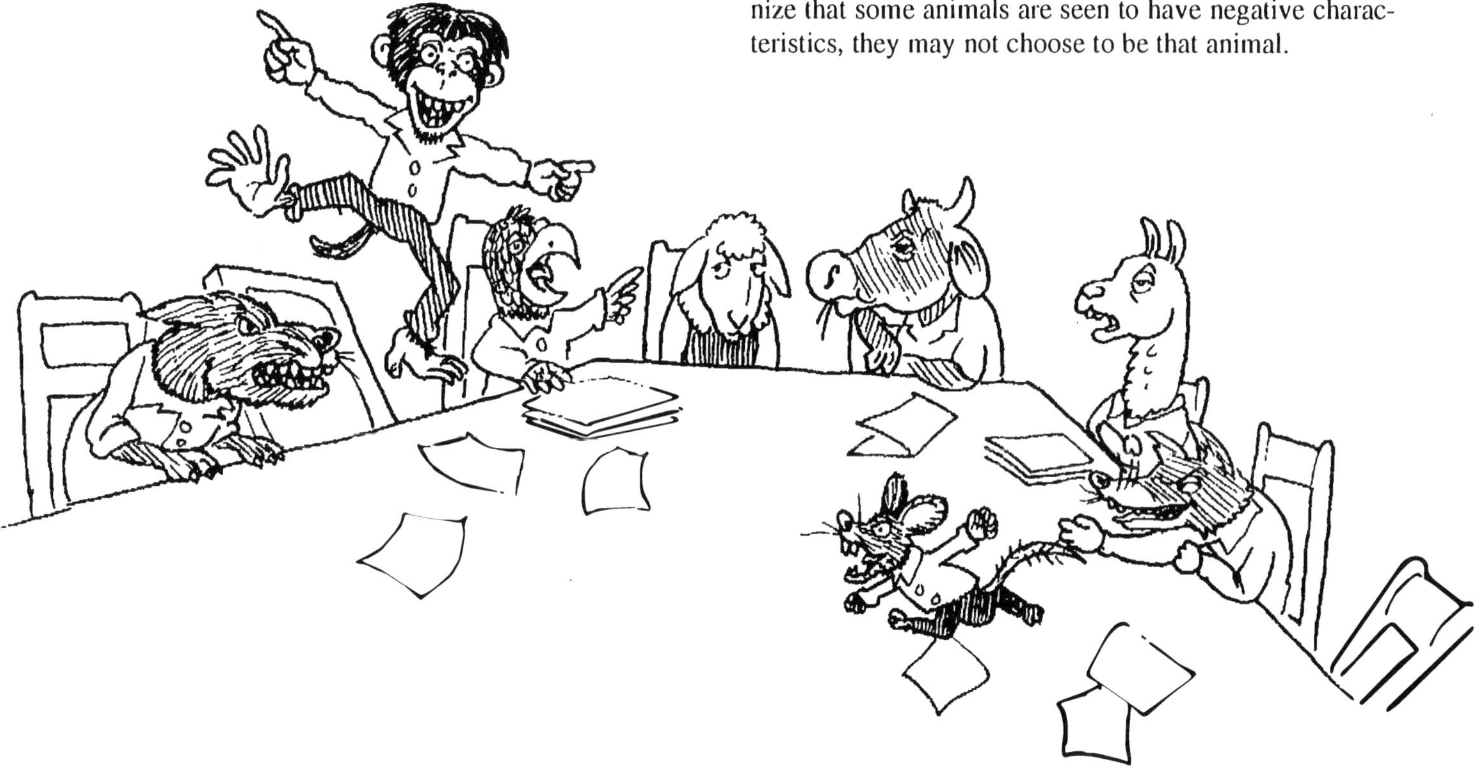

- Participants decide which animal they think they are most like when they participate in group work.
- Then everyone finds a partner who has worked with him or her at some time in the workshop. Each partner will tell the other what animal he or she thinks the partner is most like when they participate in a group. Then they analyze the characteristics. How different is the individual's chosen animal from the animal chosen by the partner for the individual?
- In the plenary as each animal is discussed, people raise their hands to show if they participate as that animal. The characteristics are listed. Generally everyone will list the positive characteristics of each animal. Or if they recognize that some animals are seen to have negative characteristics, they may not choose to be that animal.

● **Ask:**

- What is a friend?
- What is an enemy?

Talk together about friend vs. enemy.

Sometimes we think a friend is someone who only tells us positive things about ourselves, while an enemy says bad things about us. We need to have honest feedback from our friends as well as our enemies.

● Do these animals also have negative characteristics?

What are they? List them beside the positive characteristics for each animal.

Negative	Positive
gets into fights	faithful friend
very disruptive always playing around thinks he knows everything	funny to be with
Talks all the time whether he has something to say or not	has some good ideas
Quiet, bashful, doesn't participate with opinions	goes along with the crowd a calm friend, doesn't create problems
Is indifferent. Doesn't offer opinions or accept those of others	placid
Is proud, puts everyone down, doesn't think the discussion is important	Has good opinions decisive leader
Asks questions all the time trying to trip up the leader.	raises some useful questions
Opportunist. Takes advantage of the times when there is disorder to create more disorder	very intelligent has interesting opinions

● Do people also have positive and negative characteristics?

● How do the negative characteristics affect our work in groups?

● When we give feedback, why do we usually only give the positive side?

● Is that being honest with our partners?

● What value does negative feedback have for us?

> Wounds from a friend can be trusted,
> but an enemy multiplies kisses.
> Proverbs 27:6

● Ask the partners to come together again and to give honest feedback to each other. Ask them to give both the positive and the negative sides to each person. In plenary, ask everyone how they felt. Did they agree with their partner's assessment? How will this information be used in future group work?

● Give everyone a copy of the picture to take to their community. Put the most important characteristics of each animal on the back of the picture.

● This dynamic will take 1 1/2 to 2 hours. Do not use this in a short workshop where people do not have time to participate and demonstrate to others how they participate in groups.

Source: Paul Daughtery, Oxfam UK, Nepal

For more suggestions for self reflection see "Facilitators," pg. 49.

Getting rid of "me first"

Working well together also depends upon our attitude toward the group. If we always have an attitude of "Me first," or "What's in it for me?" the group will not function well. We need to develop attitudes of collaboration and negotiation in the workshop and in our organization. The place to begin is valuing the work of the group and recognizing the importance of working together.

Four *dynamics* for valuing group work:

Every person for him or herself

● Place three men and three women in the center of the circle of participants in different places apart from one another.

● Cover their eyes with blindfolds, put clear tape (or handkerchiefs) over their mouths, and tie their hands. But one person doesn't have her hands tied, and one doesn't have tape on his mouth. Next to the latter person is one who is tied really tightly. Two are tied to each other.

● Tell them: you have one minute to take all constraints off. Those who do, win a prize.

● It's always every person for him or herself.

● Ask everyone, "What did you see happening here?"

● Help people to think about what they saw happening. The one whose hands are tied undoes his hands and doesn't help others; the others thought only of themselves, not of helping others. The one with an uncovered mouth didn't speak to help the others.

● Ask the participants, "How did you feel?"

● Ask everyone: How is this like the organization? Do people think about others in the organization? You can ask one of the participants, "Did you think about helping any of the others?"

● As they answer, their ideas are written on a large piece of newsprint.

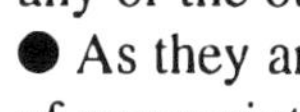

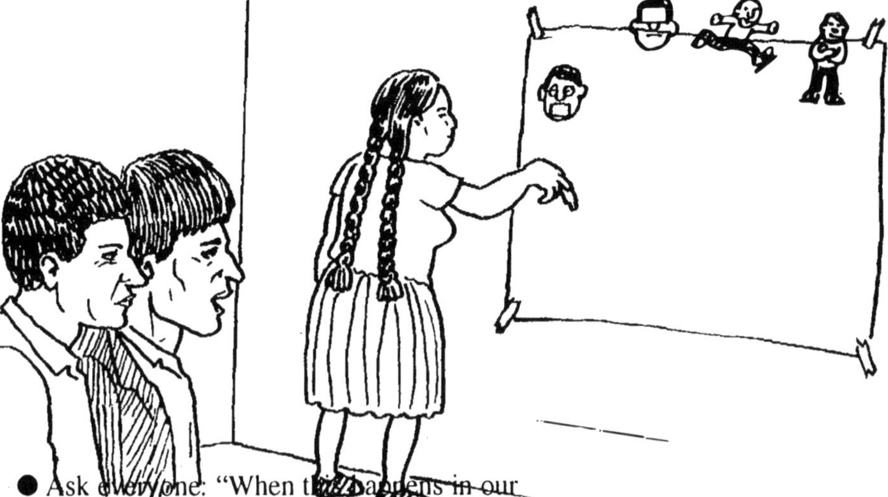

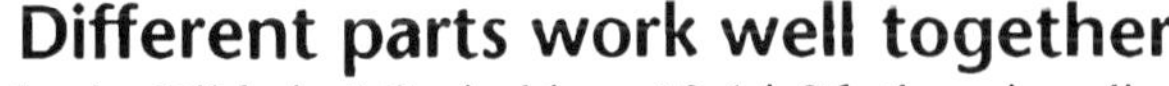

● Ask everyone: "When this happens in our organization, what problems does it cause?"

● Continue the discussion as people link this behavior to their group or organizational behavior.

● What can be done to overcome this problem?

● The organization must have solidarity to function well. We must think of others first, not only of self.

Source: C-CIMCA

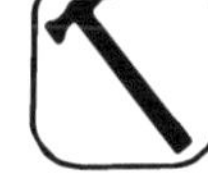

Different parts work well together

In the Bible in I Corinthians 12:14-26, there is a discussion of how the body has many parts which are different but are necessary for it to function as a whole. The parts of the body that seem weaker are indispensable, and the parts we think are less honorable we should treat with honor. The parts should have equal concern for one another. If one part suffers, every part suffers with it; if one part is honored, every part rejoices with it.

The idea that everyone who participates in an organization can bring value to the tasks of the organization is an important one for all organizations. The same applies to small-group work in participatory workshops. There is a tendency to exclude some people or think they will not help the group work. Each person brings a new and different experience and perspective to group problem solving and work.

For literate people, these verses in Corinthians are very valuable as a starting point of discussion. For people who read with difficulty, a game or role play can be used as a *dynamic* and then the verse read and discussed. An example of a game would be the above *dynamic* of untying yourself or you can have a relay race.

A relay race:

- Ask for eight volunteers. Form two teams of four.
- In each team, random members are disabled: one with an arm or leg tied, some with mouths covered, or hands tied together.
- Each person must run to the end of the room with a balloon, break it, eat crackers and whistle, then run back to the next person. The team who finishes first wins. They usually try to do the whole race without helping each other. But they see it is impossible and start to help each other to be able to finish. If they don't help, they can't finish the race.
- What did you see happening here? Does it happen in our group or organization? When it happens what problems does it cause? What force does our group have when we work together, respecting the weaknesses or problems and the strengths and gifts of all and helping one another?
- What can we do to change the way we work together?
- Make a list of the suggestions of everyone for working together.

Source: Goma K Shrestha, Pokhara, Nepal

The numbers game

Another fun *dynamic* to open the discussion about working together and good cooperation.

- Form 2 teams from everyone present. Each team chooses four representatives. Each of the four people on each team has a large number (from one to four) attached to his or her chest.
- Now put each team face to face in two lines.
- The facilitator calls out a number (made up of 1,2,3, and 4, for example, 2,143 or 1,324) and the teams have to organize themselves into that number by the count of three. The team who does it the fastest wins the point.
- Play with 5 or 6 numbers and keep score.

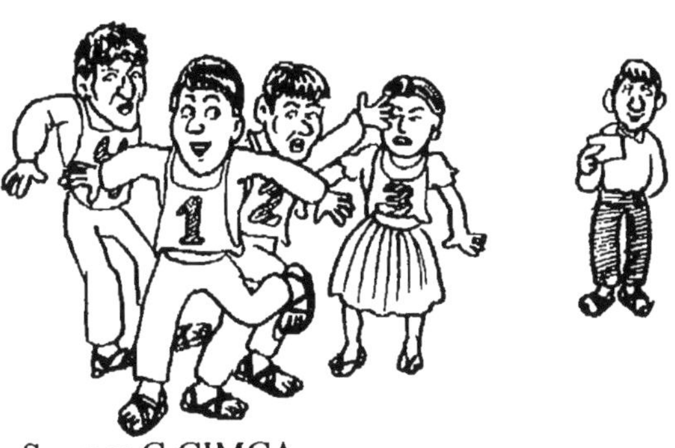

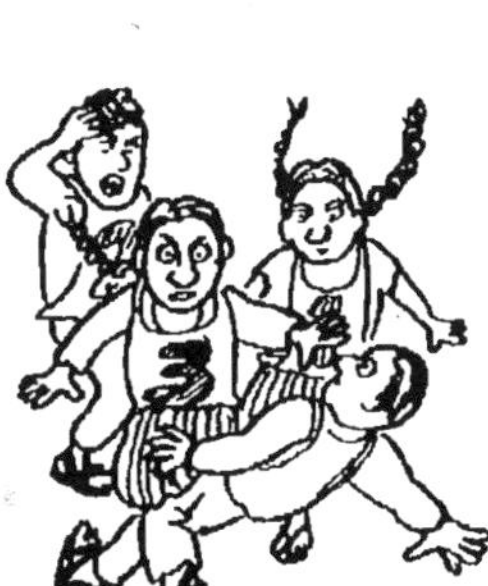

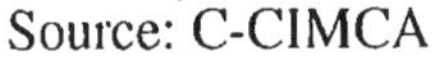

Source: C-CIMCA

- How did everyone feel? Did they coordinate well? Have small groups meet to make a list of the most important aspects of group coordination. Present them in a plenary session and make a final chart of how to coordinate and work together in a group.

Take a trust walk

● Form pairs randomly by numbering off.

● One of the pair is blindfolded the other is not. The blindfolded person depends on the sighted person to lead and keep him or her from getting hurt while they arrive at their destination.

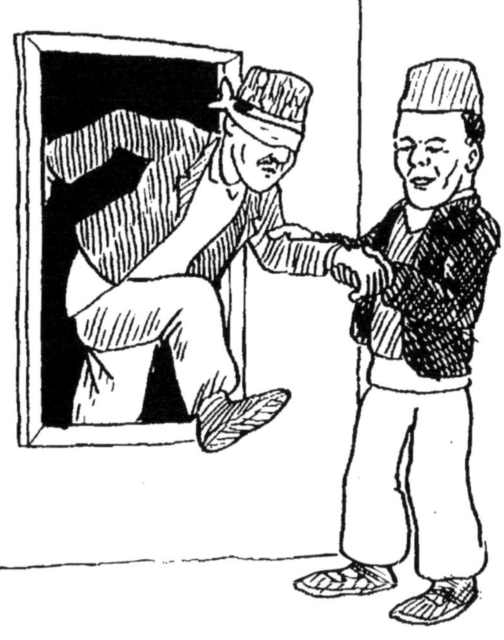

● They need to get across the room or through some obstacle course, or up or down stairs. Or you can send them all outside to walk around together for 5–7 minutes.

● Change blindfolds to the other person and repeat the exercise.

● In the plenary, people can share how they felt. They can discuss the elements of trusting others, good communication, and how much we look out for one another. People share the way this relates to their family or organization. How can they work together better? This is a very powerful dynamic for personal discovery. As each person makes a personal discovery and changes his or her behavior in the group, the group or organization can work together better.

Source: C-CIMCA, Oruro, Bolivia

How well is our organization working?

As an organization or group works and develops together, problems may appear in its functioning. Sometimes, for the initiation of a discussion about those problems, it is good to use a dynamic about organization. Here is one dynamic which works well to begin a discussion about organizational functioning. This is also a great dynamic for considering women's participation (or lack of participation) in the community organization.

The river crossing

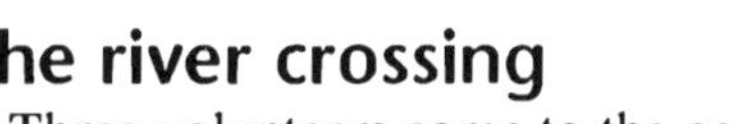

● Three volunteers come to the center of the circle. One has her eyes blindfolded, another has his hands tied and the other her legs tied and mouth covered with a handkerchief or tape. (asking for people's handkerchiefs is a good way to tie up the people.)

● These three people stand on three chairs (make sure the chairs are sturdy but lightweight).

● On the floor the banks of a river are drawn in the dirt or with chalk, or defined by two ropes.

● The three chairs are on one bank in a row.

● **The instructions:** cross the river on these chairs, without getting wet.

- The other participants should not help. Sometimes they will figure out how to do it. Sometimes the person with their mouth covered will jump their chair across, leaving the others.
- After they have tried for some time, if they do not make progress, have people make suggestions to them. If they still cannot, whisper to one who can talk that they pull one another onto two chairs and move the third chair forward into the river. Then they help each other onto the chair in the river and one other chair and put the last chair up front. In this way they can cross the river on the chairs. Don't stray too far in case someone isn't stable on the chair.
- **Ask everyone:**
  - What did you see happening here?
  - Was everyone on their team equal?
    Did they all have the same skills?
  - Could they have gotten everyone across by themselves?
  - Does our organization have people who try to do it themselves only for themselves?
  - Do we always use everyone's skills in the group to the maximum possible?
  - What happens in our groups or organizations when we don't use everyone?
  - What can we do to change this situation in our organization?

Source: C-CIMCA, Oruro, Bolivia

This chapter has discussed two important areas: Healthy Communication and Healthy Groups.

If this chapter has increased your interest and desire to facilitate better communication and better group work, please look in the "Reference" section, pg. 330 and 333 for places to find more information.

Chapter 11
Traditional management and medicine
by B.J. Lindquist

This chapter covers the following topics:

This chapter, **written by Dr. B.J. Lindquest,** focuses on the importance and application of ethnoveterinary knowledge to animal health training programs. It is a specific example of how local or traditional technical knowledge should be considered and incorporated in all agriculturally based technical training programs. The same principles suggested here can be used for animal husbandry and management practices as well as traditional tree, crop, soil or fodder practices.

Definitions of traditional veterinary medicine and practice

Some commonly used terms:

Traditional Veterinary Medicine= Ethnoveterinary Knowledge (EVK)

Ethnoveterinary means people's own cultural veterinary knowledge. This includes, but is not limited to knowledge about disease diagnosis, cause, prevention, and treatments.

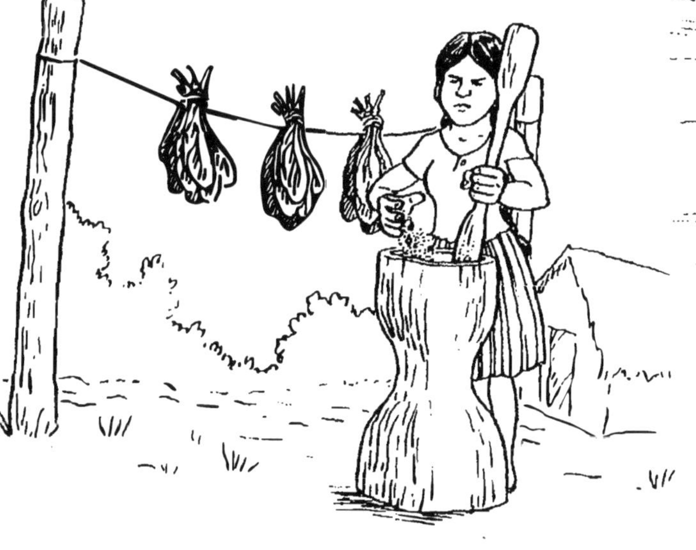

Traditional Technical Knowledge (TTK):

This is the broad body of technical information which a community or culture has developed through extensive trial and error. TTK includes EVK but also includes indigenous animal husbandry and management as well as other forms of technical knowledge in agriculture and many other disciplines.

Occidental:

In this chapter occidental is used to refer to all medicine and management practices which are not traditional or indigenous. In some places this is also called "modern," "scientific," or "western." Since TTK is also modern and scientific, and since some comes from the west, these words can be confusing.

Why is it important to include EVK in an animal health training program?

1. Understanding EVK is important so that we all use the same words.

We have talked about who makes the best facilitators of training (see "Facilitators," pg. 39) and about why speaking the same language is very important. The facilitator may be from a different ethnic group, may have a different mother tongue, or may have a different concept of disease from those he or she is working with. Even though a person facilitates in the same mother tongue as the participants, the facilitator may have received his or her own education or training in another language. As a result, the facilitator may not have correctly translated names for diseases or other words.

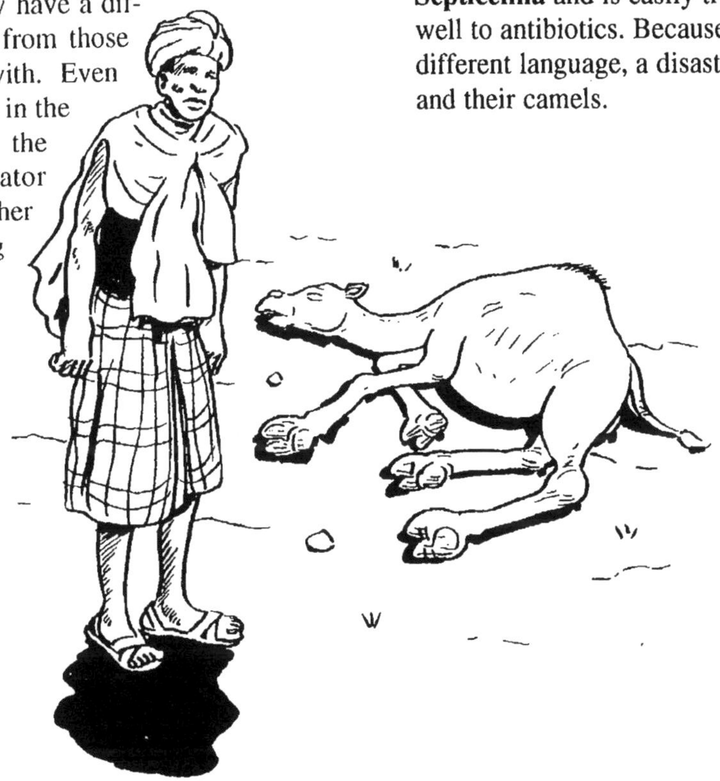

A true story:

Several years ago there was a very bad camel epidemic in Northern Kenya. The Gabra herders were familiar with this disease and called it **ganno.** They knew they did not have an effective local remedy. A Gabra animal health assistant trained in English and Swahili translated **ganno** as **trypanasomiasis.** The responsible veterinary department sent in drugs to help curb this widespread and serious epidemic. They sent a cattle trypanasomiasis drug which for camels is ineffective at best and at worst fatal. The results were not good and many more camels died, of the disease and of the drug.

The disease **ganno** is actually **Hemorrhagic Septicemia** and is easily treated since it responds well to antibiotics. Because everyone was speaking a different language, a disaster occurred for the Gabra and their camels.

At the most basic level, then, traditional knowledge is important so that when animal problems are being discussed everyone is talking about the same problem.

2. EVK is important as a foundation for training.

Grounding the training program in what participants know makes it easier to respond to their priorities of what is important and what is not. The program springs from their learning needs.

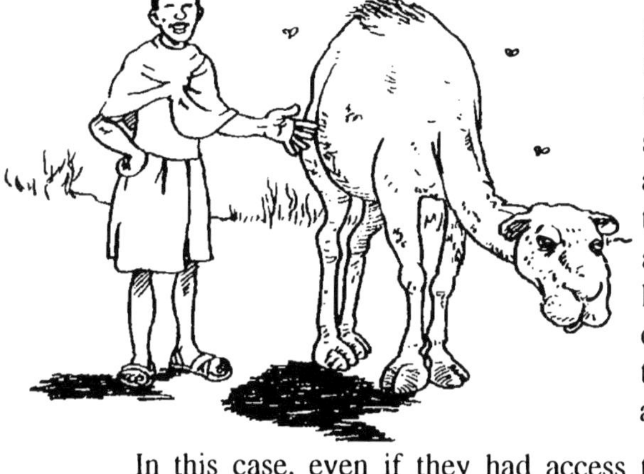

In some areas of Kenya, people do not know and do not have names for some of the signs and symptoms they see. One group of people had animals with unthrifty condition, poor hair coat, diarrhea and worms. But they did not link the conditions to each other or to the worms. In fact, they were not aware that their animals were unwell.

In this case, even if they had access to worming medicines, they would not be aware that they were needed. In planning training with these communities, it was clear that time should be spent on recognizing specific symptoms of ill health and linking these to specific diseases.

Many groups of pastoralists are very sophisticated in their abilities to recognize specific diseases. Often they are much more accurate and thorough in disease description than many occidental veterinarians. With such groups, it would be a waste of everyone's time to dedicate much time to signs, symptoms, and indicators of ill health. When the EVK is understood, training can move rapidly into prevention, management, and treatment of disease.

3. Understanding EVK is important to affirm effective traditional prevention or treatment of disease.

Local people have often been taught to feel that outsiders have "better" knowledge. It sometimes takes a great effort to show that a facilitator or program values local knowledge. If the EVK of an area is incorporated into a program, effective traditional measures will not be undermined by a workshop. They will be reinforced in the training process.

A true story:

In a program in the Samburu area in Kenya, training was begun on occidental dewormers. This was started without knowing what the Samburu had done before the advent of modern medicines. The program didn't really know if the animals had much need of dewormers.

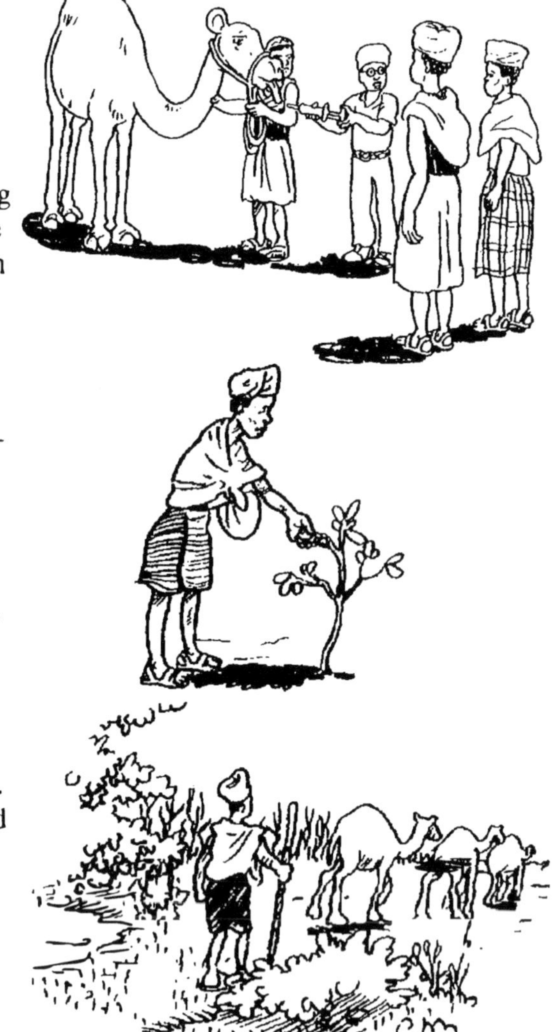

Much later, after the training program was underway, some EVK treatments were discussed. It became clear immediately that the Samburu have several herbs which they feel are very effective in controlling worms. It was also found that they know the areas in which worms are a problem. In fact, if they are concerned about worms, they will move their animals away from those areas. They understand which areas are drier and where the waters have minerals which they feel will take care of the worm problem.

The facilitators could have saved time and expense by understanding and respecting the local EVK before starting the training program. Encouraging the Samburu in their knowledge would have built their self esteem and affirmed the value of their local knowledge.

4. Understanding EVK allows the trainers and community to focus on the diseases which do not have confidently used local treatments.

This allows a training program to concentrate on specific local problems in disease and management. It also encourages solutions appropriate to the local situation.

5. Understanding EVK helps trainers understand the key differences between women's and men's local knowledge and helps them make the training appropriate to each group.

To fully incorporate women and their needs into the training program see Chapter 9 pg. 195.

In much of the EVK work which has been done in Kenya and Bolivia women knew many more herbal treatments than men. Women were also willing to try some treatment rather than see an animal suffer and die without trying anything. Women, in many cultures, do much more nursing care and they can recognize the symptoms of a disease progressing or the signs of a return to health. This can have great impact on many decisions made in planning the training program. Discuss what topics are appropriate for men and women. Invite women to share their knowledge with others.

6. Understanding EVK is important to help develop training which will reinforce and spread the body of local knowledge.

As the traditional concepts of diseases and the methods of diagnosing, preventing, and treating disease are discussed and affirmed in training sessions, people gain confidence in their own time-tested methods. They will share methods which some may have forgotten. They will teach one another methods known only to certain families or groups. Younger people will value things they may have discarded as being primitive and outdated.

As facilitators we must understand EVK and interact with it. EVK alone is not the answer. It takes more than just EVK to focus training on appropriate diseases and treatments. But local people's respect for EVK and the outsider's appreciation of it can help form the basis of an appropriately focused training program.

7. EVK is an economically sound approach to prevention, management, and treatment.

Many of the local treatments and methods are much more appropriate and economically sound than an occidental treatment under the same conditions. Thus, the expansion of the body of local knowledge contributes to economically sound animal health solutions. A training program which focuses only on occidental solutions can contribute to the loss of EVK because people devalue their knowledge.

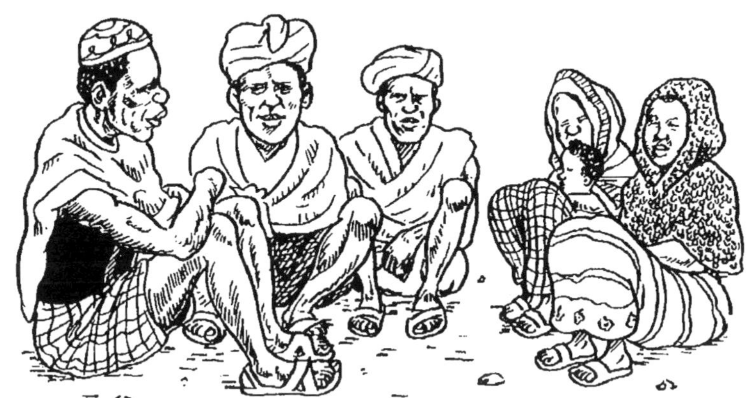

Understanding EVK: a process followed in Kenya

This is an example of a process used to help people study their traditional knowledge in veterinary medicine. It is a process which has been changed and refined by many different facilitators from different organizations. This approach can be modified for work with different peoples and areas of technical knowledge. You can change the process or *dynamics* (see "Tools," section on assessment pg. 253). You can also change the content to look at traditional practices in technical areas other than animal health (crops, forestry, nutrition, etc.).

For more information on Assessments see chapter 4 "Defining the Situation," pg. 57.

You will recognize this process as one similar to a training assessment in the tools and approach it uses.

When we use this process we make these assumptions:

- The community is already actively and participatively planning their own development.
- They have realized and embraced the importance of their own knowledge.
- They have been involved in requesting and planning their own training.
- They understand and support the reasons for studying their own knowledge.

The six steps are:

1. Brainstorm
2. Rank the diseases
3. Semi-structured interviews with an EVK question list
4. Community feedback and discussion
5. Look at diseases which are confidently treated by local methods
6. Write a disease description

STEP ONE: Brainstorm

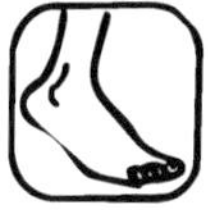

- Divide into small groups, separating men and women
- Brainstorm the names of animal diseases or problems
- Separate this list by species: all the diseases of cattle, sheep, camels, etc.
- Have people shout out the names of all the diseases they can remember.
- When the disease is mentioned it is repeated and written down on its own card.
- Go back through the list. If there is any discussion or disagreement about whether it is really a disease, this discussion should be encouraged until some consensus is reached.

For more information on Brainstorming see chapter 4 "Tools," pg. 238.

The end result is a master list by species of all of the diseases that the community is aware of. This is based on the representation by the groups of men and women. Each disease is written on its own card, indicating the species.

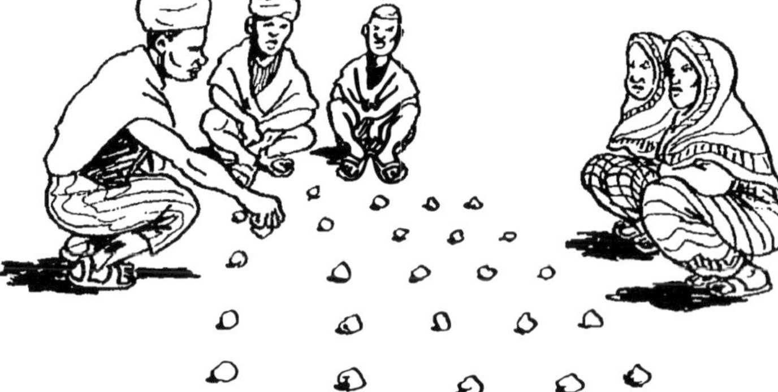

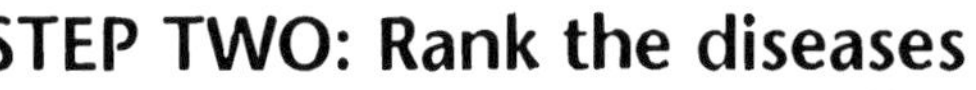

STEP TWO: Rank the diseases

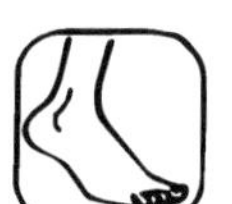

If the groups who have brainstormed still have the energy and interest, it is helpful for them to rank the diseases. They would rank them from the most common or most important to the least common or important.

For more information on ranking see "Tools,"pg. 255. Also see "Planning," pg. 90 and "Valuing women," pg. 186.

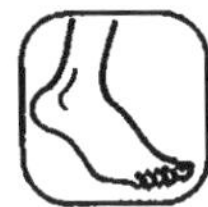

STEP THREE: Semi-structured interviews with an EVK question list

Over a period of time, various individuals of both sexes and all ages are questioned on their understanding of specific diseases. An EVK question list is used (see right) in a semi-structured interview.

For more information on how to do a semi-structured interview see "Tools," pg. 261.

- Ask each person about no more than three diseases. Most people are comfortable with the time it takes to talk about two diseases.
- Those asking the questions need to keep in mind that they are the learners. The people who are answering the questions are the experts who are being asked to share their knowledge and expertise for the rest of the community.
- The "disease information scribes" write down all of the information people give them. They do not cut off important pertinent digressions. Questions are open-ended. We have found it is best to write the answers in a notebook. This allows plenty of space for writing.
- Ask at least three (but preferably four) people about each disease. It is good to have equal numbers of men and women. Then the answers are compiled and compared with one another.

Ethnoveterinary question list

(a sample for semi-structured interviewing)

These questions will need to be adjusted for your area. Do not use it like a questionnaire. Use it as a reminder of the topics to ask about.

1. What **a)** species **b)** ages **c)** sexes of animal are affected?
2. When (season) and where (location) does the disease occur?
3. Does it usually affect one animal or a group of animals at one time? Does it spread from animal to animal?
4. What causes the disease?
5. Are there ways to prevent/avoid the disease?
6. Describe the symptoms in the order of progression or timing: **a)** What is the first symptom seen? **b)** What is the second symptom seen? etc.
7. Are there traditional treatments available? What are they? Where can they be found/ obtained? How effective are they? (always, often, sometimes, not often)
8. Are there modern treatments available? What are they? Where can they be found/obtained? Are they effective? (always, often, sometimes, not often)
9. What usually happens if the animal is not treated?
10. When did you last have an animal with this disease?
11. What happened to it? (die, recover, slaughter, still sick)
12. Are there other diseases similar to this one? How do you distinguish between them?
13. In relation to livestock and disease: What are things that women know how to do better than men? What are things men know how to do better than women?
14. What do women never do? What do men never do?

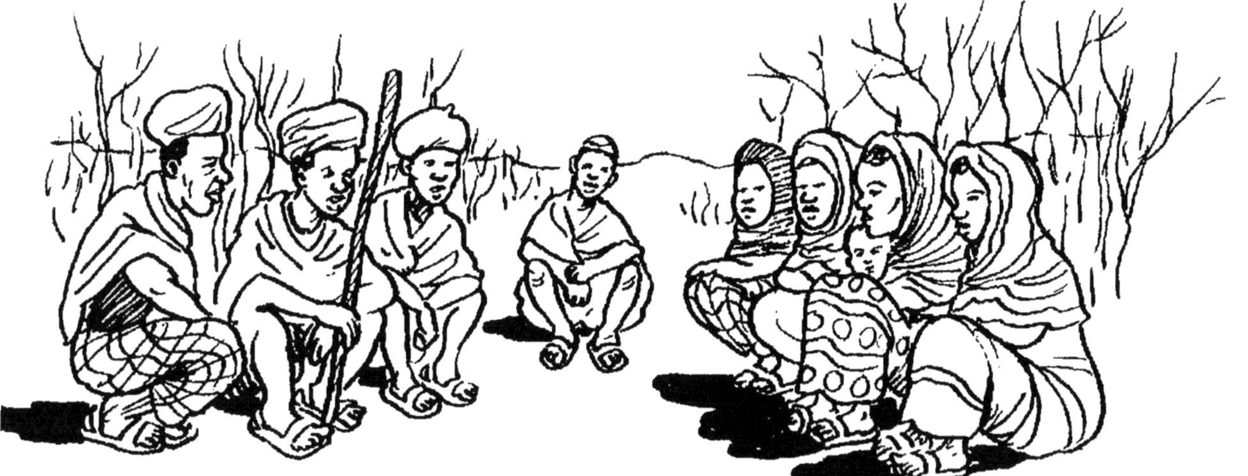

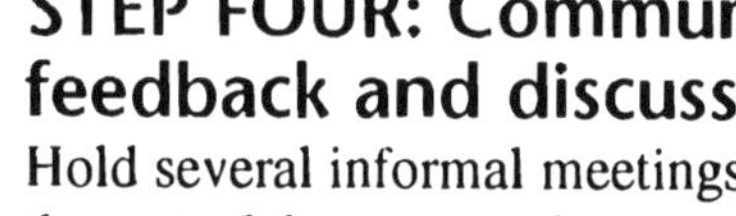

STEP FOUR: Community feedback and discussion

Hold several informal meetings with the contributors and the rest of the community to review the details of the diseases to check for accuracy and thoroughness. Any new tidbits or strong disagreements can then be noted and incorporated into the body of the information. For diseases on which there is very little consensus and lots of wildly varying information, more attention and digging is required. This is especially true if the community feels the diseases are important.

A true story:

During an EVK process in the highlands of Bolivia, the group of scribes and facilitators wanted to check their information with the community. They presented the information as a picture. The picture was the facilitator's concept of the local management calendar for alpacas and llamas. When everyone in the community began to discuss the pictures, a serious debate took place. The facilitators had represented the management calendar using the seasons of spring, summer, autumn, and winter. The people had no such concept of their agricultural year! Through the debate, the calendar was adjusted to reflect the rainy and drought seasons. The annual rituals of management were corrected.

Because the facilitators had made a picture of their concept of the local EVK the people could see what the facilitators understood. As the people saw that the facilitators did not understand correctly, they made suggestions and gave corrections. The new drawing was presented to the groups in a later meeting for their approval.

It is very important to have a good check-back process with the community!

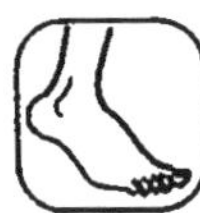

STEP FIVE: Look at diseases which are confidently treated by local methods.

This is a ranking *dynamic* to define the confidently treated diseases. This is probably more fun if done in groups, but can also be done by individuals.

Some diseases have local treatments but the consensus is that they do not work very well. Other diseases do not have any local treatment. Still others have treatments that most people feel confident are effective. This *dynamic* can be used to define which diseases need interventions if there are no local effective treatments. It can also be used to prevent undermining of local treatments. In training, confidently used remedies can be affirmed and discussed, and the treatments prepared and applied during the workshop.

- It is best to divide into groups of all men or all women. This is because for treatments, men and women will often have significantly different knowledge. In a mixed group a woman may not share her traditional knowledge.
- Put three categories on the ground: Very good treatment, moderately good, no local treatment.
- Use the disease cards from the master disease list. If people do not read or write, they can develop a symbol for each disease (for example a dry bone for a disease which always kills).
- The first card or symbol is held up, read (or the symbol defined) and given to the group.
- Ask the group if the disease has a very good local treatment, a moderately effective (so-so) local treatment, or no treatment at all. Often the participants will have a significant argument or discussion. The participants put the card in one of the categories on the ground based on the group consensus.
- Read the next disease and give the card to the participants. They put the card in its category.
- The same thing follows until all the diseases have been covered. Through the course of the exercise, some of the diseases change categories.
- At the end, name the diseases in each category out loud. Give a final chance for discussion and change.

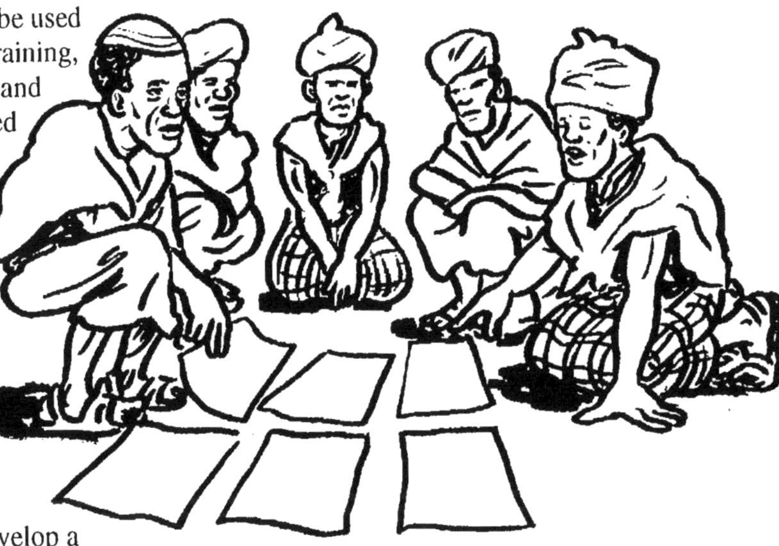

Once each category is complete, the participants can take a closer look at the diseases in one category. The participants will have a long list of diseases confidently treated by local treatments. The participants take the cards within that list and rank them. Within the category of confidently treated diseases, they rank the diseases from most to least confidently treated. This is done because medicine is an art. The confidence level will not be the same for all diseases effectively treated.

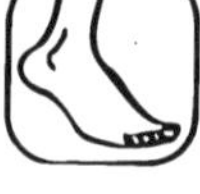

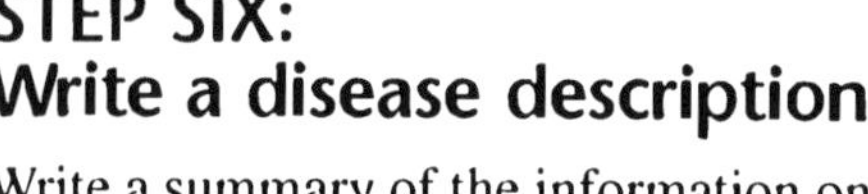

STEP SIX:
Write a disease description

Write a summary of the information on each disease. This is a compilation of all of the information gathered. It is a compact way of pulling together the information on each disease for members of the community as well as for interested or involved outsiders.

At each step, check back with the people to confirm the information. At the end, present the disease description for review.

These steps are part of a dynamic and fluid process; as the steps above feed into training, so too does training feed into the steps above…

Blending EVK with occidental medicine

Based on the six steps above and all of the information shared by the community, draft training materials can be prepared. These are focused on the highest priority diseases which all agree do not have effective local treatments. Training sessions can also be scheduled on diseases with effective local remedies or preventive measures that are not widely known. A local expert can train in this area.

Use an EVK study to choose the training topics and materials:

Thus, **the knowledge contributed by the community is used to choose the training topics.** It is also used to write the training materials. They are solidly built on local knowledge about disease. They use local people's own words and concepts about what causes disease, where diseases come from, how the animals look, etc.

Use the EVK study to train about local treatments which are harmful.

It is very important to know the local medicine and management practices which are not beneficial. This information should be included in training.

For example: For very badly infected wounds such as a hyena bite, the Gabra believe that water should be withheld from the animal. This is because they feel that the wound is already wet and "mushy." So if water is withheld, the wound has a better chance of drying out.

This has been discussed in training sessions.

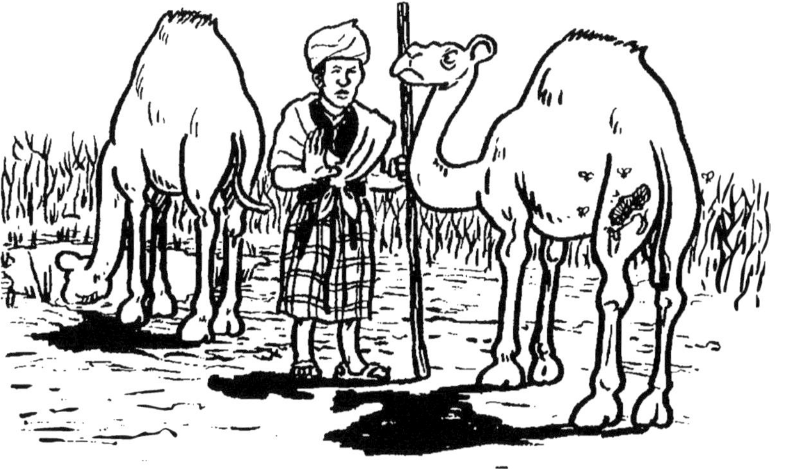

Two things from their own concept of disease helps them to understand the importance of water:

1. We talk about how the medicine needs water to travel all around in the body. If they inject antibiotics for the wound, the medicine will not travel to the wound site very fast if there is no water to help it travel.
2. We talk about water bringing strength to fight and close the wound.

Both of these concepts make sense in their world view. There have been stories of participants going home and giving water to people and animals with wounds and there being full recovery.

Use the EVK study to choose the emphasis in a workshop (prevention, management, signs, treatment, etc.)

When there is traditional knowledge as well as occidental knowledge in use, an EVK study will help to define the emphasis of a workshop.

For example:

The Gabra EVK study helped the trainers to know exactly what a particular disease was in English. The local name was *ganno ree*, literally "fever of smallstock." The people said it was only found in the highlands, always comes from the *dirandess* (amblyomma ticks), does not have an effective local treatment, and is treatable with antibiotics. That, together with the signs, pointed directly to Heartwater disease.

All Gabra herders know that it is preventable by avoiding the highlands where the ticks are. They also know to use acaricides to kill ticks if they must take their animals there.

So what remained for the workshop sessions was to:

1. Affirm their preventative methods
2. Teach safe acaricide use
3. Teach proper doses of antibiotics

Thus, traditional knowledge and modern knowledge are brought together in a useable and practical way.

Conclusions

This chapter is based on the concept that the people in an agricultural training program must know and respect local knowledge before designing a training program. Defining the local knowledge is an integral part of defining the local situation. The ideas in this chapter are relevant to the rest of the world, not just to pastoralists in Kenya. These same concepts have been used extensively in Asia and Latin America as well.

The process presented in this chapter is an example. The process can be modified by planning appropriate dynamics and a logical sequence for the people and the topic to be covered. The content can be readily changed to be appropriate for soils, crops, trees, human health, and many other areas of technical knowledge.

Caution on spreading EVK

Sharing EVK can be beneficial.

✔ When local knowledge is valued, the people continue to build on their low-cost body of knowledge. Their EVK will serve them well.

✔ As the knowledge of one group is shared with another, it helps to provide low-cost, appropriate treatments for other people as well.

✔ The intermingling of knowledge from different groups causes further testing. New techniques and treatments develop.

Sharing EVK can be harmful.

✘ Business and corporations can "steal" local knowledge for corporate profit. They claim to own the "intellectual property rights" to the local technology. This means the corporation says they invented the idea and no one else can use it without paying the corporation. Many times the corporations give no benefit to the local people who discovered the traditional knowledge. Sometimes hardship is created for the people who discovered the ideas. They must pay for the medicines and seeds they developed.

As facilitators, CLWs, and responsible administrators of agricultural programs, we should ask ourselves what our responsibility is in this situation. It is appropriate to include the discussion of this issue in the dialogue process with the community and in the training of new trainers and CLWs.

You can ask these questions and others:

- How can facilitators and program administrators be responsible in facilitating the description and use of traditional knowledge?
- How can traditional knowledge be used and protected?
- How can the intellectual property rights of local people be ensured?

In some countries, local knowledge systems for treating people and animals are parallel and sometimes integrated into occidental treatment systems. Some countries such as India and China officially recognize and respect traditional knowledge as well as occidental knowledge. As traditional knowledge becomes more widely used and accepted there will be a stronger push to commercialize it. This may bring benefits to all of society, but programs and outsiders involved in a participatory process with village people should consider their role in assuring that this use of traditional knowledge really does benefit the village people who have shared it.

Section 4
Resources, tools and references

This section is jammed with ideas from around the world about how to make your training more participatory and appropriate. Although there are many tools throughout the book, this section will jump start your idea machine during planning of assessment, training and evaluation.

Chapter 12

Tools to help people start thinking and acting

This chapter covers the following topics:

This chapter describes many tools for use in a participatory approach to training. Each tool is described in the following way:

- **Definition**
- **How It Works**
- **Pros, Cons and Other Uses**
- **Example of How It Is Used**

Essential tools for training

Small groups

Definition

This is ***one of the most powerful techniques available*** to the facilitator or organization. Small groups are formed within the training session to focus on a specific task and to foster an atmosphere of trust and sharing through participation. A small group is a forum where participants reflect on experience and teach one another as they discover new truths.

How It Works

- Place workshop participants into small groups of pairs, three, four or five people. A group of more than six people tends to exclude some from the discussion.
- Give each group a task. It may be the same task for all groups or a different task for each group. The instructions given to the small groups must be very clear and understood by all. It is helpful for the facilitators to visit each group to assure that they understand the instructions and to answer questions. The time allotted to perform the task depends on the complexity of the task.
- Sometimes it is helpful for the trainers to join a small group to listen. This will help the trainer to understand the processes of the group. Although trainers can help to clarify the task, they must not give answers or lead the group. Often the best role of the trainer is to sit quietly away from the groups and to be available as a resource.
- Each group reports their work back to all participants in a plenary session. If a group task is one of self-teaching, only a sample of the group's work will be reported back. Reflections and conclusions are drawn from all the reports.

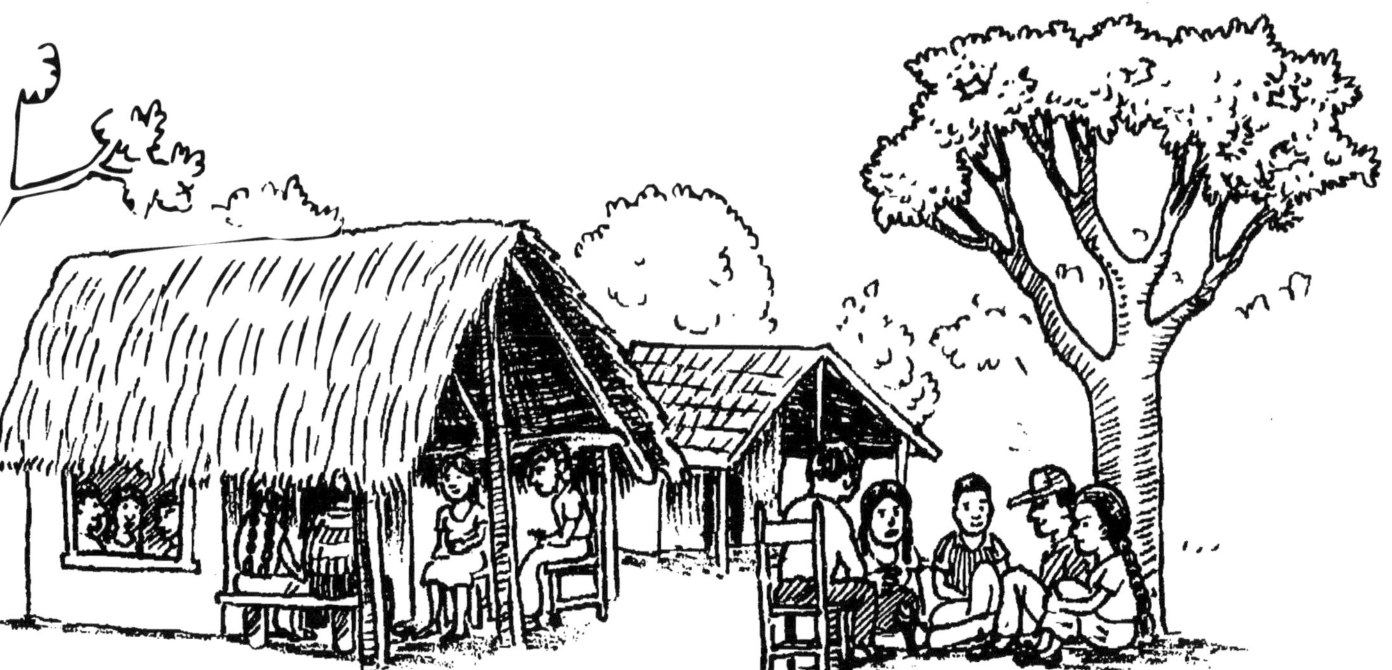

Ways to form small groups: see "Games for Group Formation," pg. 266.

Pros, Cons, and Other Uses

Form homogeneous groups–celebrate our differences!

There are times when randomly breaking into a small group does not provide enough safety for everyone to feel free to express their opinions. This is especially true with a mix of men and women, older and younger people, individuals with unequal education levels, and people from different classes or castes. At these times it may be helpful to form homogeneous groups to dialogue about the task. (women with women, older with older, etc.) This has the added advantage that those who normally do not speak up will express their opinions and be heard.

For example: In a meeting where the village is considering the criteria for selection of their Community Livestock Worker, divide men and women into separate groups (see pg. 38). Because women and men often have very different roles on the farms, their view of what makes a good CLW and what tasks the CLW should perform may be quite different.

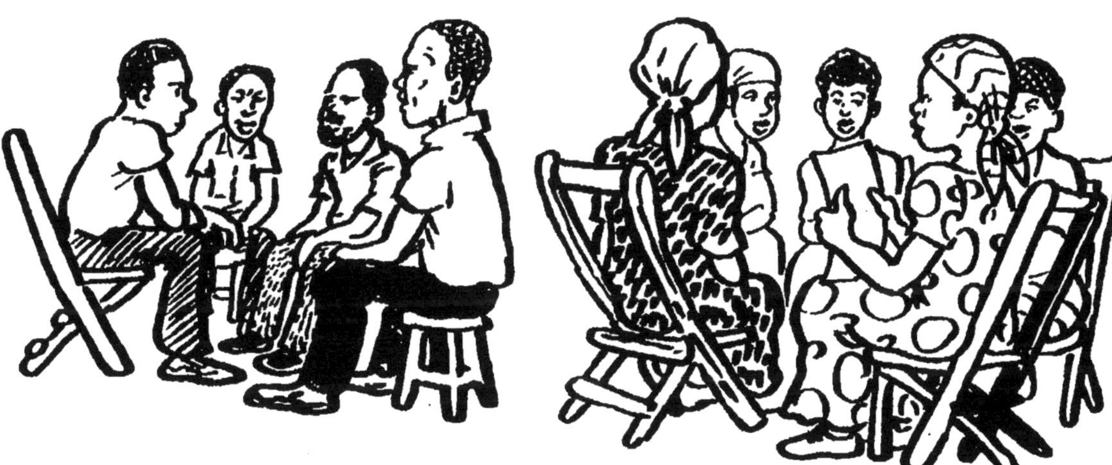

It is also good to divide into homogeneous groups when some of the people in a workshop have had more training in the program than others. This is because if those with more training are randomly mixed with those without training, those attending training for the first time may not share their opinions. They will expect the person with more training to provide all of the answers. This is only true for some tasks and activities for the small group.

It is also good to separate those with more training if they have different perceptions of the community reality. For example: A mixed group of professionals and community people would provide a very different answer to the question, "What is the community organizational structure?" than would a homogeneous group of community people and another group of professionals. It is these differences in understanding which provide the basis of the dialogue in the plenary session. The homogeneous groups can stimulate much learning from one another.

In the community's analysis of their situation, homogeneous groups are often useful. Different life experiences will provide different perspectives on the same issue. Dividing into homogeneous small groups to initiate dialogue allows us to **celebrate the differences and learn from one another.** For example, women who take care of the animals will answer the question, "What are the most serious animal diseases?" differently from men who work mostly with crops. Similarly, older women will often supply much more information about local treatments in an ethnoveterinary study than will younger women, or men. Wealthier people may have a different perception of the wealth ranking of a community than will poorer people.

Examples of How Small Groups are Used

Here are some of the types of tasks which can be given to a small group:

a. **Brainstorm a list** (cures, diseases, pastures, management techniques, etc.)

b. **Suggest a course of action** (Example: the proper way to set up a vaccination or worming campaign in a community.)

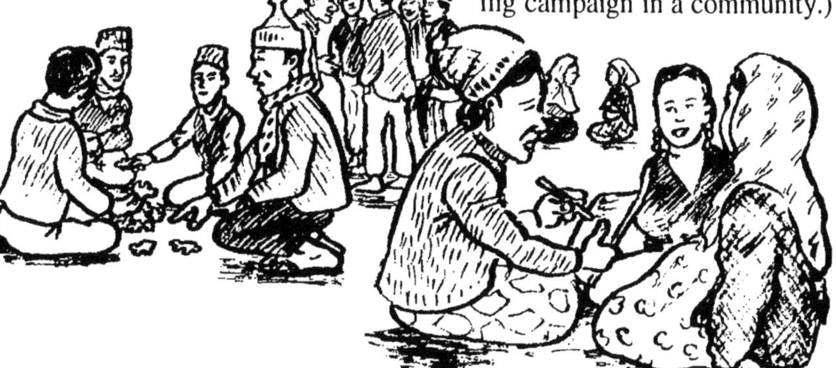

c. **Share experiences.** (Example: the best pastures for a specific management situation. Have the group prioritize three things.)

d. **Try a new technique or skill and evaluate it** (Example: how to inject an animal or how to draw blood from the tail of a cow.)

e. **Determine the most common problems** (Example: do a community map or a ranking exercise to determine the most common land-use problems.)

f. **Reflect on workshop content.** Pairs or small groups can reflect on a principle or idea from their experience or evaluate the day's work.

g. **Analyze a problem or situation.** (Example: each group is given a picture or a set of pictures which pose a problem. The group is asked to organize the pictures, discuss them and draw conclusions. We use this with the theme of community participation. Each picture is related to some situation where the community should participate to have success, such as vaccination campaigns, community meetings, support of the Community Livestock Worker, etc.)

h. **Practice.** (Example: examine and treat an animal. The group can discuss the diagnosis and treatment and report back to the group as a whole.)

i. **Visioning for the future.** (Example: landscape visioning. The small group constructs a landscape on the ground using branches, grasses, pieces of cardboard, paper or plastic. They create their model farm of the future.)

Brainstorming

Definition

In a brainstorming session everyone quickly shares as many ideas related to a theme or question as possible. New, wild or different ideas are encouraged. No idea is judged or rejected. This forms a basis for further discussion or the initial phase of another activity such as ranking and sorting.

How Brainstorming Works

- Request that one person be the recorder for the group.
- Pose a question to the group. It is important that the question is clearly understood by all. You may ask someone for an example to see if the question is clearly understood. If it is not clearly

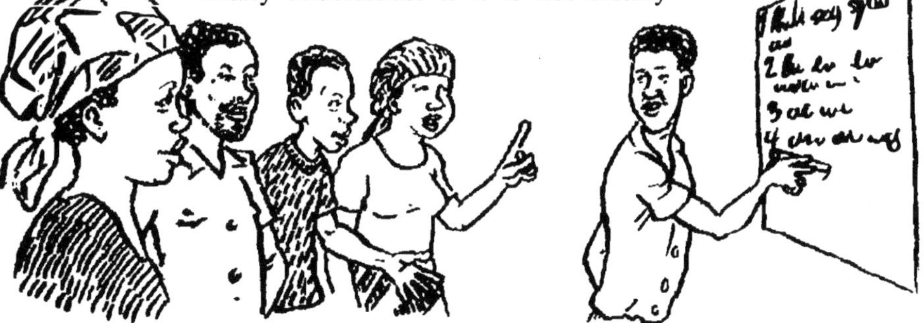

understood, have someone in the group rephrase it. The group generates as many answers to that question as they can. Everyone is encouraged to contribute, no matter how wild they think their idea is.

● There are many ways to record the answers, here are two:

1. Record a list of all of the responses on newsprint.
2. Each person writes or draws an answer on a sheet of paper or a card, one answer per card. Each person brings his or her card up front and sticks it to the wall. One advantage of brainstorming with cards is that, after all of the answers have been shared, the cards can be rearranged and organized into categories.

Hint: The temptation to evaluate each answer is strong! But in evaluating, the flow of ideas is often cut off. When brainstorming, the facilitator must encourage the sharing of a broad range of ideas without judgment of each idea.

● Once a list is formed, the list can be organized into categories. It is best not to put letters or numbers on the categories, since this might imply ranking. Shapes or symbols work well. The group names the categories when they have been organized.

Pros, Cons, and Other Uses

Brainstorming is very useful to:

- Introduce a new topic in a training workshop.
- Form a list of diseases, roles, possessions, etc. for analyzing the situation in a community for a training assessment, gender analysis, or ethnoveterinary knowledge study.
- Form a list of areas to be evaluated, list strengths and weaknesses, list criteria for choosing a Community Livestock Worker.

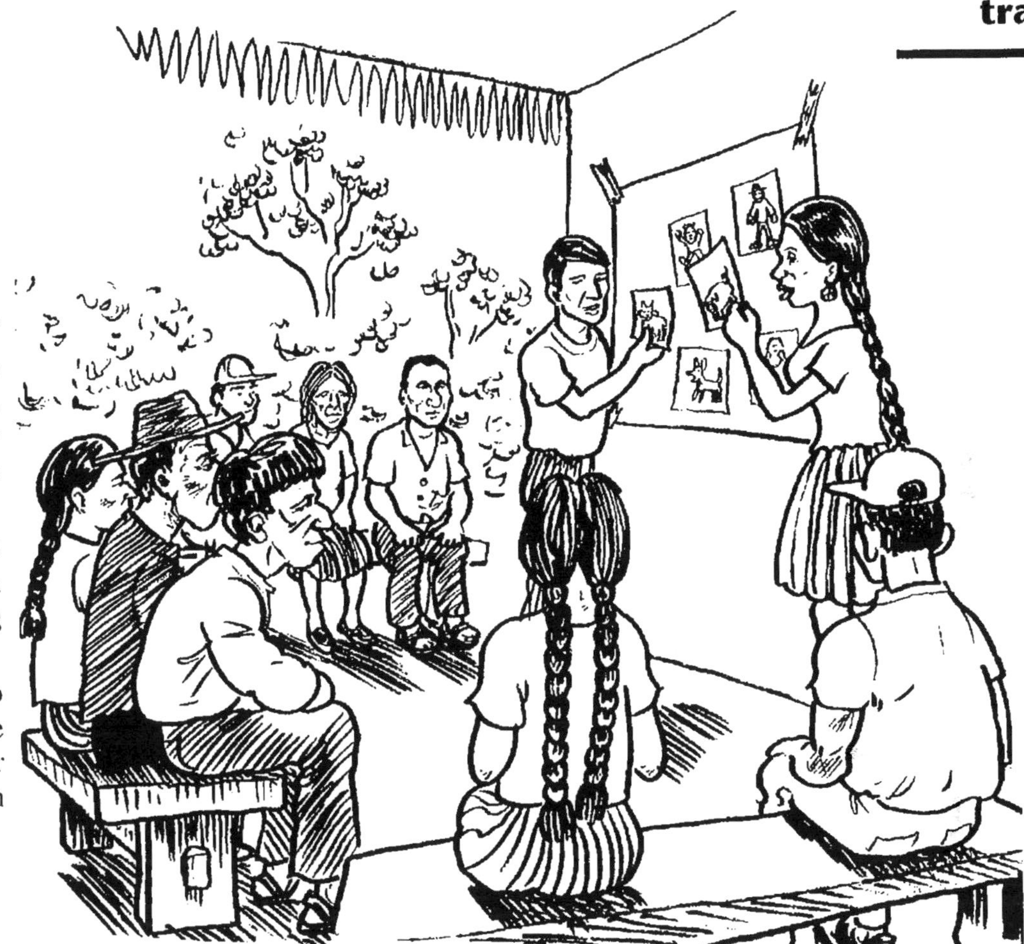

Example of How Brainstorming Is Used

For examples of brainstorming please see "Defining the Situation," pg. 68 and "Understanding EVK" pg. 226.

Practice!

Definition

Practice is the opportunity to perform a skill within a workshop. The skill for a trainer may be designing and planning and then presenting a topic in a workshop. The skill for an animal owner may be castrating an animal. The skill for a hillside farmer may be making an A-frame and using it to mark where to plant live barriers for terraces.

How It Works

For working on an animal:

- Divide into small groups. Make sure each group has an experienced person who does the skill well.
- Explain the task thoroughly, or demonstrate it.
- Make sure each person has the opportunity to practice the skill, preferably on a different animal.
- If teaching aids or animals are needed, let the participants make, get or organize them; don't do it all for them.
- Make sure there is an appropriate place and time to practice the skill. For example, is there clean grass to castrate animals on? Is there a plot of prepared land to plant trees?
- Some things to think about in deciding to do a practice session:
  - Is it safe for participants, others, animals? Include a dialogue about safety precautions and don't encourage risky short cuts.
  - Can you say how far or how long (for example, one digit deep, one liter) to give people an easy concept for measuring?
  - Is a mental calculation needed to perform the skill? How can that be shared?
  - What are the common errors made by experienced people?
- If it is a complex skill break it down into steps (see "Task Analysis," pg. 104–105.)
- Let participants know how they are doing and ask for feedback on the session to help you in the future.
- Have each small group reflect on their practice. How did it go? What problems were there? Will this work in your community? How will you apply it in the future?

Pros, Cons, and Other Uses

Someone can learn how to do a skill like vaccinating but may not vaccinate if they do not think it is necessary. **Practice should be combined with reflection to encourage a change in attitude.**

PRACTICE IS FOR SKILLS.

Practice can **teach livestock or agricultural technical skills,** such as how to measure out a dose of medicine, trim the hooves of an animal, or plant and maintain a windbreak. It can also **teach organizational and communication skills,** such as active listening, leading a meeting, or organizing a vaccination campaign.

PRACTICE IS FOR KNOWLEDGE.

Through practice we learn about how to do something, and we might learn about advantages and disadvantages of doing the skill. But it is in the reflection after the practice that we learn the most from our experience and the experience of others.

PRACTICE DOES NOT USUALLY CHANGE ATTITUDES.

Even though we practice a skill, we may not be convinced of the importance of applying that skill in our organization or animal husbandry. The problem-posing approach helps change attitudes. It is for reflecting on what we are doing now and why it might be good to adopt a different approach. In the same way, dialogue alone about a situation, without an opportunity to practice a new skill, will usually not lead to change. That is why it is so important to analyze and dialogue to determine the appropriate action, then practice the necessary skills for that action.

Remember:

Problem + Analysis + Action plan + Practice skills + Reflection = Change

A true story:

The Community Livestock Workers (CLW) of San Julian and Berlin, Bolivia observed the gradual deterioration of their community's animals over successive generations. They saw that if they could control the quality of the animals, they could control milk, meat and fiber production. They determined that, as CLWs, they should have the skill of castrating animals to assist their communities in selecting the best breeding animals. They also determined that they should include discussions about the problem and the solutions in training sessions with their communities. Because they saw the need to know how to castrate, they requested that the training program teach them castration. The new leaders of the program enthusiastically agreed.

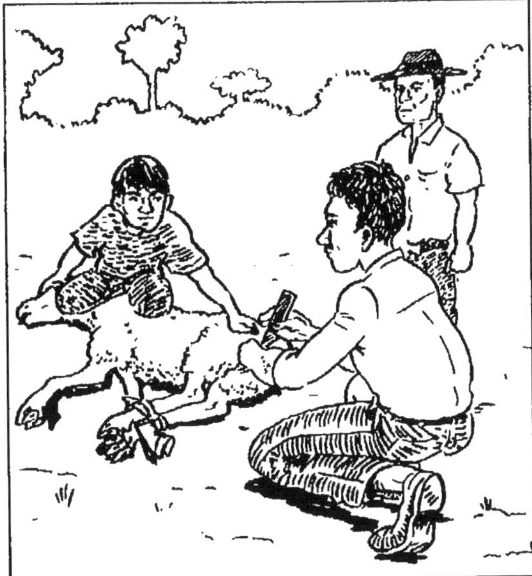

A training session and a demonstration were planned, and the CLWs were divided into two groups to watch the castrations. They decided to do demonstrations because there were not enough animals or facilitators for everyone to practice. After Don Gregorio returned home he was enthusiastic about castrating his own animals and went right out to do it. As he thought through the castration process he had learned, he realized that he did not really know how to do it and could kill his animals with a mistake, so he did not castrate his animals.

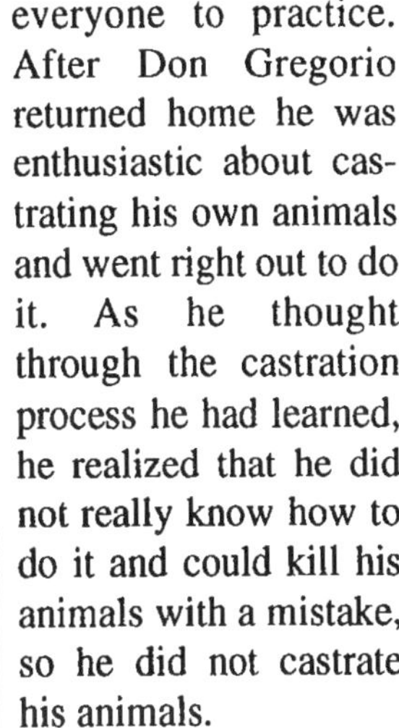

Should castration have been taught in this workshop?

In this case, the objective was that the CLW's be able to castrate at the end of the workshop. That objective was not reached, so castration should not have been taught.

What could the workshop planners have done differently?

Upon reflection of Don Gregorio's dilemma after the workshop, the workshop planners made an adjustment for the next workshop. They organized the whole group into small groups and partners. In each workshop, one small group castrated all the available animals in the community. By the end of their training, all of the CLWs had the opportunity to castrate at least one animal.

Often the decision to include a technical topic in a workshop should be based on whether or not it can be practiced.

For complex skills, people must have the opportunity to practice in order to use the skill in the future.

Ask yourself: If we teach this topic, is there time for everyone to practice? If not, can this skill be performed without practice?

If the answer to both questions is no, do not waste the farmer's time talking about the skill.

Tools which encourage dialogue

Buzz or hum session

Definition

A buzz is a short rapid discussion between a pair, trio, or small group about a specific theme or question.

How It Works

- Rapidly pair off by turning to the person next to you.
- In 2–3 minutes discuss a thought or question generated by the topic under discussion. The facilitator provides the question.
- Report back to the larger group on the results of your discussion.

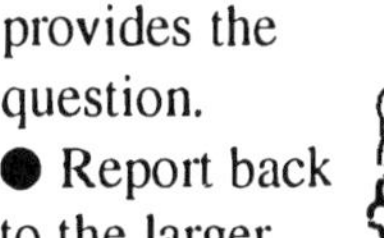

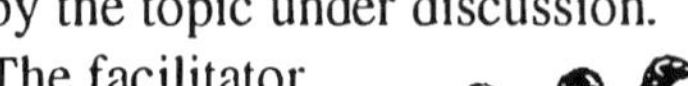

Pros, Cons, and Other Uses

A buzz session is a good way to begin a discussion about a new topic. More people will share their ideas than they would in a plenary session.

A buzz session can be used to generate new ideas about a topic already under discussion. If a discussion gets bogged down, a buzz will often generate new ideas to continue with.

A buzz session can be used to reflect in a personal way on what participants have just learned.

Feedback in the plenary from all of the groups may take time. The facilitator can request sample results, or a calling out of ideas generated.

For an example of using buzz groups, please see pg. 167.

Example of How Practice Is Used

In Uganda, every technical topic discussed in a training session is followed by a session of practice. For example; participants dialogue about land erosion and terracing and discuss the use of an A frame to terrace their sloping pasture lands. Then they build an A-frame and practice by marking the appropriate lines in a participant's field. They follow the practice with a dialogue about what they have accomplished and how it will be useful for them.

Open-ended stories

Definition

An open ended story is also sometimes called a case study or a critical case analysis. It includes the presentation and analysis of an event or incident. Some portion of the story is not complete. The open ended story always poses a problem or question. The participants discuss what might happen in the part of the story not told.

How It Works

- Usually a story has three parts:
  1. **Beginning:** Tells about a problem
  2. **Middle:** Tells about a solution
  3. **Ending:** Tells about an outcome or result

An open-ended story may leave out the beginning, the middle or the ending. Most case studies leave out the ending. The part of the story left out poses a question for the participants.

- The story or case should be taken from **a real life situation,** an experience that could happen in the village of the participants. The story needs to convey a **sense of urgency** or crisis to the participant.
- This tool can be used in many ways. It can be told as a storyteller would tell a tale, or in the form of a drama, or puppet show, or with pictures or a flannel board. The participants discuss the missing part of the story, relate it to their situation, and suggest their solutions to the problem.
- It may help to have one person tell the story and another facilitate the discussion.
- Local people can generally help the facilitators develop a story based on real life in the planning phase of the courses.
- **Be sure the story poses a question** in its open end. There are many suggestions of stories which can be used throughout this book (for examples see pages viii, 42, 125, 184, 189). **The best story, though, is one from the community's reality.**

Examples of How Open-Ended Stories Are Used

When the MIDDLE of a story is removed, it becomes a before and after story.

The participants discuss:

1. What are the problems at the beginning?
2. What were the final results (how has the situation specifically improved)?
3. What possible steps did the community take to get to these results?

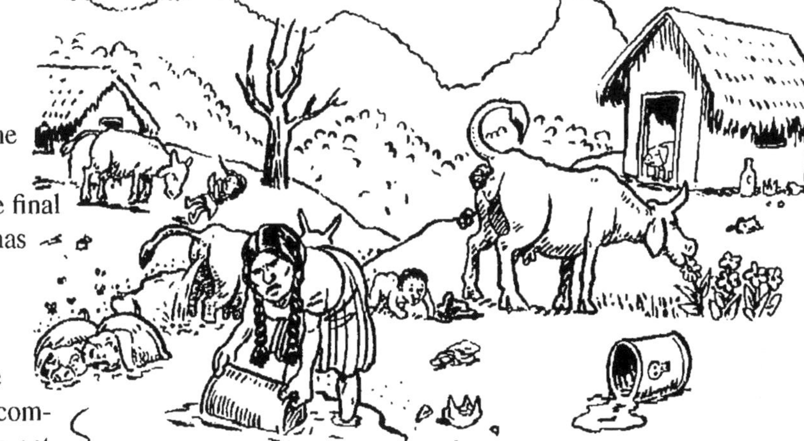

This can be used to **discuss the steps for arriving at a vision.** Once a group or community has discussed their vision for the future, the story is told. The before of the story is how things are now in the community. The ending is the vision the people have defined. They must discuss the middle. This will be their plan for arriving at their vision.

Alternatively open-ended stories can be used to **discuss a current and urgent problem** in the community. The group then envisions the possible steps to solve that problem.

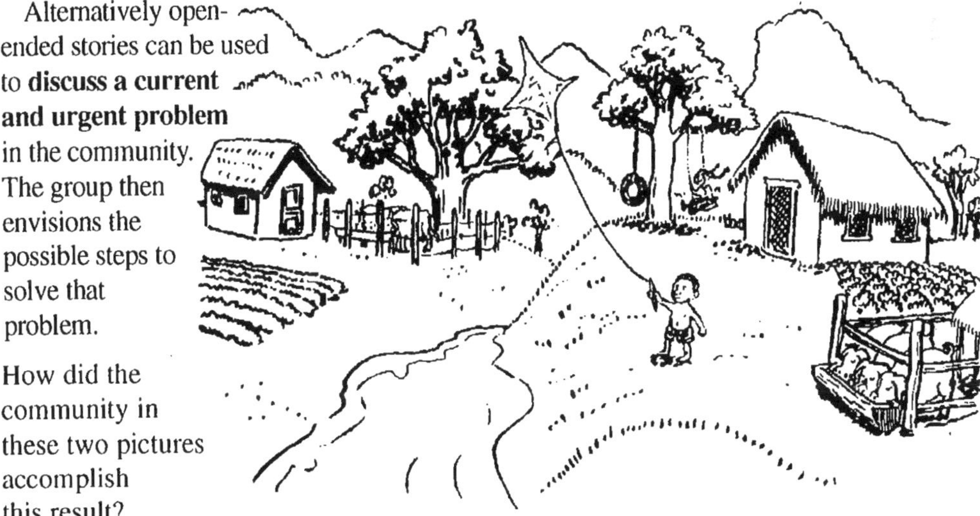

How did the community in these two pictures accomplish this result?

The MIDDLE can also be removed from a story with a NEGATIVE OR SAD ENDING. This stimulates discussion of what could have been done differently.

An example: A community sent a person off to be trained as a Community Livestock Worker. The person did very well in the workshops and really liked the training. When she returned home to her community, she worked for the community for four months. Now she lives in the community but does not help with the animal problems.

What might have happened?
What could the community have done to prevent this?
What can they do now?

When the END OF THE STORY is removed, people discuss the impact of the choices made. They also discuss alternative choices for an alternative solution. This is useful when discussing a current problem in the community. Example: The first day of a training workshop many people came, the next day fewer, and the next day still fewer.

Why did this happen?
What could have been done differently?

Example: Another story is of a person trying to cross a river where only a few stones are available. The person decided to cross alone, fell in the river and drowned.

Why did he decide to cross alone?
What could have been done differently?
What keeps the person from making those choices?

When the MIDDLE AND END are removed, a problem situation is presented without suggestions for solution. People determine if the problem is relevant for them and what solutions they want. They also define their desired outcome for the situation. This is powerful for the discussion of the social problems related to agriculture.

Role plays, puppets, and flannel boards are commonly used when the middle and end are removed from a story. In all three the participants can make a decision about the desired actions and outcome. They then use role play, puppets, or the flannel board to present their decisions to everyone. A flannel board can also be used for the larger group to discuss solutions. Figures are moved around by the participants until the board represents their consensus.

Role play

Definition

A role play or drama presents a specific case of something that causes a problem in the community. The participants visualize situations and relationships which are too complicated to explain. The role play generally is open ended, shows contradictions, and plants a question for the participants to analyze.

This tool is very versatile but sometimes used too much. It can be used for training in workshops, for defining the situation, and for evaluations.

How It Works

- There are several different uses of role plays.

1. The facilitator and/or the participants act out a current problem-causing situation. All participants then discuss the situation, its possible solutions, and actions for the future.
2. The participants in small groups define an existing problem or situation in their community, and act out the situation. The remaining participants then discuss their suggested solutions to the problem.
3. Participants who have worked in small groups present the results of their small group work in dramatic form.
4. Workshop participants present a role play to a larger community audience to inform the community and to bring about dialogue.
5. Participants practice new social skills and receive feedback from the remaining participants. Each person is given a situation. In a role play the participant shows how he or she would respond to the situation.

● Role plays are often very effective in opening a dialogue. Acting out a story gives participants some distance allowing them the opportunity to discuss the situation in relative safety, without identifying and blaming the people who have caused the problem. They can draw connections to their real-life situation in the course of defining their action plan.

● The four open questions are used to help analyze this situation with the larger group, and to allow them to draw helpful conclusions.

- What did you see happening here?
- How do you feel when it happens?
- When it happens in your community, what problems does it cause?
- What can we do about it?

● It is important that the story or problem portrayed in the role play be a current problem for the participants. It must spring from their reality if it is to generate interest.

● Role plays often show that learning is fun. There will often be much laughter, but the entertainment value of the role play should not overshadow the learning value.

Pros, Cons, and Other Uses

Hint: There is a big temptation in animal health training courses to use a role play to provide answers, as an alternative to a lecture–for example, a role play where a client farmer brings a sick animal to the animal health worker for treatment and the worker treats the animal and gives advice to the owner. As you plan a role play, ask yourself, **"Does this role play ask a question?"** A role play which provides the answers leaves no room for discussion.

Role plays are effective tools for:

- Defining a situation
- Evaluating a program
- Energizing a discussion
- Consolidating what has been learned by a small group
- Practicing skills such as history taking and interviewing.

Role plays can generate strong feelings about a topic. It is important that all role plays are followed by reflection and discussion. The facilitator should strive to create an atmosphere of trust where people can share their thoughts and feelings in a constructive way. When there are strong feelings, equally strong conclusions and action steps can be reached.

Role plays used for small groups to present their work to a plenary session can be time consuming. The benefit to the group of reinforcing the new action through a role play must be weighed against the time involved.

There are several other variations on role plays which can be used. These include:

- **Pantomime:** The role play is done silently with exaggerated actions and emotions.
- **Statues:** Instead of a role play, the small group presents their result as living statue. The other participants view and discuss the statue. The statue group can share their thinking as well.
- **Dramatized Story:** Many open-ended stories can be told in drama form rather than as a story teller would tell them. Both are very effective.

See "Helping your role plays come alive" pg. 314–317.

Examples of How Role Plays Have Been Used

1. In a role play to present the dilemmas caused by animal diseases, rabies causes a small child and a woman in two different families to die. They contract the disease from a rabid cow who had difficulty swallowing. In small groups the participants discuss what they saw in the role play. The facilitator asks if anyone has had a similar experience in their community, and what problems it caused. They discuss what could be done to prevent this in the future. Each small group presents their analysis to the plenary. In this way, the role play helps people to analyze what they think and feel about rabies and the potential effects on their family, and what they will do about it in the future.

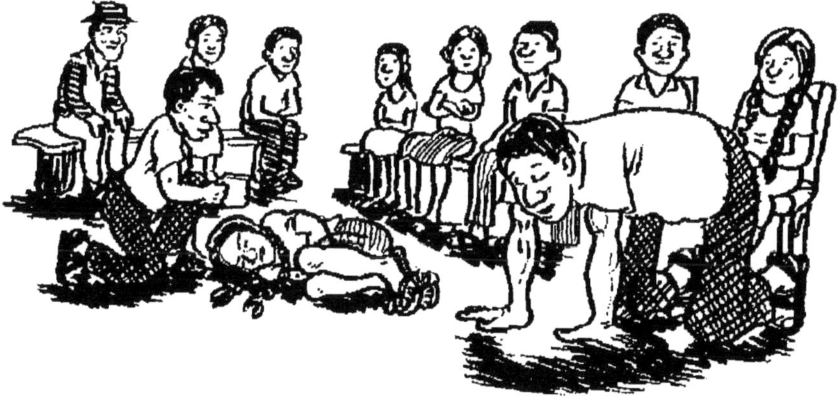

2. Each small group is given a specific case of feedback which was poorly given. Each small group presents their case in role-play form. They then discuss the case and what could have been done to give feedback in a better form. They present a role play of the feedback in a positive form. See "Feedback," pg. 208.

Source Vella 1995

Puppets

Definition

Puppets are dolls or objects made to represent people, animals, and things. They can be used to present a story or drama to a large group, acting out issues of importance to the community. As in a role play, a puppet show should leave the audience with an unanswered question to ponder. This can energize a group and generate dialogue. It is an effective way to get the community talking about an issue. (See open-ended stories" pg. 243.)

How It Works

- Hand-made puppets are more effective than those bought in stores. They can be given the features, skin color, hair style, and dress of the local people. This helps people to see themselves and their community situation in the puppet show. Puppets can be made from paper maché, plastic, old clothes, vegetables, or just about any found object. (See "Making Our Training Materials," pg. 311.)
- A role play is presented with the puppets taking the place of people and animals involved. (See "Role Play," pg. 244.) The people presenting the puppet show need to project their voices loudly. Jokes and funny characters are always appreciated.

- In small groups, or in a plenary session, the problem presented in the puppet show is discussed. Participants discuss what they saw, whether this happens in their community, what problems it causes, and what they would like to do about it.
- As in role plays, a puppet show must ask a question or present a problem without its solution. Puppet shows that pose a problem will generate dialogue.

Pros, Cons, and Other Uses

Puppets are used for the same purposes as role plays in participatory adult education. Because the puppets are not seen as real people they can deal with more sensitive issues like animal theft, burning the neighbor's trees or crops, or animals destroying a neighbor's terraces. People can laugh at the antics of the puppets but then begin a serious discussion without pointing a finger of blame. In this way, participants can begin to resolve a serious problem without blaming and getting emotional. As in many serious problems, if the problem can be separated from the emotion about the problem, it can be discussed with greater clarity. Once the problem is defined and discussed, the participants can suggest solutions to act upon.

If the puppet show is used to initiate serious discussion, it is best used in a workshop situation with a limited number of people.

Puppet shows can also be used for:

- Motivating a community about an organizational program or meeting.
- Generating a discussion among school children about a problem upon which they can take action.
- Giving suggestions. Sometimes, the "wise puppet" character can offer suggestions for discussion among the group.
- Energizing the participants.
- Assessment, gender analysis, and evaluation.

Hint: If a puppet show is used for a large gathering, it is often difficult for everyone to hear. A puppet show will probably not generate a dialogue among a large gathering of people, but it will attract attention and draw people to a meeting.

Examples of How Puppets Are Used

1. In one show in Bolivia a cow puppet had signs of warts. Two farmers discuss the symptoms they see together in plain terms. The owner says she is going off to get the Community Livestock Worker to help her with the cow. The puppet then turns to the CLWs and asks them questions about her cow, the warts and what she should do. They answer from the audience. A facilitator can encourage discussion between the puppet and the CLW's. One of the participants writes the symptoms and treatments for warts on newsprint.
2. In the selection process for CLWs, a puppet show is used to illustrate the problems a CLW can have once he or she begins to work in the community. They discuss some of the things which cause the CLW to be discouraged and stop working. The puppet show serves two functions:
   - it draws the whole community into a discussion about the selection of their CLW;
   - it brings out one of the most common problems with CLWs – attrition due to discouragement.

Flannel boards

Definition

A flannel board was traditionally made of flannel material with pieces of cloth which stuck to it. Now, the term refers to any large board to which small objects can be stuck. The objects can be manipulated by the participants to express the concept or story and the solutions they desire.

A flannel board is useful for training, defining the situation, and evaluation.

How It Works

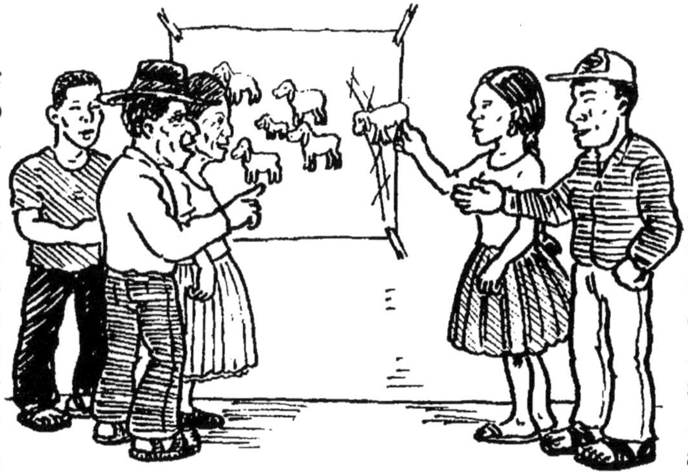

- Introduce the *dynamic* and its purpose to a group of no more than ten people.
- Objects made of paper, cardboard, plastic, cloth, or wood are stuck by tape or paste to a wooden board, blackboard, plastic board or even a wall or the side of a vehicle. Any of these boards or walls can be covered first with a piece of cloth as a background.
- The participants should physically control the objects to be pasted. For example, small pictures of antibiotics and diseases can be given to people or drawn from a hat. They match the appropriate antibiotic to the disease it will cure.
- If the objects are sheep, trees, water, etc. participants put the objects on the board to show their farm management system. If they are pictures of different people doing tasks, have the participants organize them. If they are flexible people, give them to the participants to move and define the story. As people place objects on the board, they discuss their decision to place them where they do. They tell why they belong there.
- Participants should be involved in the reorganizing and reordering of the objects once they are all on the board. Consensus should be reached by the group as to their correct scenario.

Pros, Cons, and Other Uses

Flannel boards are very useful to generate discussion, if used properly. The participants should always control the outcome. Since flannel boards usually use a prepared set of pictures or objects, they can limit spontaneity. It is a good idea to have blank cards or extra drawings or sheets so an extra picture or idea can be added by a participant.

Flannel boards can also be used for a group of people to tell a story, identify a problem in their community, or explore alternative solutions to a problem. The participants are given a set of people and objects to move around the board. People are made from thick paper or thin cardboard to look like local people. Other objects such as houses, animals, crops, trees, and possessions are also available. The objects and people are spread on the floor. Ask the participants to make a picture which shares a current problem in the community. Alternatively, ask the participants to suggest a solution to a current problem in the community. The story created by the group can be used to trigger a deep analysis of the problem or solution.

An Example of How Flannel Boards Are Used

Small drawings of sheep, trees, water troughs, etc. were given to a small group. The drawings showed ewes and rams of all ages, some healthy and some with physical deformities. The group was told that this was their herd of sheep. They needed to make a decision about which animals to raise and what management was needed.

This led to a lively discussion of culling, breeding selection, castration, and separating males from females. Each small group presented their resulting herd to the large group. They each gave their reasons for their decisions about how best to maintain the flock.

Drawing and discussion

Definition

Drawings are made jointly by groups or by individuals as they discuss an issue. When a group discusses and draws, they can discuss each new item added by an individual. When individuals draw, the pictures can be compared, contrasted, and placed into categories to aid in coming to conclusions.

Drawing and discussion is often used for defining the situation, for focusing on an issue or topic for training, and for comparison in evaluation.

How It Works

- Divide into small groups – no more than 3–4 people per group.
- Each group receives drawing materials–newsprint and markers or crayons or pastels.
- Explain the purpose or focus of the drawing to the groups. They need to understand they are not being asked to produce works of art. Explain that the importance is in the discussion.
- As the groups discuss, they may talk about the placement or size of the object they are drawing. This may indicate its relative importance. Homogeneous groups are probably best so that people will discuss freely. Some groups sit in a circle and make individual drawings all around the page. Others make one consolidated drawing.
- Once the drawing is complete, the group analyzes it. What does the drawing say to them about the issue being discussed? What new things have they learned from each other?
- Each group interprets their drawing in the plenary. Discussion and conclusions follow.

Pros, Cons, and Other Uses

This tool is most useful in a culture with a strong visual tradition. People may not feel comfortable drawing at first. Help them to understand that the dialogue and learning is the purpose, not creating a work of art. If it is so disconcerting to people to be asked to draw that they do not relax and discuss the issue, perhaps this technique is inappropriate for the local situation and culture.

Hint: In some groups where the decision is made to make a single group picture, the group may charge one person with the task as the chief artist. In this case, it is easy for the group to become distracted or bored, and not all participate in the outcome. Emphasize the importance of the discussion and the participation of all.

An Example of How Drawing and Discussion Is Used

In a study of local knowledge, a group of elderly women were asked to draw the management calendar for their alpacas and llamas. They included all of the ritual aspects of management related to the local festivals. They defined the local management as integral to their spiritual ritual. When they finished their drawing they discussed how these management practices had changed through the years. They defined areas where they were no longer maintaining the same quality of management due to social changes. They pinpointed these areas as important areas for a training workshop to discover how they could still apply good management, given changing social and economic conditions.

These women were elderly women who generally had little voice in the community. They usually would not participate in large group discussions. They became quite animated in their discussion and the sharing of their ideas.

Pictures and posters

Definition

A picture or poster as used in participatory training is also often called a code. The picture illustrates a real community situation. It encodes a problem. The picture leaves a question in the mind of the viewers, which leads to dialogue and action.

Posters can also be the result of group work. The group has a discussion about a topic and decides to present their results to the larger group in pictorial form. As a result of a workshop, a group may decide to create a poster for teaching or inspiration in their community.

How Pictures and Posters Work

As a *dynamic* starter of discussion:

● In a plenary session, or in small groups, participants analyze the content of the picture. They decide if it presents a real situation. They determine what would be the best action to take to solve this problem.

As the result of group work:

● This is similar to drawing and discussion in that the group defines the content of the poster through dialogue. However, instead of using the drawing to stimulate the discussion, the group draws a poster to present their results.

● If a poster is to be displayed in the community, the people must decide on the content, presentation, and location. If there is a talented local person, she or he should be recruited to draw the poster based on the community's design. If an outside artist is hired, he or she can respond to the direction of the community. An outside artist will often create interest and excitement in the process and the discussion of the poster's content.

It is helpful, when designing a picture to ask yourself, "Does this picture ask a question or pose a problem for discussion?"

Pros, Cons, and Other Uses

Many times a picture code developed by local trainers is more effective than a code developed by an artist. Although the local drawing may seem crude at first, it is generally an excellent representation of the real situation. Trainers can develop their drawing skills over time. (See "Making Our Training Materials," pg. 289.)

When local trainers create their own picture codes, they feel they are able to do it at any time, and they do not depend on an outside artist to create their materials. Sometimes when an outside artist is used to create pictures local trainers feel they cannot make their own picture codes for use in other training sessions.

Hint: It is easy when doing technical training related to crops or livestock to make pictures of answers. These have all been seen: Symptoms of diseases of crops or animals, pictures of treatments, chemicals, or instruments to apply them, a sick animal and a healthy animal with the appropriate treatment, life cycles of parasites, anatomy, appropriate spacing of plants or trees in farm systems, appropriate forms of terracing, etc. Although in some cases these may be appropriate, they are usually inappropriate for participatory training.

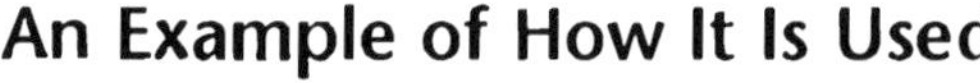

An Example of How It Is Used

One particular code designed by the local trainers in Bolivia drew much discussion. It depicted a common problem. The woman responsible for herding the sheep fell asleep under a tree. The sheep got into the neighbor's corn and destroyed it. The neighbor discovered the sheep and went after them with a machete, while the shepherdess slept.

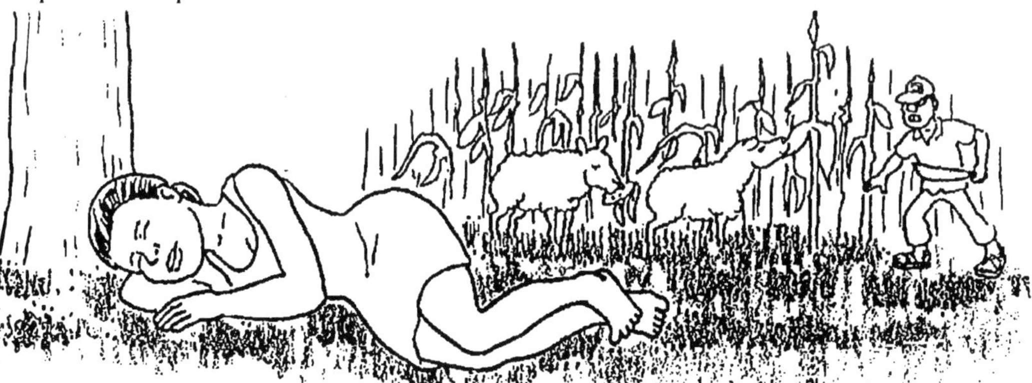

This created a lively discussion about proper management techniques and a plan of action for the future.

Sayings

Definition

A local saying or proverb is used to generate a discussion about a specific situation.

How It Works

As the group is discussing an issue or a situation, the facilitator inserts the proverb to deepen the discussion. The proverb is used to create a dialogue about the human aspect of a situation. It is a quick way to focus people's attention on an issue, energize the group, and bring a local context to the discussion. It also can be used to reflect on larger universal truths and principles.

Examples of How Sayings Are Used

This proverb has been used in Kenya to discuss changing village resources, jealousies over resources, and planning for the future:
"He that doesn't have anything doesn't fear anything."

These Kenyan proverbs are used in different planning situations:
"Stomp on the fire before it gets close."
"It doesn't help to put the stick up after the banana has fallen."

This Haitian proverb is often used in discussions of group or organizational work:
"Many hands make light work."

This Bolivian proverb is used to discuss the participation of all:
"He that doesn't cry, doesn't suck."

Here is a proverb to reflect on creation and ecology:
"May you find the treasure, but leave it in the field."

Source: Josephat Ngaira, Mission Moving Mountains, Kenya

Puzzles

Definition

A puzzle is a picture or object that has been cut into many pieces. In participatory training the picture or object when put together poses a problem or a question, and generates discussion of that problem or question.

How It Works

- Participants are divided into small groups.
- Each group receives a full set of loose pieces of a puzzle.
- The small group must put the puzzle together and discuss the question posed by the picture or object.
- When discussion has finished, all participants look at each puzzle. The group explains their puzzle and shares the results of their discussion.
- The plenary discussion formulates conclusions from the work of the small groups.

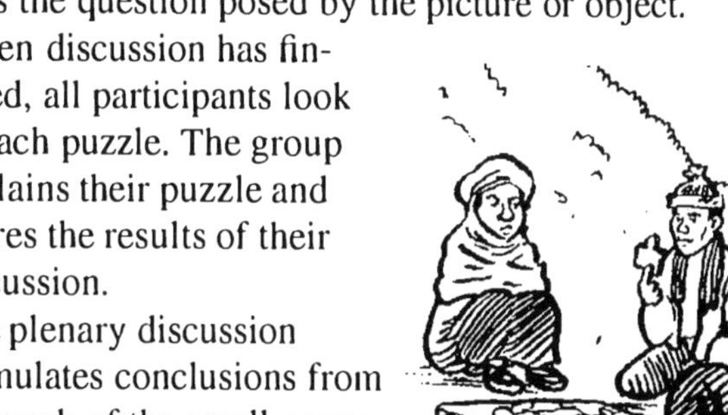

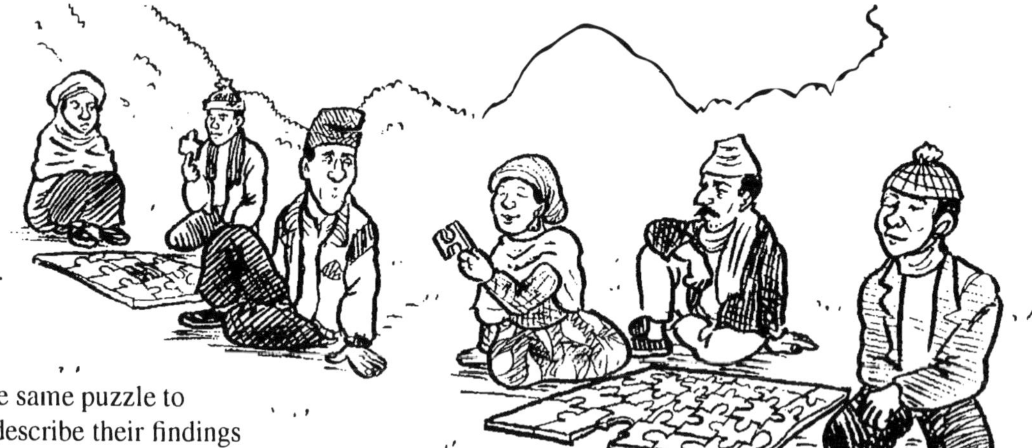

Examples of How Puzzles Are Used

1. Each small group receives the same puzzle to discuss. In the plenary they describe their findings and suggest solutions.
2. Each small group receives a different puzzle. The pictures illustrate different problems related to a similar topic. For example: the intermediary and their effect on marketing. In the plenary, each group shares their analysis of the different aspects of the problem. The whole group comes to consensus on the issue.
3. Each group receives a different puzzle in an envelope. One group is missing pieces and cannot form their puzzle. Another group has extra pieces for the group missing pieces. A third group is missing pieces entirely. The participants must look for their missing pieces and negotiate with other groups for them.
   In the plenary, each group shares what happened in their group. This dynamic with puzzles can be used to discuss different aspects of team building such as: shared resources, the importance of collaboration, the difficulty of completing a task if all of the resources are not available, the frustrations caused by lack of resources, and the importance of the participation of all to complete a task.
   Source: Tom and Dee Yaccino (MCC 1993)
4. Puzzles can be used to form small groups. If there are to be four small groups, there are four puzzles. Each participant receives a random puzzle piece. They must find the other people with the pieces to their puzzle, put the puzzle together, and discuss the picture that is formed. The resulting groups become new working groups.

Tools for assessment and evaluation

All of the tools of assessment are also great tools to generate dialogue. They each have their uses in training workshops as well.

Mapping

Definition

Drawing or making a map in a small group encourages a thorough discussion of the area being mapped. Maps can be of a farm, community, or larger area. They can represent how things were in the past, how people see them now, or what they would like to see in the future. Thus they can be used for defining the situation, setting a future vision, or evaluation and comparison.

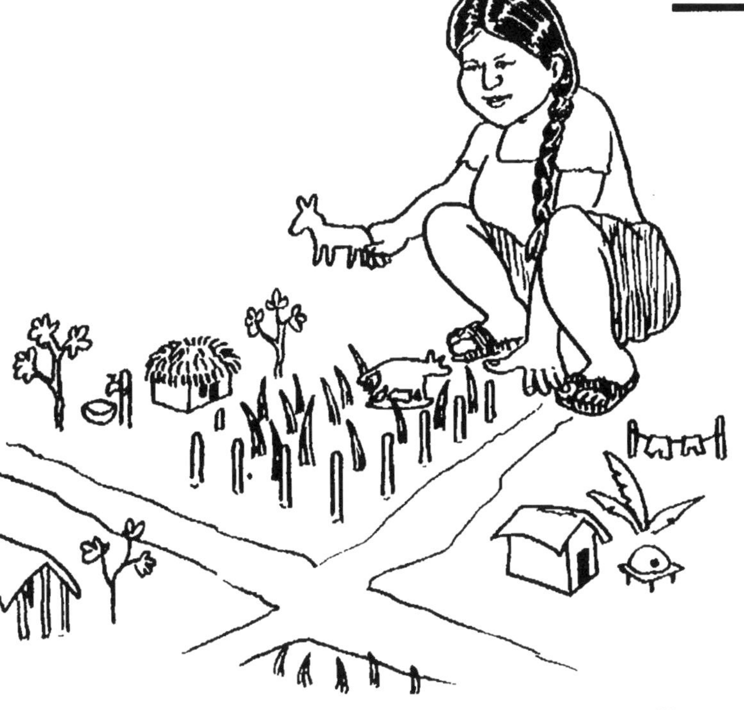

How mapping works

- Divide into small groups.
- Explain the map each group will create. The map may be of their farm or community. It may be focused on some aspect of farm or community life such as infrastructure, crops, trees, etc.
- The maps can be outlined on the ground with sticks or rocks, or drawn in dirt or sand. Maps can also be drawn on paper with markers. In a windy area with people who are not familiar with written maps, paper can be placed on the ground and heavy objects such as rocks used to outline the land.
- People become very inventive with a map, using available materials to make it more alive, if it is on the ground. For example, they might put in grasses and branches to illustrate pastures and forest, make houses from sticks, show wells or other water resources with cans or by wetting the map, etc.

Hint: When drawing maps with markers the group will appoint an artist. There is more of a tendency for one person to take over.

- Give the group a set amount of time to complete their map.
- Once the maps are completed (which may take around 45 minutes), give the participants an opportunity to stroll by each map.
- Each group presents and explains their map to everyone. In the plenary session, draw conclusions about the current situation in the community and the things the people would like to change.
- Each group makes a large paper copy of their map to leave in the community.

Pros, Cons, and Other Uses

Sometimes the activity of making the map distracts participants from the discussion and dialogue. It is important that people realize this is not a competition but a reflection of their thoughts and feelings.

A community map could be used as a part of analyzing the community's current situation. Once the map is made, the group discusses what they like and dislike about the community as it is now, and identifies problem areas they would like to change.

This can be followed by a map where the group envisions their future. They share what they would like the community to look like after five or ten years. Once the future vision map is made, they discuss the steps to reach that vision.

A map can also be used to focus on one specific area of community life. For example, the map could describe the current livestock situation of the community; which families have livestock, where they graze or how they are managed, what the marketing strategy is, etc. Or the map could focus on the current organizational situation in the community. What organizations/infrastructure exist and what are the problems? If the map is used to focus on one area, that area can be covered in greater depth.

Community land-use maps are a powerful tool. They are helpful in monitoring community forestry and watershed areas. For example, a community may draw a map of crop lands and realize there is better production in the bottom areas than on the hillsides. This can generate a discussion of what can be done about the erosion. Periodically returning to the map and recording any changes seen is useful in monitoring.

Maps can be used to demonstrate and discuss the different ways men and women view the resources and infrastructure on their farm or in their community. When made by separate groups of men and women and discussed jointly, they point to who controls the resources and which resources are viewed as most important by men and women.

Maps are very effective tools for people to envision the future they desire. People can make a plan for the use of their land and production for the future. Or a map can include the infrastructure changes desired for the community. Maps can be used to consider future reforestation and land-use planning by a community. Once the plan is made, the steps needed to reach the goal are discussed. The map can lead to a good discussion about the necessary collaboration to accomplish common goals.

Tip for the facilitator:

Please let the people make the map! Too many times the facilitator has been impatient and taken the pen from the hands of the people to make the map as he or she sees it. Keep asking yourself, "Who is holding the pen?" If you are, give it up! The same applies when a map model is transferred to paper for the facilitator's use. Please be sure to include all of the information placed on the map by the participants.

Examples Of How Mapping Is Used

This is an example of how a mapping technique was used **to focus and direct a whole workshop on farm planning:**

The participants bring samples of each soil type on their farm. They name each soil type (using their local names) and place some of it on the map of their farm in the correct location. They fill in other things on their farm as it is now. This includes areas under cultivation, pasture, resting areas, and infrastructure (house, well, animal shed, etc.)

Participants discuss each soil type, what will and won't grow in it, such as forages and other crops. This discussion springs from their experience. The facilitator may suggest some alternative crops as well.

Participants discuss protection of certain areas, such as water, wetlands, forest, and how these fit the ideal farm.

Participants decide on their goals for the future–what they want for their family, themselves, and their farm in the next ten years.

They make a map of their future farm based on an understanding of the use of each type of soil, their goals for the future, and protection of fragile areas. For an example of using mapping in the visioning process see page 76.

In some community level workshops mapping is used **as an evaluation tool** to sum up the workshop:

In the early stages of the workshop participants are divided into small groups. Each group is told they have formed a cooperative and have purchased a set amount of land. We use the same land area most farmers would have on their small farms.

Each group is asked to draw a map of the farm as they would like it to be developed by their cooperative. They draw this first map on paper with markers. Most groups will make the map based on their current management goals. These maps are shared and briefly discussed, but not discussed in depth. The maps are used to identify problem areas, to make a list of workshop expectations, and help guide the workshop facilitators.

On the last day of the workshop, the participants again form their cooperatives. This time they are asked to make a map model on the ground to design how they would like their land in the future. The groups will reflect on all of the things they have discussed during the course of the workshop. Their new maps will reflect the thought processes and attitude changes brought about by the workshop. They will see for themselves the things they have learned and value for the future. This is a synthesis activity where participants gain a greater confidence in their new knowledge and a commitment to apply it on their own farms.

Ranking, sorting, and rating

Definition

An activity where participants can prioritize a set of items. They can also evaluate items against one another, or score an item against a list of criteria. Creating these simple charts also creates dialogue about:

Why people make certain choices

How many people in the community make a certain choice and

What the specific choices are.

The reasons for the choices are recorded and compared.

This tool helps to gather information for assessing training needs or defining the current situation of the community. It can be used in the process of investigating local knowledge or for a community's analysis of their gender-based roles. It can also be used as an evaluation tool. This tool is also very useful in training situations to analyze thoughts and feelings about an issue.

Ranking

How it works

- The group or community brainstorms a list based on a specified topic, for example, common cattle diseases, duties of animal caretakers, the uses of trees.
- The list is written down the left side of the chart. In some cases, people will make a picture or use a symbol for each item, rather than writing the name. Make sure each symbol is understood.
- In a small group people rank the items according to a specific question. For example, "Which disease is the most serious?" "Which is the least serious?" or "What person fulfills each role in animal care?" or "Which tree is the most important?"

See "Valuing women" pg. 186, and "diseases confidently treated" pg. 229 for an example.

- Each person will rank each item with pebbles, leaves, or piles of colored sand. More pebbles would be most common, no pebbles would be least common.
- The dialogue is related to the topic being discussed. If it is the most serious local diseases of cattle, there may be a dispute about which is the most serious. The group can form a list of why one disease is more serious than another. This way they define their criteria for judging the disease. Different people will use different criteria.
- This type of ranking can be used to determine the relative importance of topics in a training workshop. (see "Planning," pg. 90.)

An Example of How Ranking Is Used

A community in Paraguay had invited a veterinarian and his team to discuss their serious animal management problems. The veterinary team divided the community into homogeneous groups (older women, older men, younger women, younger men, landless youth).

Each group decided on the five most common and serious problems with their animals. Each group chose a symbol to represent each problem or disease (for example, a dry bone meant dying animals).

Each group presented their symbols to the whole community. They put the symbols in a line on the ground in the middle of the circle. As each group finished presenting their symbols, someone in the larger group had to say what each symbol meant.

Finally there was a line of 20–30 symbols and they had all been repeated several times.

Each person was asked to pick 6 small leaves and vote for the three most common and serious livestock problems they had. They put three leaves with the most common, two with the next, and one by the third most common.

The village elders counted the leaves by each symbol and gave a tally on the ground next to each symbol. The results were confirmed by discussion in the plenary. The community then chose to request training on each of the five highest priority problems with the livestock in the community.

Source: Dave Bremner

Sorting

How It Works

The community has a number of items to be sorted into categories. In a small group they can sort the items and discuss why they feel the arrangement to be correct. They make a decision as a group and present it to the plenary. Sorting when it is done privately is also a way for individuals to add or correct information in a study of traditional management. The differences between the individual's thoughts and the community's response can be discussed.

Pros, Cons, and Other Uses

Can you see how these tools could also be very useful *dynamics* at the initial stages of a training workshop to help focus on the most important diseases or problems with their animals? Remember, the participants brainstorm the list–not the facilitator!

When doing a participatory assessment, a facilitator will often write down the list of ideas generated onto paper for the future. Be sure to include all of the ideas the people have generated, not just the ones you as facilitator think are important.

Sometimes with ranking and sorting *dynamics* it is better to divide into small groups to do the activity. Also, everyone should put down their rocks at the same time. This is because one influential person can control the whole exercise, as happened in China:

You have a list of diseases here. Which is the most important?
The cows are always most affected by diarrhea all year.
I agree!
My cow doesn't ever have a problem with diarrhea, but he is the CLW and he knows best.
What more can we say?

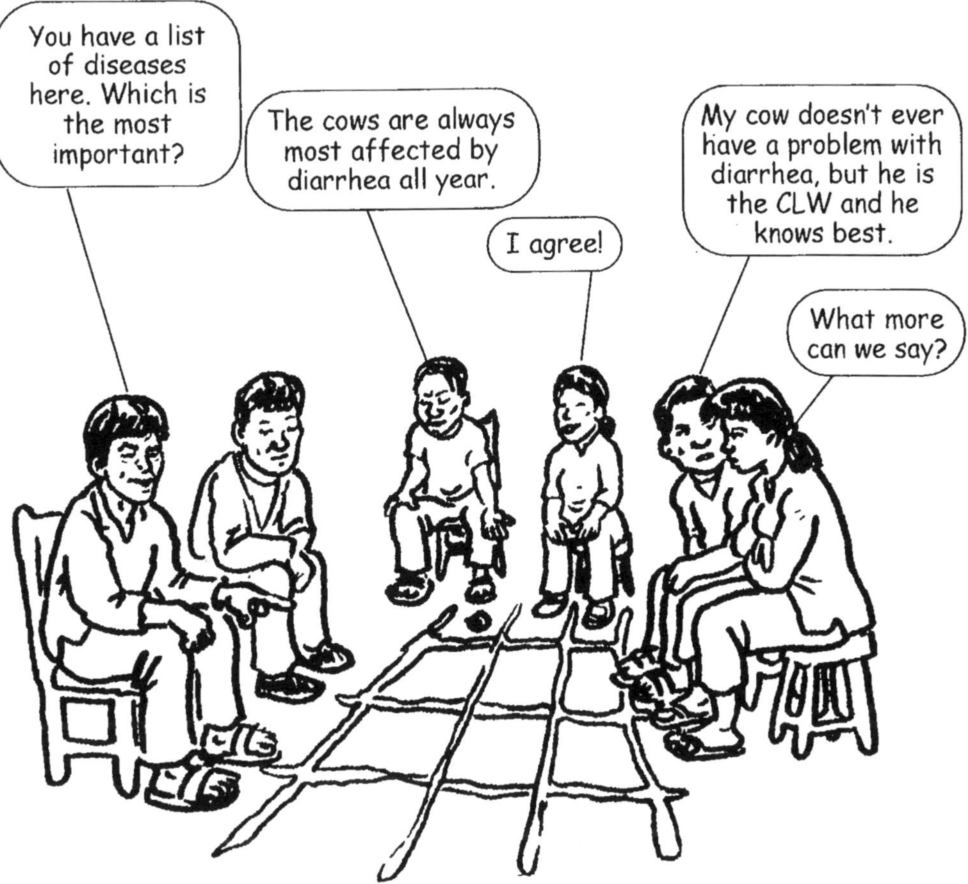

From this *dynamic* nothing more than the opinion of the Community Livestock Worker was learned. His opinion was important, but the other people did not contribute their answers.

P.S.: The facilitator changed her strategy to allow the participants to put down their stones first. After everyone else voted, the Community Livestock Worker voted. Then the group analyzed the results.

An Example of Sorting

In an evaluation of a training program two years after a week-long workshop, the people wanted to know which topics had been most beneficial in the workshop.

Each of the topics were written on a separate piece of thin cardboard.

They had three categories on the ground (but they could have used baskets as well): most often used, sometimes used, not used.

Each small group sorted the topics into these categories.

As they discussed the most valuable topics, they found that all of the topics of prevention and management had been used often. Most of the topics in disease recognition and treatment had not been necessary. They discussed how healthy their animals were because they applied the good management techniques learned during the workshop. The sorting stimulated a very valuable discussion for the community and the evaluation.

Rating

How It Works

- The set of items to be rated is on the left hand side. They may be in the form of pictures to facilitate the discussion. For example, there might be a picture card for each animal species raised in the community. A set of criteria is placed across the top of the chart. Or each question can be asked individually as the group responds.
- Animals can be in pictures on cards. You can make a chart on the ground, and participants can rank the animal according to each criteria by placing 0–5 stones under each of the criteria for each animal.

most important

easy to raise

easy to sell

most diseases

Source: Irene Christensen

Pros, Cons, and Other Uses

It is important that people understand that the discussion created by forming the chart is more important than the final chart itself. Although the information from the chart will help the community in it's analysis, the discussion used to create the chart will often point out the difference in the criteria people use to judge things.

Ranking, rating, and sorting are valuable assessment tools. They are also a lively way to initiate a dialogue in a training workshop. For example, in a discussion of sheep management principles, the participants listed all of the management tasks (e.g., castrating, separating, culling, foot trimming, etc.), then they discussed who did each task, how often, and the relative importance. This led into a good dialogue about the importance of regular herd management for better production.

If pre-designed materials are used for a ranking or rating activity, (such as pictures or symbols or charts) it is important to pretest the materials. This ensures that everyone understands the materials and is rating on the same basis. It is also important to include blank cards for extra pictures or symbols the participants define as important to their ranking chart.

Rating can also be used to help people to explore their feelings on an issue. For example, women and men assess their participation in the local organization:

Three pictures form three categories on the board. One picture shows a woman who is too timid to enter a group meeting. The second shows a woman who goes to the meeting but is too timid to speak out. The third picture shows a woman actively participating and sharing her opinion in a meeting.

Place a plastic jar or a large envelope under each picture.

Everyone rates their own participation in the group by putting a leaf or stone into the jar under the picture which represents her situation.

The process of making the decision to vote causes people to analyze their participation. This dynamic opens a good dialogue about why people do or do not participate. It is especially useful for women to discuss the barriers they feel to participating in the local organization. A list can be made of these barriers and strategies can be designed by the participants to overcome them.

Seasonal calendars

Definition

A seasonal calendar is drawn on the ground or on paper. It uses local rainfall patterns to define the seasons. In this way, differences in ways of naming times of the year are overcome (for example, within one country there may be different names for seasons or months) and commonality is reached through rainfall.

Various local materials such as leaves, stones, seeds, sticks, or colored sand are used to add details to the calender. Anything which varies over the course of the year can be discussed using this calendar. Such calendars are used to discuss the occurrence of disease in crops or animals, times of the year when there is abundant and less fodder, times of the year when people are more or less occupied for project planning purposes, relative task load of men and women.

The seasonal calendar is a useful assessment tool for the community, for training needs, for gender analysis, for investigating local knowledge, and for evaluation.

How It Works

- Divide the participants into small groups. It is often helpful to have a facilitator in each small group to understand the discussion involved. Each small group will make their own calendar.
- Participants begin making the calendar by representing the rainfall on the ground in a straight line across the top. The group uses sticks broken to different lengths, or small pebbles in a line (more for times of greater rainfall). Put the longest stick down for the month with the most rain and build the rest of the calendar months by amount of rainfall.
- Once the rainfall is described across the top of the calender, the list of things to be discussed is listed down the left hand side.

These areas and others can be discussed on a seasonal calendar.

- Fodder use and availability: On the left of the calendar you can list, or have participants make a picture of, each of the types of fodder. Participants put rocks, sticks or colored powder in the season when the fodder is available. More of the object means there is more pasture in that month. Or if you have leaves or samples from the different pastures and fodder trees in use, put those in the calendar.
- The seasonality of animal disease: For each disease listed, the participants put a counter into the space representing the time of the year it most occurs. If they use pebbles, they might put five pebbles at the time when the disease happens most, and one pebble when the disease happens least.
- Time use of men and women in their work (analyzed in separate groups).
- Marketing of animals and animal products: purchase, sale, and prices.
- Seasonality of crop production and crop related tasks.
- Men's and women's work roles and work loads.
- Seasonal income and expense.

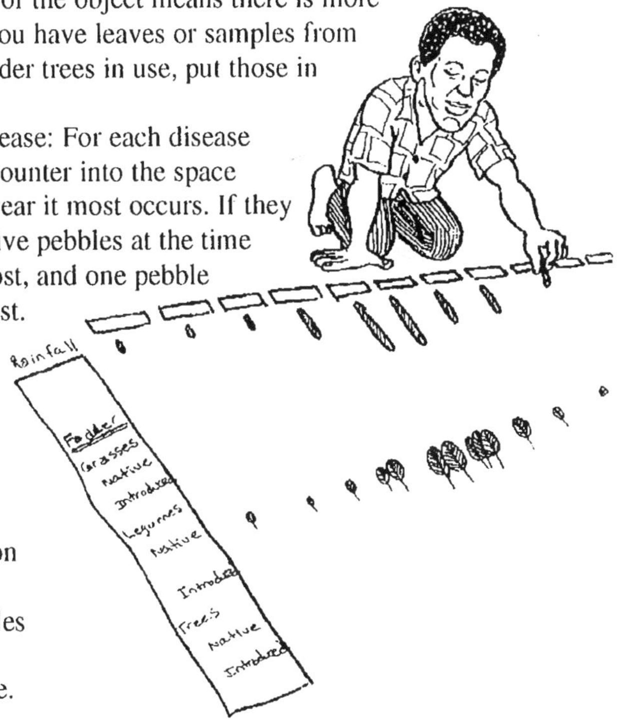

- A seasonal calendar can help people set priorities as to what areas to cover at which times in a training program. The analysis of the calendar is the most important aspect. Villagers can draw many conclusions from the visual presentation of the seasonal calendar.
- It is important for someone – either a facilitator or participant – to replicate the calendar in a drawing. This will give the participants and facilitators a point of reference for later discussions and planning. Try not to simplify if the simplification changes the meaning.

Pros, Cons, and Other Uses

Hint: Limit the number of items on one calendar. Don't put so many things on the calendar that people lose interest in making it or it becomes difficult to analyze. Separate calendars can be compared to one another for more information.

Tips:

Keep the groups small. The group needs to be small so that one person does not dominate the activity.

Make sure the activity is short enough so that people have time to analyze it.

Write down the comments. The facilitator or a chosen participant can note comments and discussion on a large piece of paper during the development of the calendar. As each group presents and explains their calendar in the plenary, a rich analysis begins.

An Example of How a Seasonal Calender Is Used

A seasonal calender used for a beekeeping program:

- Participants bring the leaves of all the plants which grow and flower around their houses.
- Participants put the leaves on the seasonal calendar on the months when the plant is flowering.

This shows when there is no nectar for the bees. They can then discuss which crops and trees are good for planting during which months for the best nectar for the bees.

This can lead to an excellent discussion from which the farmers make their decisions about what to plant and when to plant it for good bee nutrition and maximum production of honey.

Seasonal calendars can also be used with other constants rather than the rainfall. For example, crop production and prices can be analyzed to aid farmers in planning decisions and possible diversification of crops. The tasks done in different agricultural roles by men and women or young and old can be the constants. These calendars are very helpful for gender analysis. They can be used as an evaluation tool for analysis of daily activity before and after a project. The activity levels can be compared to daily and monthly income.

For a further suggestion of using a seasonal calendar please see "A note on gender roles" pg. 71.

Semi-structured interviews

Definition

A semi-structured interview is a guided dialogue. The interview can be of individuals or small groups. It is not an interview with a rigid questionnaire. An interviewer uses a mental or written checklist of initial points to discuss. The checklist is used to initiate the interview and to cross-check answers from different people. New lines of questioning arise during the interview, following up on answers or comments on previous questions.

The semi-structured interview is used in defining the situation, investigating traditional knowledge, and evaluations.

How It Works

- Facilitators, CLWs, administrators, or anyone with a desire to understand the local situation can learn to be a good interviewer. This is an informal interview. Although a short list of questions may be used, it is not a questionnaire. The interview results in dialogue about an area of interest to both the facilitator and the participant.
- **What the participant needs to know:**
  - The purpose of the interview: It should relate to the participant's goals and values.
  - The ways in which the information will be used.
  - That they are qualified to answer the questions.
  - The length of the interview. (Do not take longer than one hour)
- **What the interviewer needs to do:**
  - Communicate respect, trust, and a desire to learn in attitude and actions.
  - Arrange a place and time when the participant feels comfortable.
  - Start with a question about something that can be touched or directly observed.
  - Do not ask rhetorical or leading questions.
  - Be sincere, do not flatter unnecessarily.
  - Never suggest the answer.
  - Thank the respondents for their participation
- A short checklist of questions can be used to initiate the interview. Also, many assessment tools can be used. An interviewee can make a seasonal calender, rank, rate, or sort items or make a map. All of these tools help participants to visualize the situation they are sharing information about.

Pros, Cons, and Other Uses

If a long and specific list of questions is used to initiate the interview, it will often become a question-and-answer session. The more rigid the questions, the less spontaneous the answers and dialogue will be.

Sometimes a question will not be clearly stated or well understood. There is a great temptation to rephrase with an example. Often the example will lead toward a specific answer and the information gained may not be accurate. Questions which are open and concrete will generate dialogue. (For more information on asking open questions see "Implementation," pg. 132.)

Some of the tools for semi-structured interviewing described in RRA and PRA literature are quite formal. A technique called herder recall makes an inventory of the whole herd history over the past year. This is done to examine the productivity and problems in the herd. It classifies the animals by age, sex, class, pregnancy or lactation. Then births, deaths, sales, and purchases are discussed. Sometimes the resulting information is very complex. It appears to be more for information gathering for scientists use than as a tool for community analysis.

The same is true for a technique called progeny history. In this technique the history of the offspring of all the adult female cows is collected. The information is placed on a time line. It is used to calculate productivity in terms such as fertility, mortality, and calving intervals. These are terms which scientists use. Most of the information collected in this way is not readily useable by the community in an analysis of their livestock production. Perhaps some visual tools could be developed to make this information useful for the community.

Some uses of semi-structured interviews:

- *Chain Interviews:* These are a series of interviews from group to group or person to person. Each person or group is an expert in a different stage of a process. For example, in marketing milk, interview men who milk the animals, women who process and sell the milk, intermediary people who buy and sell the milk products, and consumers of the products.
- *Critical Incident:* The interview is used to explore the causes and effects of an event such as flood, fire, drought, or conflicts over land. The interview explores how the family or group coped or did not cope with the situation or how the conflict was resolved. Different versions of a critical incident can be discussed in small groups or with individuals. This will give a clearer overall picture of a situation for discussion by the larger group and for planning to overcome difficulties and resolve conflicts.
- *Family or Herd History:* This interview is a way to check the cases of individuals and families against information provided by the larger group. It is useful in the women's or men's analysis of their tasks and their use of time. This information can help broaden the dialogue in a community's gender analysis process. The history of the offspring of a herd or flock is used to define the productivity of a herd over time and the major problems in production. Usually this is done by asking about the history of the offspring of the adult female cows.

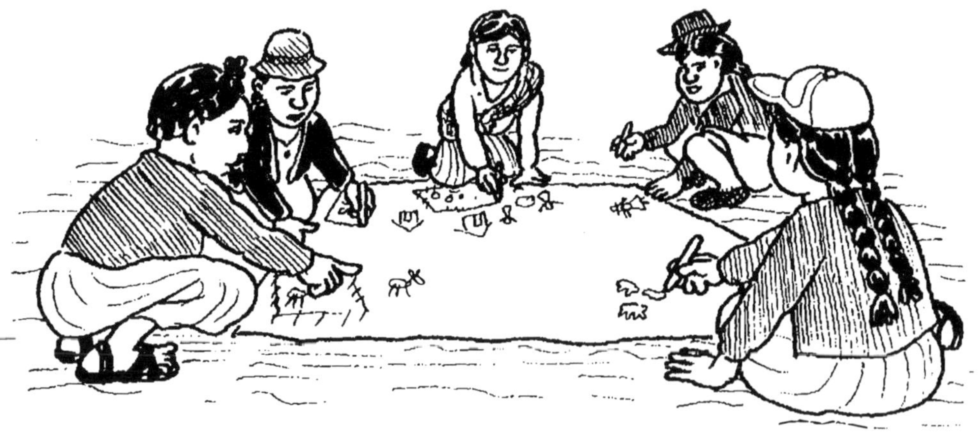

An Example of How Semi-Structured Interviewing Is Used

For an example of the use of an Ethnoveterinary Question list, please turn to "Traditional Medicine and Management," pg. 227.

Warm-ups: creating an atmosphere for participation

Forming pairs for interviews

Definition

There are many entertaining ways to form pairs and get people moving, talking, and meeting one another early in the workshop. Once the pairs are formed the interview task is explained. The interview task is related in some way to the content of the workshop or expectations participants have for the workshop.

How It Works

- One of the games described on the next page is played by all of the participants. The end result is that random pairs are formed.
- Each person interviews his or her partner with questions such as:
  - What is your name?
  - Where are you from?

  If the focus is on expectations, they can ask:
  - What are your expectations for this workshop?

  If the focus is on an aspect of the workshop they may ask:
  - What is your experience with animals? (or crops, or trees, etc.)
  - What would you most like to accomplish with your animals in the next year?
- After five minutes of interviewing each other, the partners sit together in the circle. Go around the circle and have each person introduce their partner to the plenary group. Each person also shares their partner's answers to the interview questions. They need to summarize the information in one minute for each person.
- If the purpose is to gather expectations, each shared expectation is written on newsprint as each person is introduced to the group. If the focus is on animal problems, these could be recorded. The list of expectations or animal problems can be used to inform the workshop.
- After each person is introduced, he or she receives a name tag with their first name in large letters.

Pros, Cons, and Other Uses

An important aspect of this dynamic is that pairs introduce their partner. Because they are not introducing themselves, there is less pressure, and people are thinking about the other people, not what they will say.

Hint: The greatest difficulty in this method is limiting the time of each response. If each person takes a long time, people get bored. Let people know the time limit. The facilitator can model this by presenting a partner and giving an example of a summarized introduction.

The list of expectations can be used at the end of the workshop as one form of evaluation, to check back to see if expectations were met.

Examples of games to form pairs

Example 1: The other side of the money

Upon arrival, everyone receives a coin made of paper or thin cardboard. On one side is the face of a regular coin, the highest denomination coin there is. On the other side two names are written, (note that each pair of names will appear on two coins) the name of the person receiving the coin and one other name. Once everyone has arrived they must find their partners by checking out everyone's coins.

Example 2: Animal pairs 1

Have enough pictures of different animals ready so that each person can receive half of an animal. Mix up the halves. Each person draws a half from a hat or other container. Or they can be put face down on the ground and everyone can take one. Everyone has to find the other half of the animal and introduce themselves to their partners as above.

Example 3: Animal pairs 2

A set of cards, each with the picture of an animal, is placed face down in the center of the circle. Each animal appears on two cards. Everyone chooses a card and then has to make the sound of and act like the animal on their cards and by so doing find their partners and introduce themselves as above.

Example 4: The round about

- Count off everyone present in twos (one, two, one, two)
- The ones form a circle and the twos form a circle around the ones.

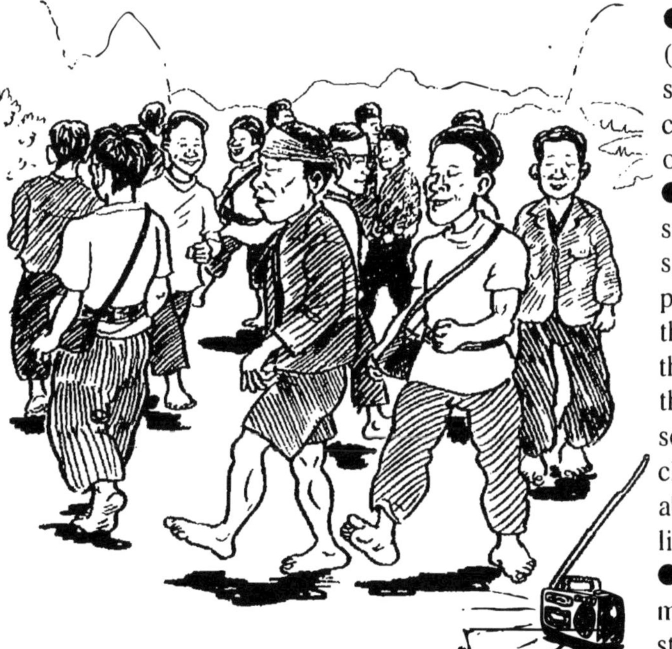

- Start some music (radio, tape or a song) and each circle moves in the opposite direction.
- When the music stops, each person speaks with the person in front of them. They share their name, where they are from, and something which challenges them about raising livestock.
- After a couple of minutes the music starts and the circles turn again. When the music stops they introduce themselves to a new partner. Keep doing this 4–5 times. When the last pairs are introduced everyone sits with that partner. They share their expectations for the workshop. Then they introduce each other to the group.

Source: Tecnicas Participativas para la Educacion Popular

The imaginary animal

Definition

A game for learning everyone's name for a group of participants who are nervous and unknown to one another.

How It Works

- Everyone stands in a circle.
- The facilitator begins and explains that he or she is holding a chicken. The facilitator shows the size and the weight of this imaginary chicken and lets the wings flap a bit. Then he or she asks all the participants, "Do you see the chicken?"
- The facilitator explains the dynamic: You must pass or throw the animal to another person in the circle, but first you must say the other person's name. This person receives the chicken, says another name and passes the chicken to that person. If you don't know someone's name, ask them first.
- After a bit the facilitator can say, for example, "It is no longer a chicken, it is a pig." The gestures for receiving and passing the object must be in accordance with the weight, size and character of the object. The person who receives the animal can change it as well, perhaps to a lion, and so on. This game is a good opportunity to loosen up a group who doesn't know each other, combining the introduction of names with creativity and theater.

Pros, Cons, and Other Uses

This game can be applied to anything the workshop is about. For example, if it is about forestry, the things passed can be tree seedlings, tools, a contract between the community, etc.

Source: Que Tal Si Jugamos

The web of names

Definition

A game to introduce everyone and relax the group.

How It Works

- Everyone stands in a circle. The person who begins holds a ball of yarn. She holds on to the end of the yarn and says her name and an expectation she has for the workshop. Then she throws the ball of yarn to another person. That person catches the yarn, says the name of the person who threw it and his own.
- He holds a piece of the yarn and throws it on to someone else across the circle, again saying the name of the person who threw it and his own name, continuing on until everyone has said their names and a great spider web is created. To undo the web, everyone must say the name of the person who threw it to them, their own name and the name of the person they are throwing it back to. They go along undoing the web this way.

Source: Tecnicas Participativas para la Educacion Popular

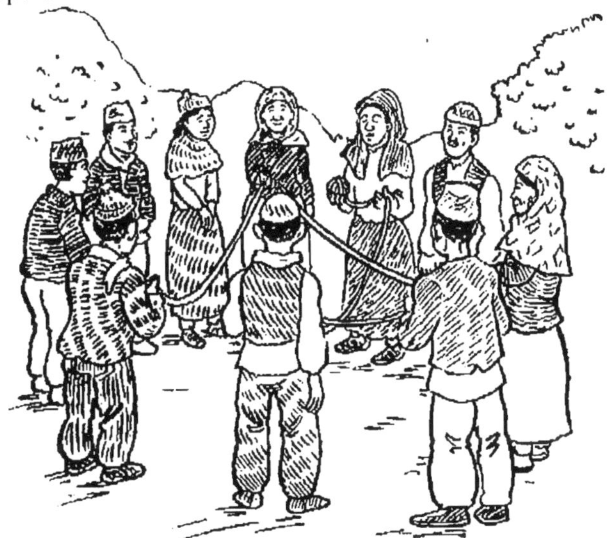

A found object

Definition

A warm-up using found materials which helps people to begin thinking at the symbolic level. They relate their feelings about themselves to their group.

How It Works

- Divide everyone into working groups of 3–4 people. Ask the participants to find an object, inside or outside, which symbolically represents their work in the world, who they are.
- An example might be a cup of rainwater to show that the person encourages others to grow. Or it could be a stone, providing a solid place and foundation for the family.
- Within 10 minutes they return to their group and introduce themselves to each other. They explain their symbols and why they chose them. Share some of the symbols in the plenary.

Pros, Cons, and Other Uses

If this is a training of trainers or CLW's, have them discuss the purpose of a warm up, the need for external materials in *dynamics,* and the levels of training. It is easy to share what we do with other people. It is a bit harder to share with others what we think. It is the hardest to share what we feel with other people. This dynamic reaches the level of what we feel about ourselves.

DO

THINK

FEEL

A variation: Provide sticky name tags and colored pens, pencils and sticky colored papers with scissors. Each person can create a name tag with a symbol which represents how they feel about themselves – for example, a drawing of a bird to show the freedom to seek after a personal vision.

Source Vella 1995

Games as energizers and teachers

Games for group formation

Definition

These are a set of simple games to aid in the formation of random groups. Since small-group work is integrally important to participatory adult learning, as is laughter and fun, these games are aids to creating a good learning atmosphere.

How It Works

Each game will get the larger group moving or thinking as they form new small groups.

Counting off

- Everyone stands or sits in a circle. Participants will count off from one to seven. As each person says their number, they turn their head toward the right and the next person. They must count off loudly and quickly.
- The person who has the number seven does not say "seven." He or she only turns his or her head to the right rapidly and silently. The next person begins again with one.
- We try to get this going as fast and loudly as possible. Anyone who says a number incorrectly or says seven, loses and later has to pay a penalty with a song or joke or dance.
- Once this has been done several times, the group can count off to form small groups, counting from 1 to 4 or 5 or 6, depending on the number of small groups desired.
- Once people have played this game with vigor, they tend to count off in the future with vigor.

Choose one of these

- In each variation, participants choose an object, usually a picture or a word, from a hat, the floor, or a small box. There are as many identical objects as the number of people needed for each small group.
- This can be used to form permanent work groups for the duration of the workshop. These groups then retain the identity of the object they have chosen.
- **Numbers:** The simplest is to choose pieces of paper with numbers (for example, 1 – 4 from a hat to form four groups.)
- **Pictures:** Pictures of four different kinds of animals or bugs, tools, medicinal plants, forage trees, crops or something with significance culturally. These are placed in a box, bag, or hat, and people draw one.
  The pictures chosen should relate in some way to the workshop content. They can be used several times over the course of the workshop for group tasks. Then you can refer to the groups by the name of their object: "Would the honey bees please come to this corner or do this task."
- **Words:** written on a small piece of paper. The words relate to some aspect of the workshop.
- One of the tasks given to the groups is to explain the significance of their object or word to a plenary session. For example, in one workshop which was centered around group organization, four traditional words from the local language were used. Each word represented a different form of working together. One was *aine*, a Quechua word describing the collaborative work people do when they harvest together for one another. Each group then had the name of a collaborative way of working together. They had to discover the significance of the word and explain it to the larger group. This *dynamic* served as a way to focus on the

importance of culture, word meanings, and local language.

- **Go fish:** Small drawings of four kinds of fish with loops on them are placed on the floor in a "pond." The participant receives a fish pole (stick), line (twine) and hook (bent paper clip).

  Each person fishes a fish from the pond. All of the fishes of one type form a small group.

  This can form a part of a preceding *dynamic* which involves participant's responses to questions. Each fish will have a question written on the back. As people get their fish, they read the question and answer it for the whole group.

  The questions are focused around a specific topic under discussion and are open questions. For example, questions about management of newly placed seedling trees, or questions about how to make a seedling bed for a vegetable garden could be used. These open questions initiate a dialogue among the participants.

  After the *dynamic* related to the questions is finished, all the fishes of one kind can join together and form a new small group.

Noah's ark

- Everyone is told they are different animals on Noah's Ark. There is a big storm and the Ark is about to sink. The leader is Noah.
- Noah will shout to the group how many life boats there are. The group must then form itself into equal groups to fill the lifeboats. They must get close to each other in their lifeboat.
- For example, Noah says there are three boats. Everyone divides into three groups. Then Noah says there are two lifeboats. Everyone divides into two groups. You can play this several times, changing the number of lifeboats each time.
- The last time Noah says there are X lifeboats, he says the number of small groups he wants for the task. These final groups are the small groups which work together on the new task.

Source: Roxana Vega

Get off my back!

- To form four groups make pictures of four different animals. Each person has one animal picture taped to his or her back.
- The person has to try to guess which animal is on their back. No one may speak. Everyone can use pantomime to help the other people discern the animal on their back.
- As people discover which animal they have, they form a group of that animal.
- This can also be used to open a discussion about the importance of verbal and nonverbal communication.

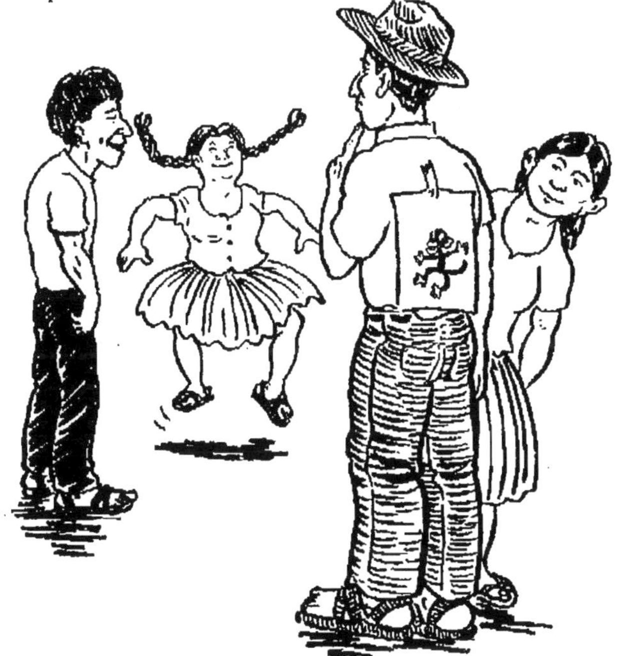

Games for evaluating and sharing

Definition

Each of these games is a fun way for a group of people to begin discussing a serious question. They can also be used to discuss a series of questions on a related topic.

These tools work well in situations of training, assessment, or evaluation.

How It Works

- For each game there is a set of prepared open questions.
- The game is usually played with the whole group of participants present in a workshop or meeting, up to 25 people.
- Depending on the purpose of the game and the topic, there may be discussion of the answers or a simple sharing of the person's experience without discussion.

Examples of these games:

Spin the bottle

- If the group has more than ten people, they can be divided into two teams and the teams play against one another. The people form a seated circle.
- A bottle is placed on the floor in the center of the circle. One person spins it. When the bottle stops, the person it points to answers a question.
- We use this to have Community Livestock Workers share interesting or difficult cases they have seen. One person describes the case and what he or she did, and then everyone discusses it.
- It can also be used in a situation where there are many questions, such as about pasture or disease management, or land use, or a community forest. The questions are put into a hat, and the person the bottle points to chooses a question and answers it. The question is discussed by all. Be sure to include some fun cards, such as: "Sing a song," or "Tell a joke."

Come over to my side

A game for encouraging Community Livestock Workers (CLW) in their work.

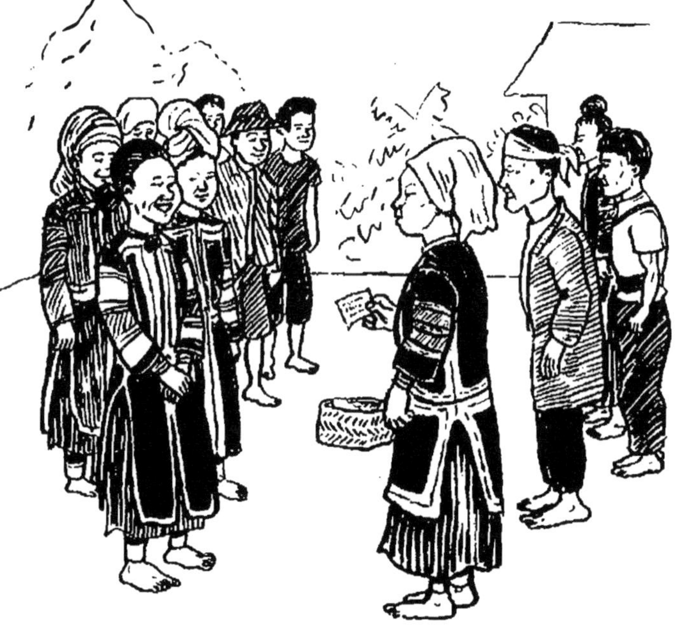

- The participants form a line on one side of the room. The facilitator has a basket with questions. The facilitator faces a CLW and draws a question and asks it. The CLW answers the question and moves beside the facilitator.
- Then the CLW on the side of the facilitator stands in front of a CLW and asks her a question. When she answers, she moves to the facilitators line and asks the next question.
- Another facilitator or participant will write on newsprint the answers of the CLW's. They can be organized into successes and problems.
- After the game is played, discuss the results. Discuss the high value of the work that is being done. Give time for the group to problem solve and encourage the others in their problem areas.

Some of the questions which have been used:

- What work have you done with your community organization?
- What difficulties have you had in your community with your work?
- How many animals have you treated and how many got well?
- Last month did you have a problem with an animal?
- They say medicines have arrived in the medicine shop that we don't know about. How can we learn about them?
- Bring a blue flip flop with you.
- Give a back rub to another CLW.
- When an owner comes with a sick animal and you don't have time to look at it, what do you do?
- If someone comes from another community to ask you to go treat their animal, will you go?
- How have you shared what you've learned in these workshops with your family?

Roulette

- A spinner wheel with different color sections is made (See "Making Our Training Materials," pg. 318). Questions are prepared ahead of time on colored paper or on white paper with one side colored to match the spinner colors.
- Participants sit in a circle. Or they sit in teams. Go around the circle, each person taking a turn to spin the spinner. Or each team sends a volunteer to spin the wheel.
- When the spinner lands on a color, the person who spun chooses a question with the same color.
- The person reads the question out loud and answers it from his or her experience. If this is a team game and the person is stumped by the question, the team can discuss the question and answer it.

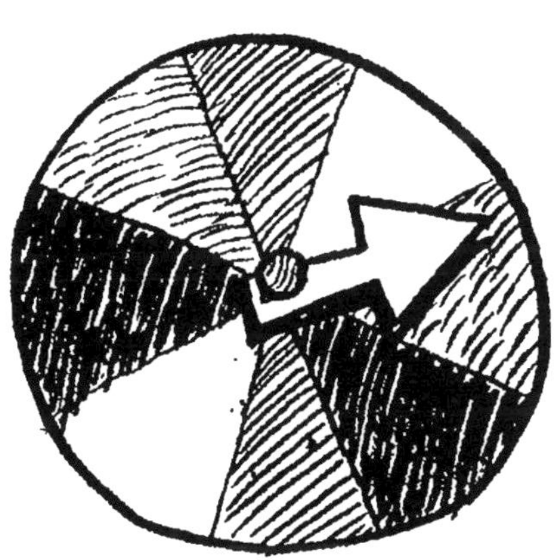

The well of "They say"

- With this *dynamic* a box is used and has statements in it which all begin, "They say..."
- Divide into teams. Each team sends a volunteer to reach into the well of "they say" in turn.
- The person draws a statement from the well, and the team decides if it is true or false and why.
- The other team must decide if the answer given is correct or not in the village context.
- If the other team agrees that the answer is correct, the team who answered receives one point.

Examples of statements used:

- They say there is a trained Community Livestock Worker here, but he does not help with sick animals.
- They say women are not allowed to attend community meetings here.
- They say there is a CLW here who is a woman and that she is very good at making sick cows well.
- Be sure to include some fun things like "Sing a song" or "Tell a joke."

This dynamic must be carefully used. The statements are drawn from an assessment process involving the community and represent situations people in the community have outlined as difficulties and achievements. But the statements can be leading in nature and not allow free dialogue. People need to understand that the discussion created is the important part of this dynamic, not the points given to each team for a correct answer.
Source: C-CIMCA

Musical ball

Play music and pass a ball at the same time. When the music stops the person explains some aspect of the day's material.

Tape toss

Toss a roll of tape or a stick or whatever is handy to a person. That person then tells something he or she learned today. He or she tosses the tape to another person who does the same, and so on.

Questions

Everyone takes a slip of paper with a question about the previous day's topics. Some papers say answer the question, others say ask someone else. If the person doesn't know the answer he or she can ask someone else. Some papers say win a prize (you could have some treat or sweet as prize) or pay a penalty. Make it fun. The person comes to the front of the room and follows instructions correctly but with lots of joking and laughing.
Source: RDC Nepal

Games for review

Definition

When people are learning new technical information it is often helpful to review the new information together. These five games are from the Rural Development Center in Nepal for their CLW training program.

Diseases and animals

- Put pictures of all of the animals studied on the wall up front. You can also add one or two not studied.
- Have ready a set of cards with the names of the different diseases studied in the workshops – some with duplicates if they attack several species.
- Distribute the cards among all the Community Livestock Workers.
- In turn, everyone puts the disease on the animal who gets it. In the discussion, everyone decides if the cards are correctly placed.

Source: RDC Nepal

Fever exchange

- Go around the circle counting off the people. Instead of saying 1, 2, 3 say the names of the three medicines used for fever: Penicillin, Terramycin, Penadur (Benzathene Pen).
- The first participants in the circle say the names of the medicines. Then the same three medicine names are repeated around the circle.
- The leader stands in the center of the circle. There is one less chair than the number of participants. When the leader says Penicillin, all the Penicillins have to change places. If she says Terramycin, all the Terramycins have to change place. If she says FEVER, everyone changes place.
- The leader runs to take a chair. Each time there is a new leader.
- You can change this game to fit the situation and the thing being learned.

Source: RDC Nepal

Concentration

- A set of cards is made (usually 18 – 20). Half the cards have names of diseases, half the cards have treatments for the diseases. Each disease card has its paired treatment. Put the cards on the floor upside down in the center of the circle.
- Go around the circle or play in a small group. Each person turns over two cards to try to match the disease with the treatment. As they remember where the cards are, people will turn over matching cards. When they turn over a matching pair, they can keep them.
- Continue around the circle until all of the pairs have been removed. Each person holding a pair can give a brief description of the disease and why the treatment is used.

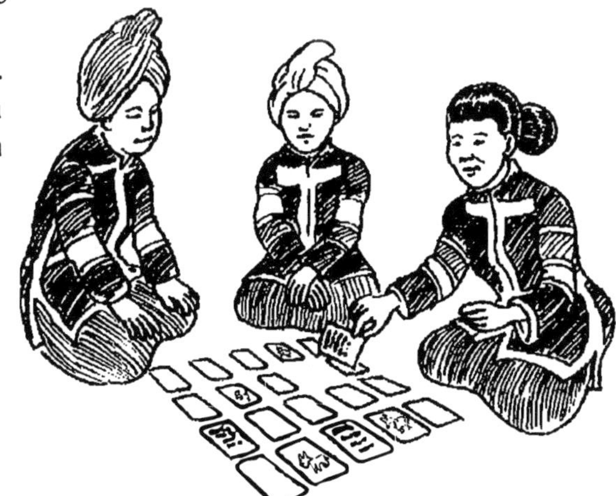

Quiz contest

- Form everyone into three teams. Each team can have a name such as liver fluke, pneumonia, round worms.
- The three teams are on one side of the room. The facilitator is on the other side.
- Each group selects a leader and the leader answers.
- The first team leader draws a question from a small basket, and the facilitator asks the first team the question. The team has a set amount of time to answer. The team consults its members for the answer. Each correct answer gives a point for the team. This game is only for subjects and questions for which there are right and wrong answers.

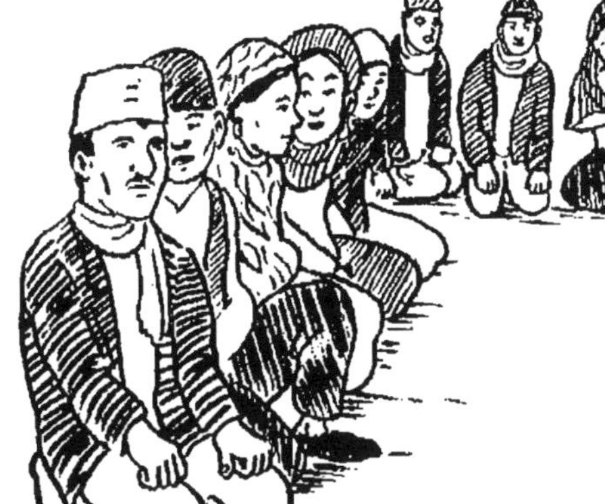

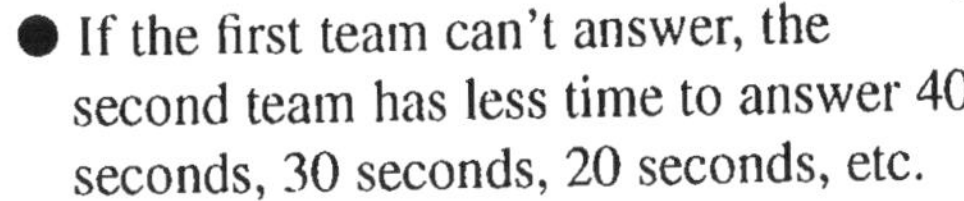

- If the first team can't answer, the second team has less time to answer 40 seconds, 30 seconds, 20 seconds, etc.
- Once the first question is answered, the second team draws a question, and so on until all the questions are answered.

Source: RDC Nepal

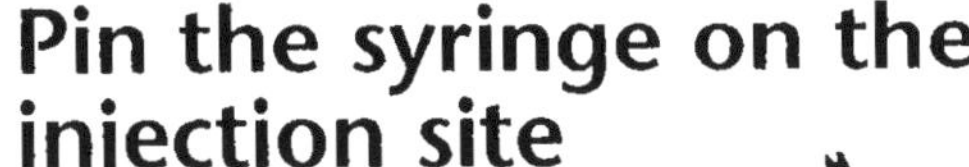

Pin the syringe on the injection site

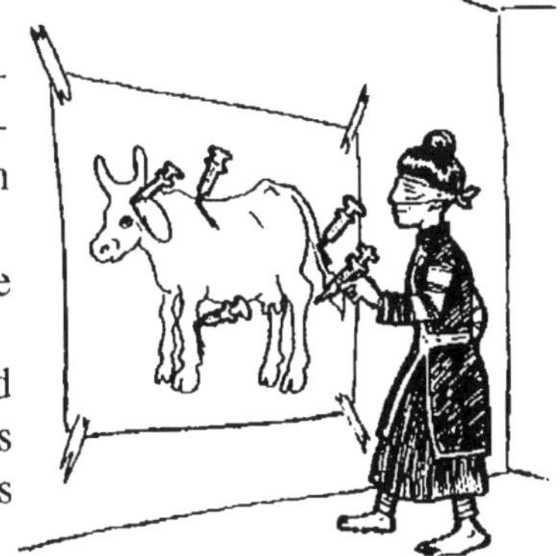

- Blindfold a person who volunteers. The person has a cardboard syringe and there is an animal drawing on the board.
- The blindfolded person pins the syringe on the animal picture.
- After several people have pinned on syringes, the group discusses the correct injection sites for this animal.
- They move around the syringes to show appropriate sites and remove the inappropriately placed syringes. Source: RCD Nepal

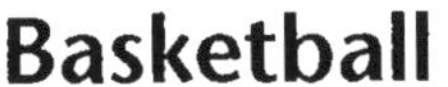

Basketball

- One large basket in the middle of the room has several small balls with the names of anti-inflamatory medicines on each one. Around the room are 5 – 7 smaller baskets with the names of different diseases on them. The object of the game is to take a ball from the big basket and throw it into the small basket for that disease.

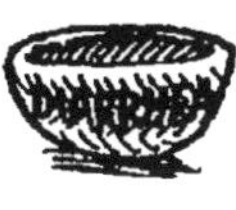

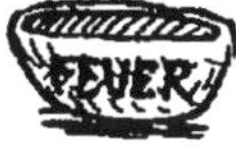

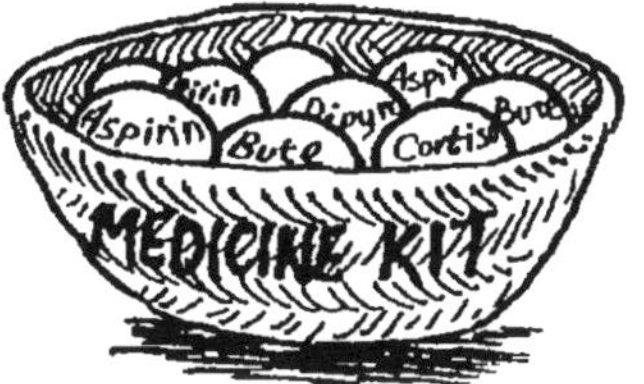

- Everyone judges if the ball has entered the correct basket. Can this anti-inflamatory be used for that disease?
- Discuss the good use of anti-inflamatory drugs.
- This game can also be used for antibiotics and diseases.

Source: Mark Bounds

Other games for learning medicine use

Helping Health Workers Learn is a manual with excellent games and dynamics to learn the use use of antibiotics. We have adapted many of their dynamics for use with livestock diseases and drugs.

It is important to use only medicines available locally when teaching about antibiotics or other medicine use. If medicines are taught which then cannot be purchased by the participants, they will not be able to use their training.

For teaching concentration in medicines

Definition

This *dynamic* shows people How a medicine such as teracycline can be used in different concentrations.

It helps people begin to calculate the concentration of a medicine to be able to give the appropriate dose to an animal.

How It Works

- On a table where everyone can see: have three empty glasses; have three tablespoons of sugar, one next to each glass.

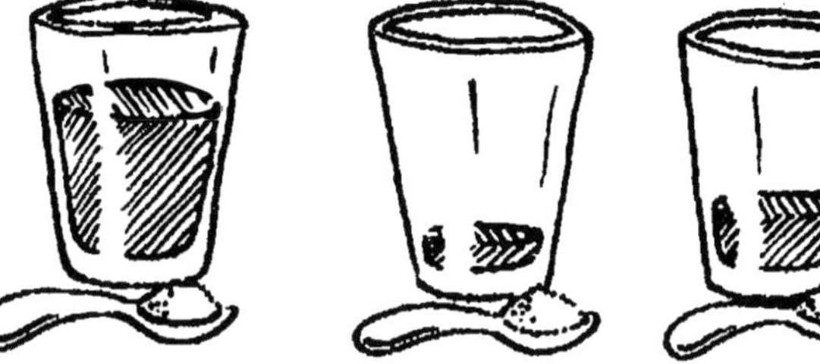
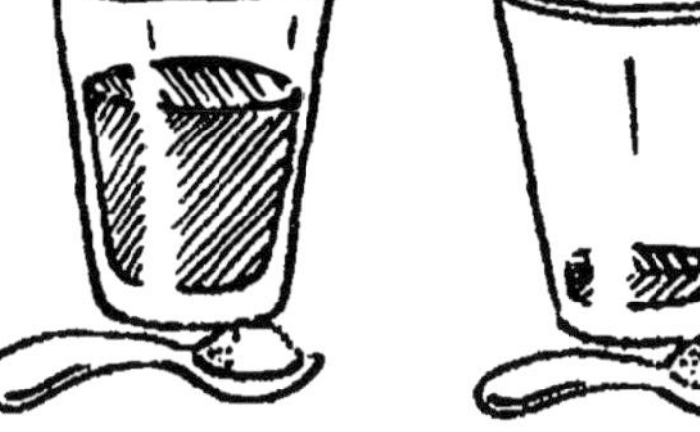
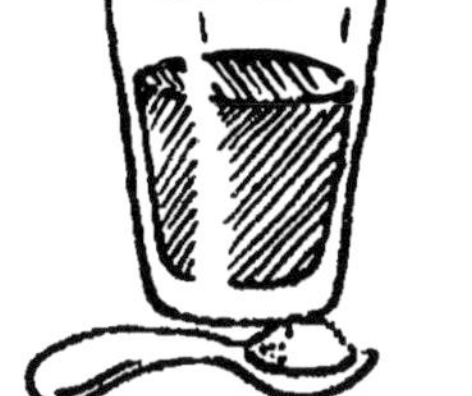

- Into each glass put the tablespoons of sugar. Next pour tea or lemon in water into each glass. The first glass receives a small amount of liquid. The second glass is filled half way. The third glass is filled up.
- Stir all three glasses.
- Three volunteers drink the three glasses of liquid.
- Ask the people, "Who drank the most sugar?" First ask the people who drank the liquids, then ask the remaining people. Have them discuss it. Almost always people will say the person who had the sweetest tea drank the most sugar.
- This is a very good place to begin a discussion of concentration of medicines. You can repeat the activity again and they can see all the glasses have the same amount of sugar. Once they have agreed on this, you can use three bottles of the same medicine in different concentrations to discuss the concentration of medicines purchased.
- In our local markets there are constantly varying sources of medicines. One week tetracycline may be sold in one concentration and another week it may be different. It is important for people to understand the concentration of the tetracycline to buy wisely and use the drug wisely.

Fun and energizing games

Definition

An energizer is a quick, fun way to get people up and moving when they have been sitting too long to be actively participating. These games are helpful when people are tired, just after lunch, or as a break in the middle of a long session where much concentration is needed. They should not be over used. The best energizers are ones which also relate to the topic being discussed in some way.

Examples of How They Are Used

Here are some examples of different energizers.

Different ways to walk

- With the participants in a circle, ask each one to walk to the other side of the circle, one at a time. Each person has to walk differently to get there. Someone could walk like an elephant, or like a cat, or hop, or skip, etc.
- This energizer can start a discussion about the many ways which exist to reach the same destination. The same work can be done differently by different people but the end result is the same.

Source: Goma Shrestha, Nepal

Tie the *auyao*

An *auyao* is the cloth Bolivian women carry their babies in and wrap up other loads to carry on their backs. In most countries there is a corresponding wrap and a way to tie it (you can also use a rope or belt).

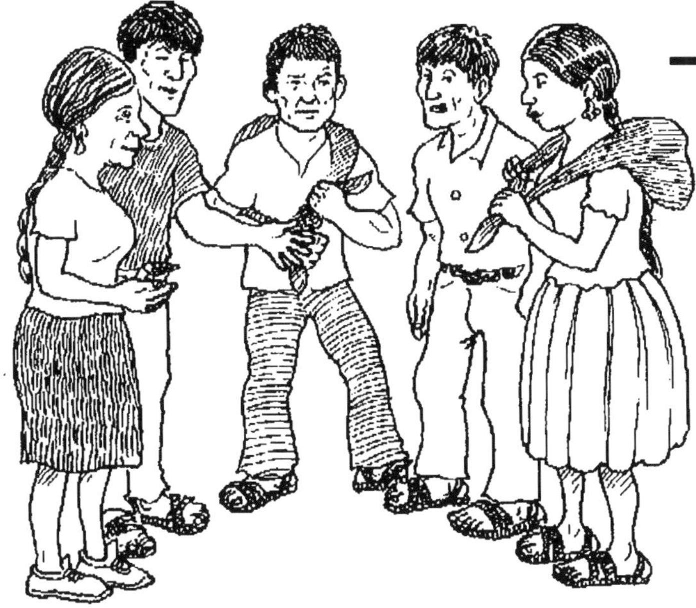

- The participants stand in a circle.
- Give each of two people at different places in the circle an *auyao*.
- The person who receives the first *auyao* has to tie one knot in it, untie it and pass it to the person on her right.
- The person who gets the second *auyao* has to tie a double knot in the auyao, untie it and pass it to the person on his right. The two *auyaos* will travel at different speeds around the circle.
- Tie and untie as fast as you can and continue to pass the *auyaos* around the circle.
- Whoever ends up with the two *auyaos* at the same time loses. You can play this game two or three times.
- People will go faster and slower to affect who receives the two *auyaos* together.

Source: Lina Maria Nivia Obando, Columbia

The people say

This is Simon Says with a twist.

- The leader says;"The people say pat your head," and everyone pats their head.
- The leader says, "The people say hop on one foot," and everyone hops on one foot.
- When the leader says, "Raise your right hand," the people who raise their right hands lose because the people didn't say to raise their right hand.
- Do a round slowly at first, so the participants get used to it. Then start to give the instructions faster. Gradually eliminate all the people except a winner. Or play a round and have all the people who lost pay a penalty.
- This is a fun way to talk about working together. It is easy to act without thinking about what the community has decided to do.

Source: C-CIMCA, Bolivia

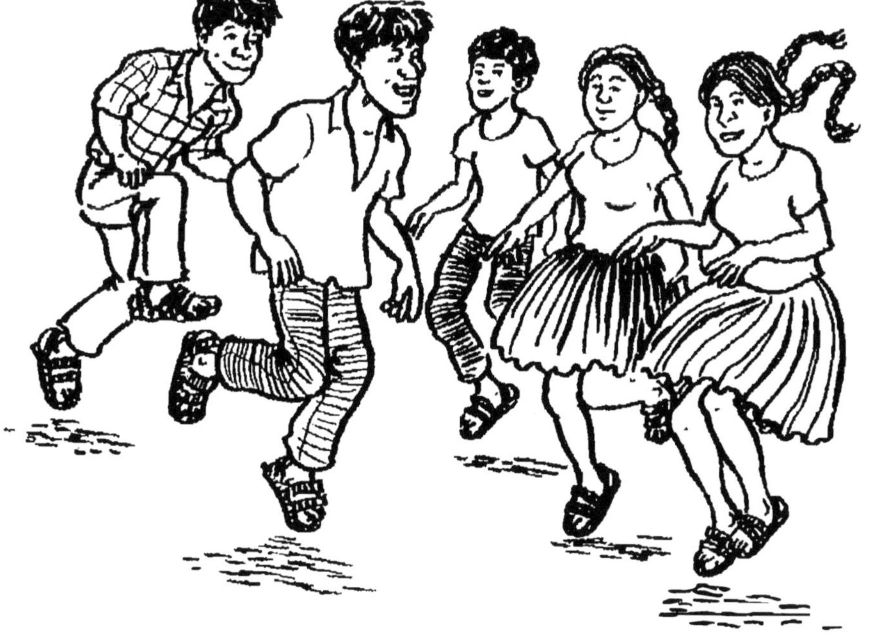

I pass the scissors crossed

- Ask for two volunteers. Tell the volunteers the secret of the game.
- Everyone sits in a circle, the volunteers interspersed with the other participants.
- Use one pair of scissors. The leader begins and passes the scissors to the person on her left. She tells the person how she is passing the scissors: for example "I pass the scissors crossed," or "I pass the scissors open."
- The person on the leader's left tells how he is receiving the scissors and how he is passing them on to the person on his left. They keep passing the scissors around the circle.
- The secret of the game is that players are supposed to describe the way their legs are situated when they receive and pass on the scissors. A player's legs may be crossed, open, or closed.
- Initially the leaders and volunteers will pass the scissors in the same position as their legs, open, closed, or crossed. The other people in the circle will think they are talking about the scissors. But gradually, the volunteers will pass the scissors in a different position from their legs and the people will notice the difference.
- As each person passes the scissors and tells how they have received and passed them on, the leader will say if they are correct or not.
- This game is just relaxing and fun.

Source: Carlos Tello

My right side is waiting for

- Everyone sits in a circle. Everyone in turn chooses to be a different kind of animal. Each person says the name of the animal and remembers it.
- There is one empty chair or space in the circle, to the right of the leader.
- The leader begins by saying, "My right side is waiting for the elephant." And the elephant must run to sit in the chair.
- Whoever is to the left of the now empty chair says, "My right side is waiting for (an animal name)."
- The leader counts off to five each time. If the person who sits next to the empty chair doesn't respond rapidly, he or she loses. Also, if the animal called doesn't respond rapidly, that person loses.

Source: Victor Alvarez

Fruit basket turnover

This game is an energizer as well as a way to get people to mix with each other. Everyone ends the game sitting in a different place.

- Form a standing circle of all of the participants.
- A leader goes around the circle and gives everyone the name of a fruit. There may be several apples and several papayas. Each person remembers his or her fruit.
- The leader says, "I'm going to the market to buy apples." All of the apples change places. The leader says, "I'm going to the market to buy pears." All of the pears change places. The leader continues this for several more fruits. Then the leader says, "Fruit basket turnover." All of the fruits change places.

An alternative way to play:

- All of the fruits stand in a circle in front of their chairs. One chair is removed. The leader begins to walk around the room. She says, "I'm going to the market to buy papayas." All of the papayas begin to follow the leader around the market. Then the leader asks for each of the other fruits. Eventually, all of the participants will be following the leader.
- The leader says, "I spilled the basket!" Everyone scrambles for a chair. The person who does not have a chair loses.

Board games

Board games are games played by a small group of people using a pre-made board. They often also use a die for determining how far to move pieces, a small item (rock, stick, or plastic toy) for each person to move around the board, and cards with questions to generate discussion.

Board games can be very helpful in initiating a discussion or reviewing a topic. They are used for assessment, training, and evaluation. Most traditional board games can be modified to be played in a training context.

Some commonly used board games:

The road to our vision

Definition

This is a game to help small groups analyze their future vision. In the game the people progress down the road to their vision for the future. Along the way they take positive steps and find pitfalls in working toward a common vision.

How It Works

- This dynamic is for a small group of 4–6 people.
- Each space on the road is a different color. Three or four colors are used. For each color there is a stack of questions and a place on the board to put the questions.
- Each player chooses a token. If tokens are provided they should each be different (plastic toys or animals work well). If people get their own tokens from inside or outside the room, they should each be different (match stick, pebble, seed, coin, etc.)
- Players roll the die and the highest or lowest number goes first. The first player rolls the die and moves his or her token forward on the road the corresponding number of spaces.
- When their token lands on a space, the person draws the top card from the pile of the corresponding color. The player reads the card and does what the card requests. If it is a question, the player gives an answer. This answer begins a discussion of the topic by the group as a whole.
- When the topic has been discussed, the next person takes a turn.
- If you don't have dice in your area see "Making Our Training Materials" for how to make one, pg. 319.
- Remind the players that the questions are for initiating discussion. The aim of the game is not to arrive at the finish first!

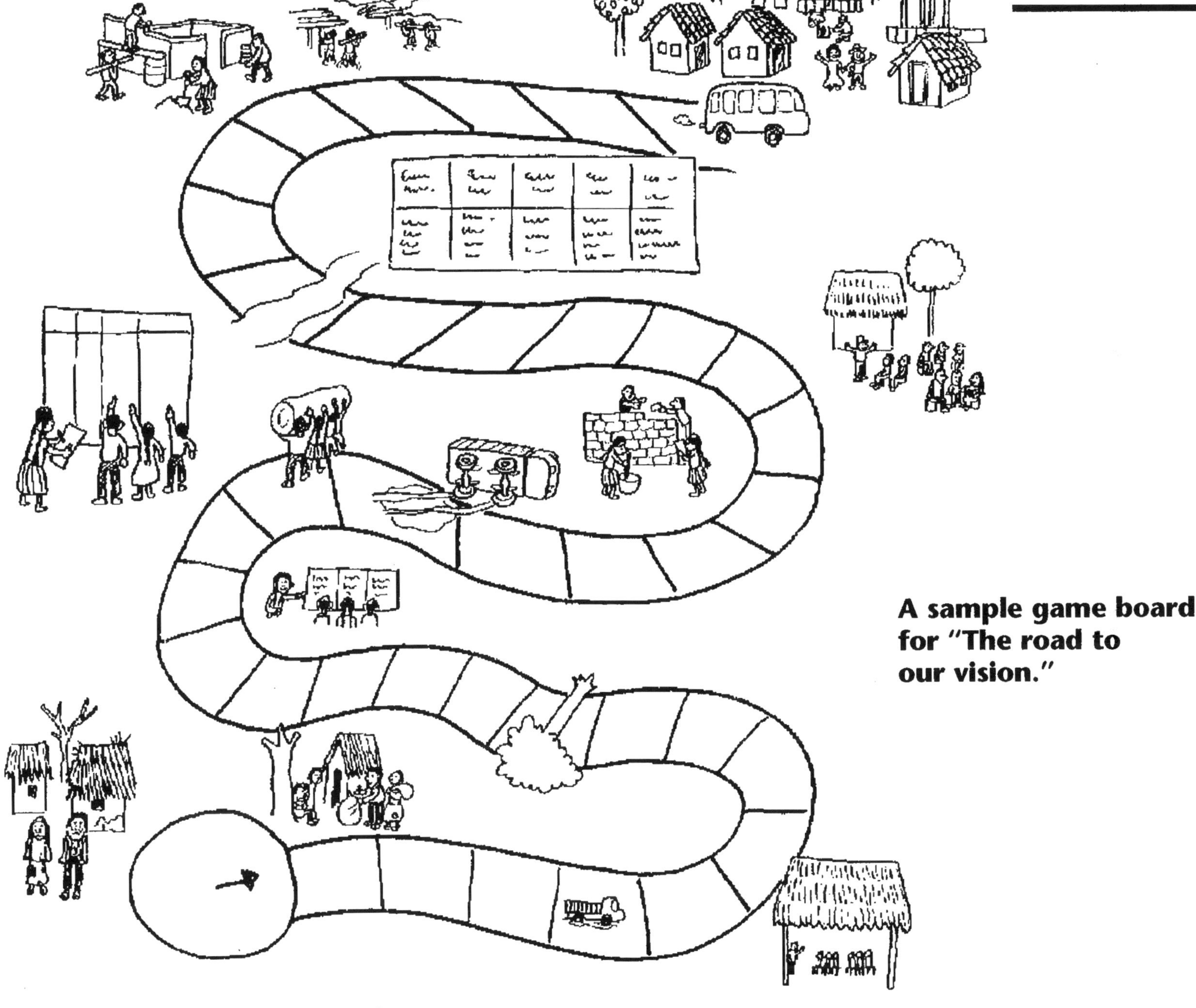

A sample game board for "The road to our vision."

Board Games

- The questions should be related to the reality of the local situation and the vision people have been talking about for their organization. They can be from all categories: economic, social, political, spiritual, cultural.

  Some examples:

  - What should the job of our organization be in goat production?
  - How should our organization help the members in selling their animals or animal products?
  - What would you like our community to look like in 10 years?
  - What would you like your farm to be like in 10 years?
  - How can our organization help you to accomplish your 10-year goals?
  - How should our organization be involved in community health care?
  - What should our organization do about schooling in our community?

  These are some ideas. The team of facilitators will help to make the appropriate questions.

For more information on defining the vision see "Defining the Situation," pg. 73.

- Some of the cards should also have pitfalls on them.

  Some suggestions:

  - Your organization has a fight about who should be the next president. Everyone is mad. What can be done?
  - Your neighbor did not control his fire and your new tress all burned. What can be done?
  - The river flooded your best pasture land. How will this affect you in working toward your vision?

- On the game board there are also several pitfalls. The first is, "Truck mired in the mud, lose a turn." The second is, "Tree down in the road, lose a turn." The third is, "Truck accident, lose a turn."
- Some of the cards used should also have fun things on them. One might say, "Tell a joke." Another might say, "You are happy to be moving toward your vision. Whistle a song and jump ahead two squares." Be creative as you invent your version of the game.
- Once the games have been played, a plenary session can draw conclusions about defining the vision. Then each small group can begin the work of defining the vision of the organization.

Pros, Cons, and Other Uses

One of the drawbacks to this type of *dynamic* is the tendency for participants to engage in superficial discussion in order to reach the finish first. It is important for participants to understand that discussion is the reason for playing. The time taken after the game to discuss in small groups is also essential. Once the group's creative juices have started, they will have many more ideas for setting their organizational vision.

A game such as this one is good to use in a "game night" with participants. They can have fun playing the game while they discuss a serious issue. This could prepare them for the following days work. So they have fun, relax, and learn at the same time.

These games should always be field tested before they are used in a workshop. They should be tested for clarity of the questions and intent of the game. If a question is not clear, throw it out and start again!

Developing this type of game can be challenging and helpful for CLW's. Once they have played the game, they will be able to write more effective questions to use in their community. Create a space in the workshop time for the CLWs to make their own games.

This type of game board can also be used in an evaluation. A small group can analyze where they have come down the road since they began their project. It has also been used to generate discussion about traditional knowledge and oral history.

We also used the game board described above to generate a discussion among CLWs about their work in their communities. The questions focused on what they had accomplished to date and what was left to be done. It was a good starter to a discussion which ended in a listing of problems and accomplishments with CLW work in their communities. The CLWs gained self-appreciation as others honored their work in their communities. They also established a set of recommendations for how to overcome the problems they faced.

Pigs in the pen

Definition

A board game used to focus discussion on a specific technical area. The same board and tokens can be used for different games by changing the questions asked. Players progress around the board and try to put their token in the home base area.

How It Works

- This game can be played with up to four people or four teams.
- Each player has a token which he or she places on the board in one of the four places labeled "Start." Each start area is a different color.
- The first player rolls the dice and moves his or her token to the right around the board based on the number rolled.
- There are four piles of questions based on four different areas of the topic. In this example, the topic was pig management. The four areas were nutrition, housing, genetics, and disease.
- After the player has moved, he or she draws a card from any one of the areas. The player answers the question. The group then discusses the answer and comes to consensus on the answer to the question.
- Once consensus is reached, the next player rolls the dice, moves his or her token, and chooses a question. Continue around the circle until all players have had a turn.
- Each player must move his or her token completely around the board and return to their start. From their start there is a set of six spaces leading to the home base. Players must enter home base on an exact roll of the dice.
- Home base is in the center of the board. For this game, our home base had a drawing of well cared-for pigs in a good housing situation.
- After the first person arrives at home base, the group should discuss their results from the game. They can make a summary presentation of their work to the plenary session. They can summarize in each category of questions.

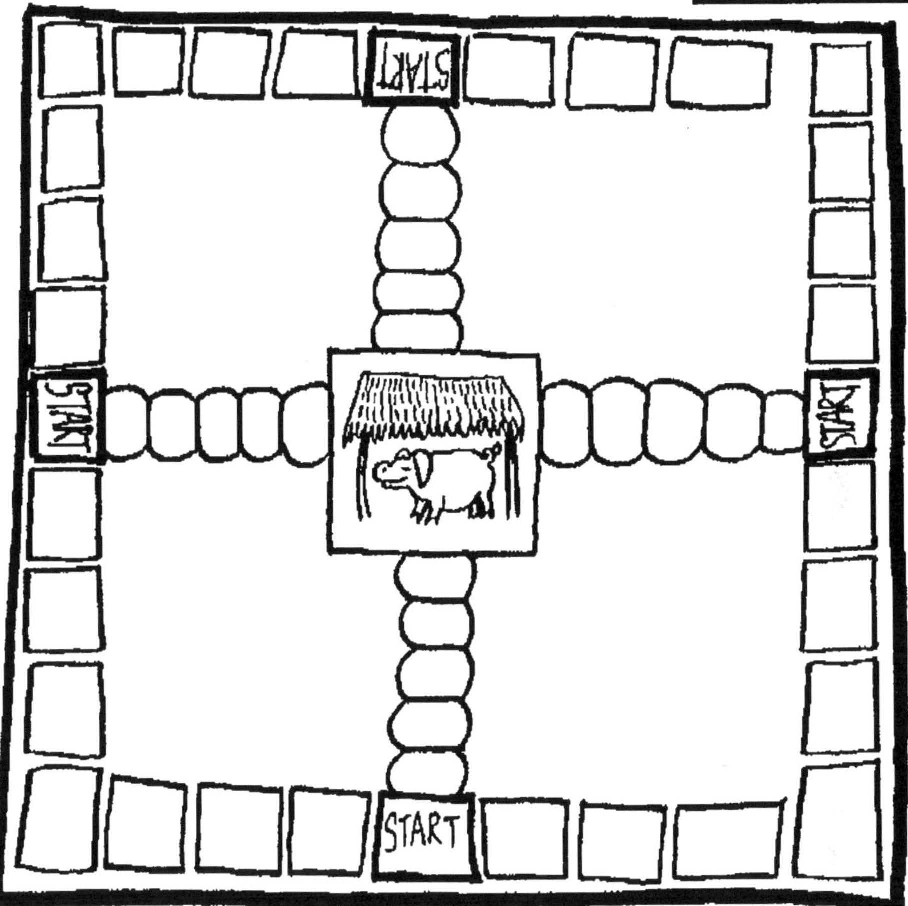

- An overall summary should be reached in each area. If there are gaps or questions, a further discussion can focus on those areas.

Pros, Cons, and Other Uses

As for all games with questions, the questions here should be field tested before the game is used in a workshop. Do not try to standardize the questions. The questions for each game must be tailor-made to fit each situation.

This game is very versatile. It can be used to generate discussion about a social issue as readily as a technical topic. Its greatest value is in the discussion created. This type of game can be used for assessment, training, or evaluation.

Our land

Definition

This is a type of mapping *dynamic* in a game-board form. It is used by a community in the process of decision-making about land use. People have the opportunity to experiment with different land-use scenarios and to discuss the problems and fears they have about the changes.

How It Works

- If you pre-make the board the background should look like what is commonly seen in the countryside of the community. The composite map people have made of the land surrounding their community makes an even better board. This would be a copy of a land model drawn onto a large paper with the current land uses and improvements removed.
- On a pre-made board, there are blank spaces for the game cards. The game has a stack of cards depicting different types of land use possible in your area including (with pictures):

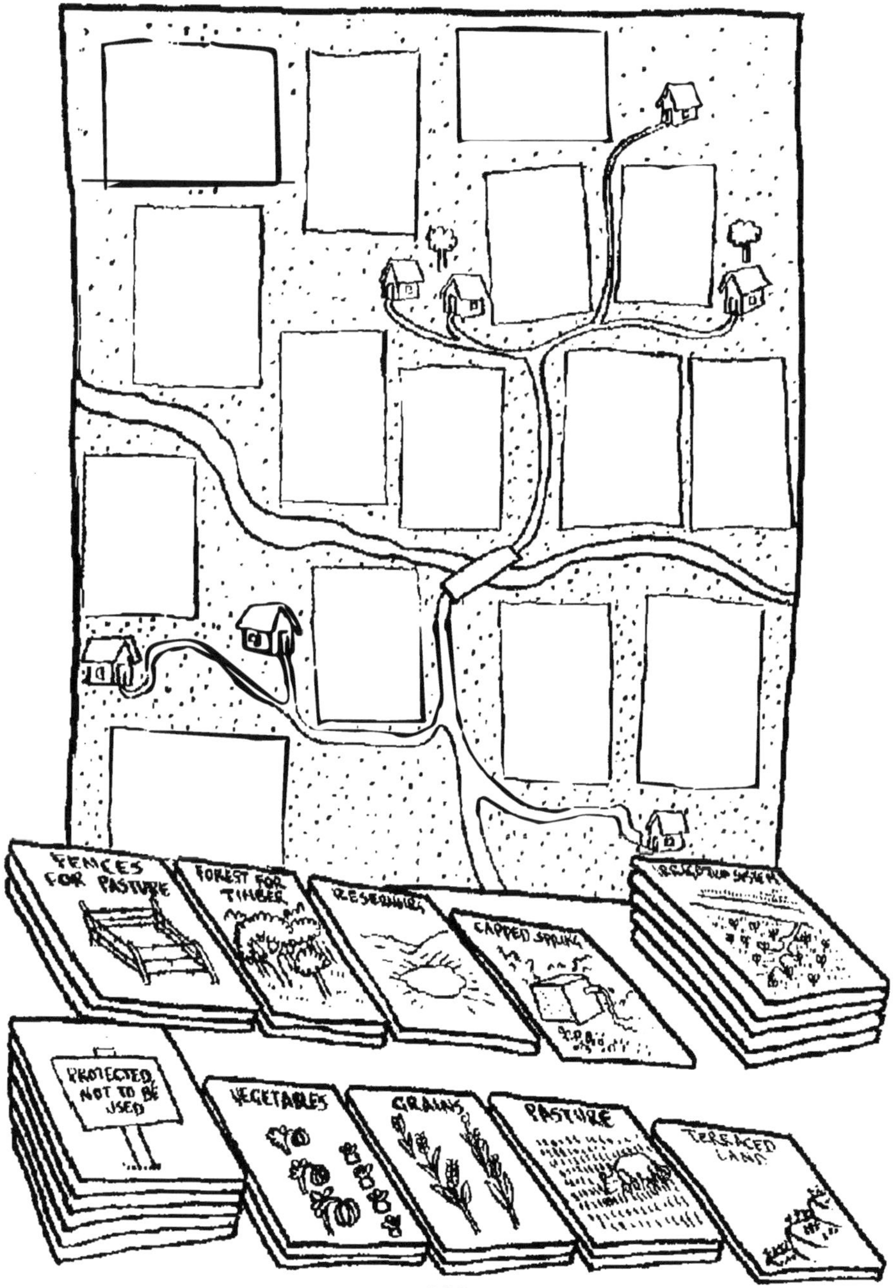

  6 with a sign that says "protected, not to be used"
  3 farming of vegetables
  3 annual crops such as grains
  3 pasture land
  2 terraced land
  3 fencing for pasture
  3 forested land for timber
  2 reservoirs
  1 capped spring
  5 irrigation systems
  Or the appropriate cards for your area
- There is also one community card to be placed on the map where the community center is located (if there is one).
- The game is for 4–6 players. The idea is to design the best land-use plan for their community. The players first put the community card on the map where it is currently located.
- The players decide together who will begin. The first person begins by placing a protected area sign as he or she feels is appropriate.
- Each person continues, putting the protected area signs in appropriate places (such as watersheds, steep hills, timbered areas, streams or rivers, etc.)
- After the protected area cards have been placed, the people take turns placing the land-use cards where they think is appropriate, one by one.

- After all of the cards have been placed on the map, each person in turn has an opportunity to move a protected area sign.
- Then each person in turn has two opportunities to move a land use card.
- Now discuss the map which has been created. As a group, you can decide if the map is a good one or if there is a better logic to changing or moving some of the cards. Reach a consensus as a group.
- In the plenary, each group presents their ideal land-use map. Discuss the problems involved and their possible solutions. It is possible to go from the game to developing an actual land use plan for the community area.

Pros, Cons, and Other Uses

This *dynamic* is a starter to a discussion on land-use planning. When a pre-made game board is used, the participants can discuss the various aspects of land-use planning a bit removed from their own context. If a pre-made board is used, it is important for the group to discuss the relationship to their own situation after they finish the game. Sometimes, if land use issues are difficult to discuss, this will open the door. After this game has been played, it would be appropriate for the small groups to then make a model map of their best land-use plan for their area. (See "Mapping," pg. 253)

Source: modified from CISTAC

Educational criteria

(Or discussing our work)

Definition

This game uses a board with six categories of statements. Each participant rolls a die and chooses a statement from the category corresponding to the number that comes up. The individual decides if the statement is true or false, and the group records the answer. This is a game for the training of trainers. Trainers can discuss the different aspects of education and educators.

How It Works

- A group of up to eight people plays this game sitting around a table. The board is placed on the table, and all the cards for the six categories are placed in their respective places.
- There are also three spaces on the game board which begin empty, they are: Agree, Disagree, and Question Mark.

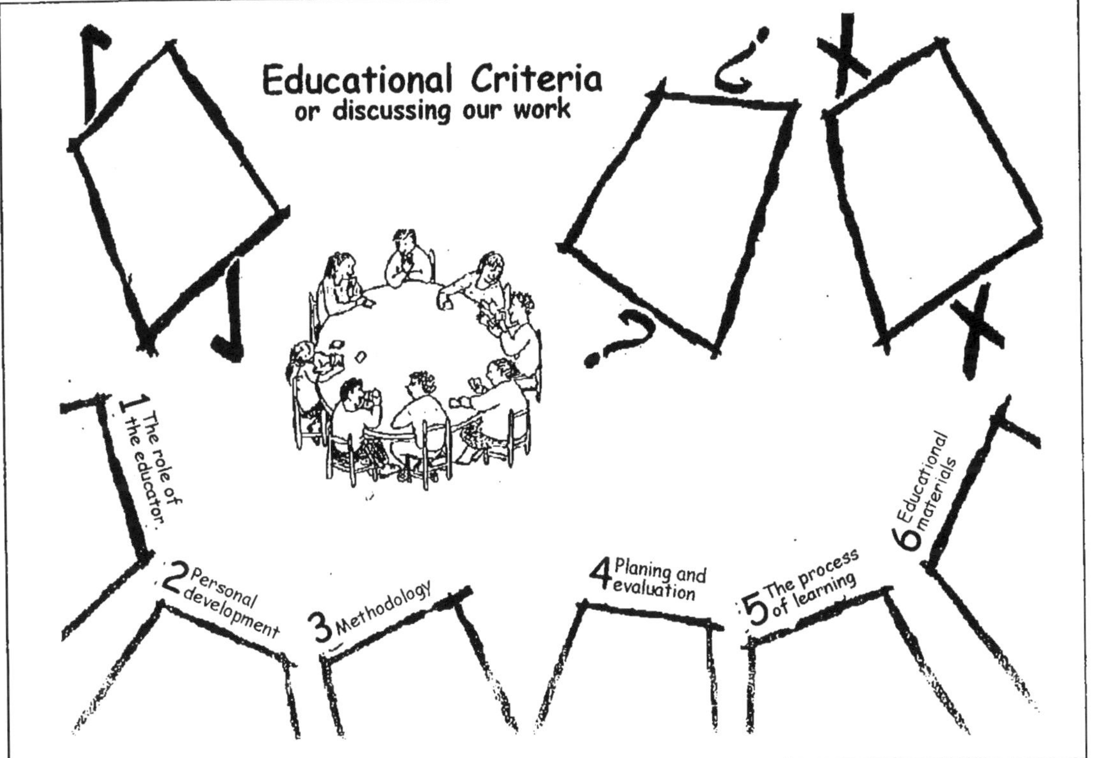

- Participants roll the die to see who begins. The highest number goes first. The first player rolls the die. If it falls on 3, he or she takes a card from category 3, methodology. The player reads the statement from the card.
- The player decides if he or she agrees, disagrees, or is not sure, then places the card where he or she thinks it belongs. The group then discusses how they feel about the card. If the group arrives at consensus, they place the card in that pile. If they cannot agree, the card goes on the question mark pile.
- Continue on around the circle, each player rolling and responding to each statement. This game can be played for a specified amount of time, or until all players have had a specified number of turns (perhaps 3 or 4), or until all the cards have been read.
- When the group finishes, they should summarize their results in the plenary session. The issues in question can be discussed by the whole group.

Examples of the Statements Used in This Game

There are 60 statements in this game, 10 for each of the six categories. Each category has some statements which are clearly true and some which are clearly false. There are some which are clearly ambiguous, to generate dialogue. In addition, each category has one fun thing which the person drawing the card must do.

Include one fun thing in each category:

- Get on a chair and call like Tarzan. The monkey Cheetah will applaud you.
- Pantomime how you get up in the morning.
- Tell a joke. If no one laughs, tell another.
- Recite a poem, dedicating it to someone in your group.
- You are a famous orchestra director, direct a brief piece. All the rest of the group will cooperate with you.

Pros, Cons, and Other Uses

Because this board game is not competitive and there is no winner, it tends to be a very good generator of discussion. But also, because it is noncompetitive, people may lose interest in playing the game if it takes too long. A good balance should be reached by field testing the game and by the attentive facilitator. The field testing of the statements used is very important. They should be clearly understandable and expressed simply.

Source: Cecilia Yanez and Osvaldo Almarza Centro de Investigacion y Desarrollo de la Educacion (CIDE) Erasmo Escala 1825 Santiago, Chile

CATEGORY	STATEMENT
1. Role of the Educator	In training, the educator must be able to satisfy all of the needs of the group.
2. Personal Development	When conflicts arise in the group it is best to solve them individually, outside the group.
3. Methodology	In the formative process, lectures are irreplaceable.
4. Planning and Evaluation	An evaluation is a moment of learning for all participants in the educative process.
5. The Learning Process	All learning implies change.
6. Educational Materials	It is better not to use educational materials because it takes lots of time to make them.

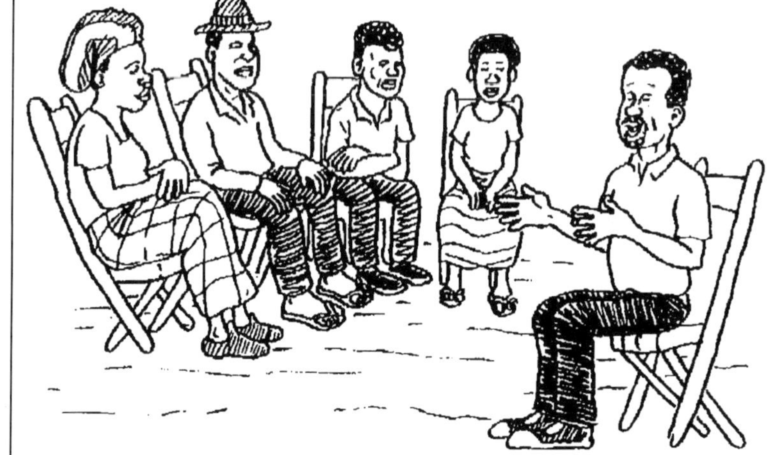

Card games

Definition

These games use a set of 20–25 cards which have been developed to initiate discussion about a certain topic. The same cards can be used to play several different games. These are usually for literate people but can be very effective.

How It Works

Cards for a Sustainable Farm Systems game – see the cards on the following page.

Three ways to play this game with a small group (up to eight people):

1. **Put all the cards face down on the table** scattered around.

- One person starts by picking up a card and telling everyone what he or she thinks about the statement. Is it true or false. What can happen if this is done? If it is not done? Or what should be done in this situation?
- Give each person the opportunity to state his or her opinion about the card. Discuss the topic and arrive at a conclusion.
- Have each person take a card in turn and respond, then discuss the response.
- Blank cards can be included to express things that have happened or that people know about on this subject which are not included in the other cards. The blank cards can be interspersed with the others.

2. **Put all the cards face up on the table** and give the participants time to choose the one they think is the most important or that they can identify with from their experience.

- Once each has selected a card, they take turns around the circle. Each person shares his or her experience, and the group discusses it, asking questions to clarify what has happened. Suggestions are given to each person from the group.
- After all have discussed their experience, the group makes a decision about the three things they would like to suggest to all regarding sustainable farm systems.
- In the plenary, each group proposes their suggestions and they are discussed. The plenary session results in recommendations for farm systems establishment.

3. **Put all the cards face up in front of the participants.** Give them time to read them all.

- As a group, they choose the one card most important to them and with which they can best identify. Based on the card, the group decides what the past was which created this situation, and what the future could be (or a possible solution).
- Once the history – past and future – is decided, the group prepares a drama to represent it to the rest of the groups.
- In plenary, each group presents their drama and discusses the problems and their solutions. The whole group makes decisions about what can be done to prevent these problems or to solve them.

Pros, Cons, and Other Uses

Can you see how version 1 could be used with different cards with a discussion of pig management or perhaps common diseases of cattle, or appropriate pastures? Any of the card games could also be used for other social issues such as the situations which arise in a marketing program (for example for marketing cheese or eggs), or good and bad leaders, or organizing for community animal health care. They can be very good discussion starters. Each small group should be given a task related to this game so the plenary session results in useful conclusions for all.

Card Games

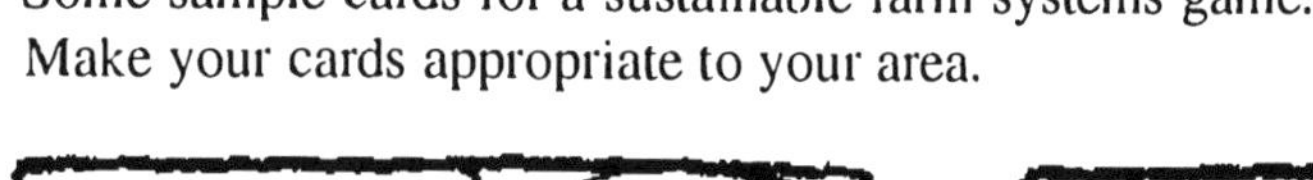

Some sample cards for a sustainable farm systems game.
Make your cards appropriate to your area.

I THINK THAT MEN UNDERSTAND MORE ABOUT FARMING AND SHOULD MAKE THE DECISIONS ABOUT THE FARM PLAN.
I AM NOT SO SURE ABOUT THAT.
WHEN I LOOK AT THE HILLSIDE OF MY LAND, I SEE EVERY YEAR THE PRODUCTION GETS WORSE.
WHAT SHOULD BE DONE ABOUT THIS?

I HAVE A LOW AREA OF GROUND WHICH FLOODS EVERY YEAR, BUT THE SOIL WON'T GROW ANYTHING WELL, I KEEP LOOSING EVERY TIME I PLANT RICE THERE.
WHAT CAN YOU DO ABOUT THIS?
AFTER I MADE MY FARM PLAN, THE RIVER FLOODED MY LAND AND DESTROYED MANY OF THE TREES I PLANTED. I DON'T BELIEVE THIS PLANNING WORKS.
WHAT DO YOU THINK ABOUT THIS?

THIS YEAR A FIRE FROM MY NEIGHBOR'S LAND DESTROYED ALL OF THE TREES I HAD REFORESTED ON MY HILLSIDE. THIS IDEA DOESN'T WORK.
WHAT CAN BE DONE ABOUT THIS PROBLEM?

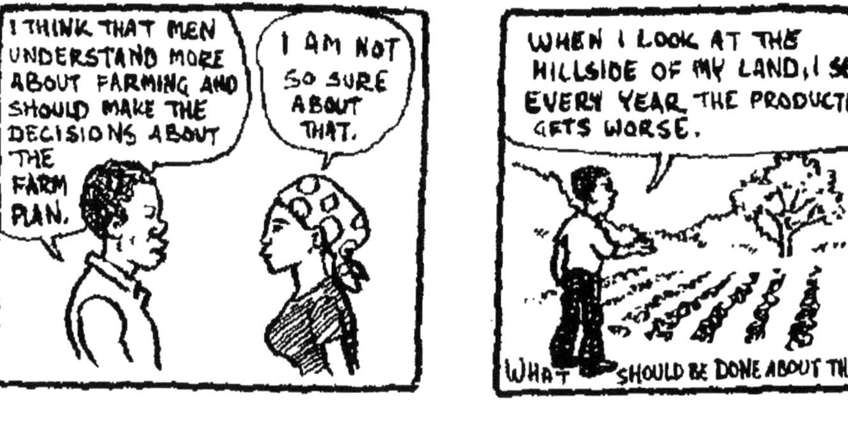

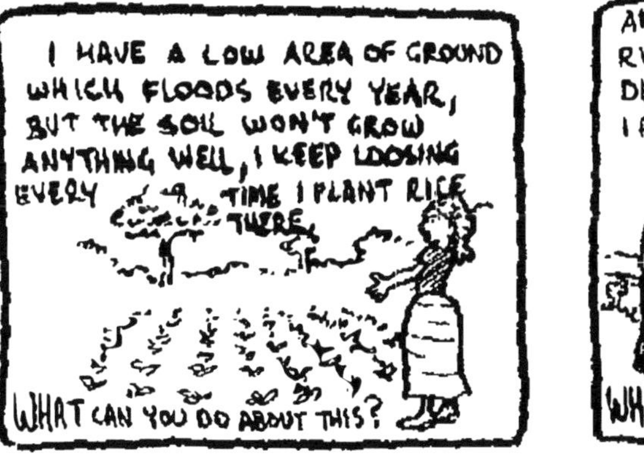

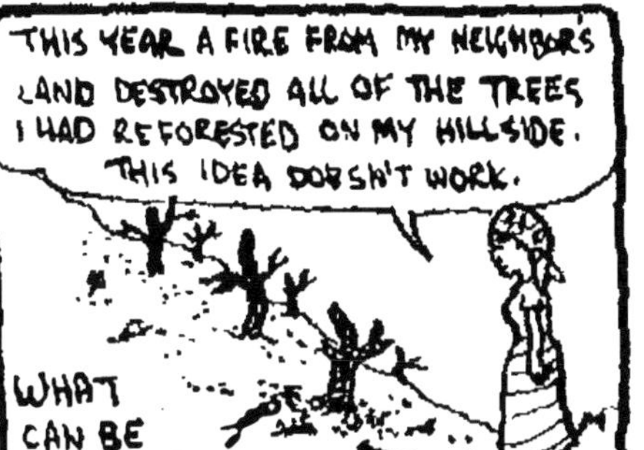

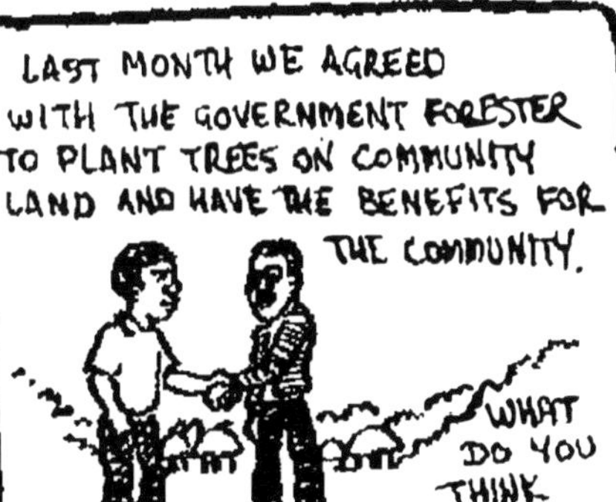

OUR ORGANIZATION MEETS ALL THE TIME BUT NEVER ACCOMPLISHES ANYTHING FOR OUR FARM SYSTEMS.
WHY DOES THIS HAPPEN?

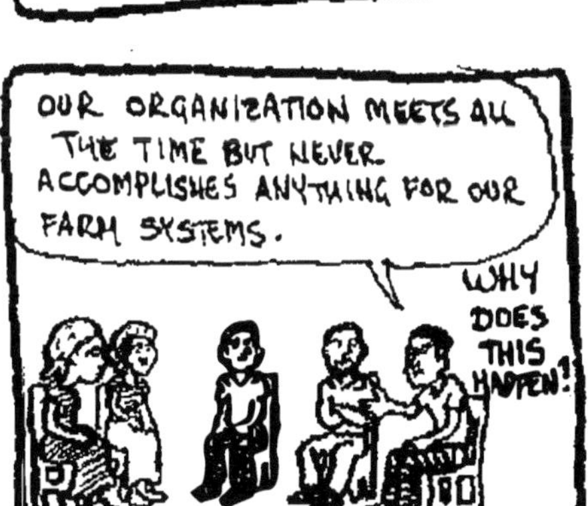

Add some more. You will need 20–25 cards.

The treasure hunt

Definition

In this game small groups go on a treasure hunt. There is a treasure for the winning group. But the greatest treasure comes from the small group work to organize a set of cards which they have gained through the treasure hunt.

This game can be used with any topic which has a series of actions to complete. It energizes the groups to dialogue about the series of actions and the order in which they should take place.

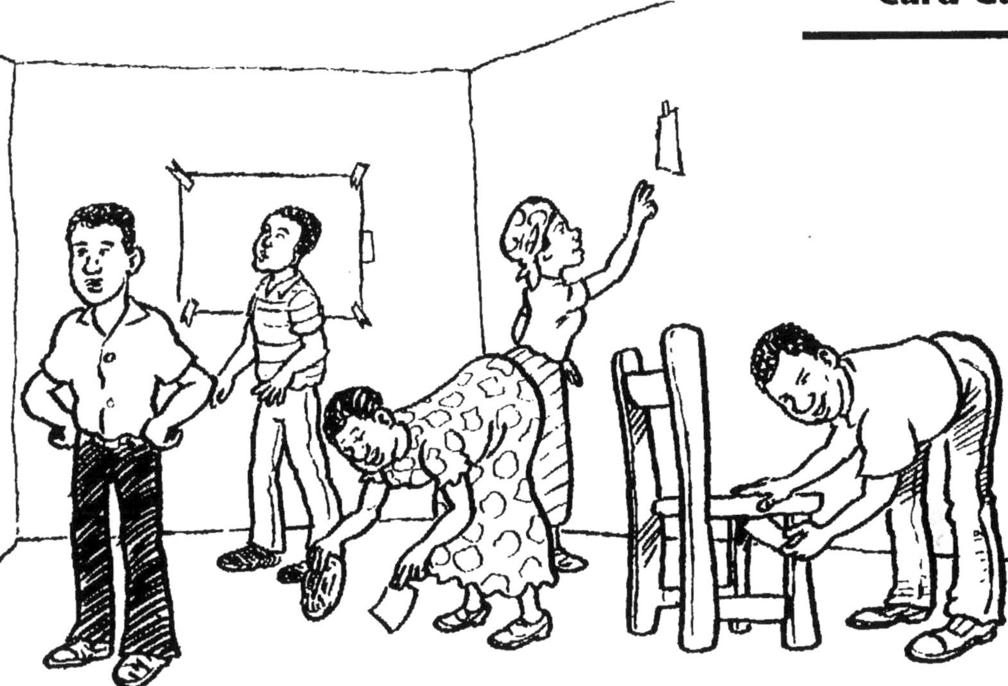

How It Works

Here is an example used to discuss how to organize a community vaccination or worming campaign.

- Divide into small groups. Each group receives a color (green group, red group, yellow group, etc.) For each group there is a set of papers of the corresponding color hidden around the room or training area.
- When the leader says GO, everyone looks for their set of papers. The first group to find all of their papers wins.
- There should be a prize for the group who wins, something they can all enjoy and or share with the others (like a bag of candy or fruit or crackers).
- Each group then takes their papers and organizes them in the order they feel one should follow in organizing a vaccination or worming campaign.
- We have used this list:
  - Talk to the community president
  - Discuss campaign at community meeting
  - Talk to government agent
  - Visit house to house
  - Do community training on the disease to be prevented and the importance of vaccination
  - Community meeting to organize the campaign
  - Buy medicines
  - Have the campaign

  We add in a few extras like:
  - Hunt a fly
  - Wear a cap of the institution
  - Consult with local NGOs
- Also include a blank card so the group can add in a step they feel has been left out.
- Each group has a set amount of time to do the task.
- Each group presents their order in the plenary session. Together everyone discusses the proper order for the papers. Together the participants arrive at an order they feel is the best for their future work. Each step should be clear for all present.

Pros, Cons, and Other Uses

Usually most groups will try to work in all the papers as steps, even those which are irrelevant to the campaign. When these show up in the order, it is a good opportunity to talk about group decision making and creativity in thought and planning, as opposed to blanket acceptance of what a trainer or organization says. It creates an opportunity to encourage those who thought critically and eliminated the inappropriate papers.

This can also be used to discuss whether a community that needs the vaccination should wait until an NGO comes to help them, or do it themselves. The idea in this game is for a community to think about their own independent planning of a vaccination campaign. This is so that they will not be dependent on an NGO or the government for future vaccinations. We use this in areas where NGO and government services are very sporadic. This way the community will be assured of regular disease prevention for their animals.

Also, the groups who hunted the fly can be asked about manipulation and the way some activities distract us from our purpose or goal (that of organizing the campaign), if we don't think about them well before we act.

The sequence will vary from country to country depending on the laws. If the country requires that only a certified vaccinator can vaccinate, you must include the steps of coordinating with that vaccinator. In this discussion you can also dialogue about the problems involved in a campaign and the solutions to those problems.

The treasure hunt can be used for any activity which has steps to complete it. The same game can be used to discuss the steps for planning and implementing a community training or an organizational project such as well drilling.

To make the game less directive, have the participants brainstorm all of the steps to completing an activity. Make up the cards for each group based on the brainstormed steps and add in a few extras. Go on the treasure hunt. The groups define the proper order of the steps as above.

Source: Adapted from Alforja

Chapter 13
Making our own training materials

This chapter covers the following topics:

Some tips for making training materials

As you plan your training events and *dynamics* think about these things:

✔**Make your own training materials,** or better yet, **make them with the training participants.**

✔Use locally available, **low cost materials** so local trainers see they can make their own training materials as well.

✔Try to use **real objects** or animals and plants rather than drawing them.

✔Design training materials so they **build on the knowledge people already have.**

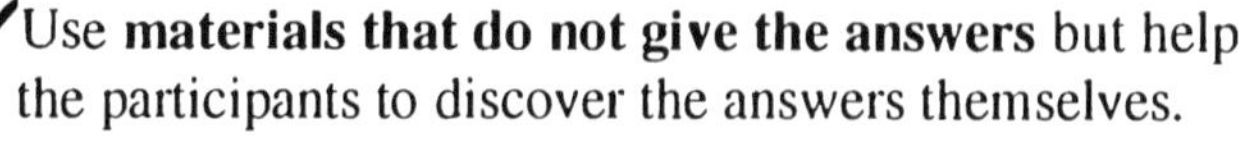

✔Use **materials that do not give the answers** but help the participants to discover the answers themselves.

✔Develop materials which express the local reality.

✔Give time in the workshop for making new teaching aids and applying creativity and imagination. Use the materials the students develop for future workshops.

✔Use fairly **simple training materials** so the participants can go home and use them in their community.

✔Field test the materials, especially written ones, before you use them, wherever possible.

Learning to make and use pictures

Illustrations can be effective, inexpensive, and easy to reproduce.
They can be a tremendous aid in communicating well.
It is important that your drawings say what you intend them to say!

Types of drawings

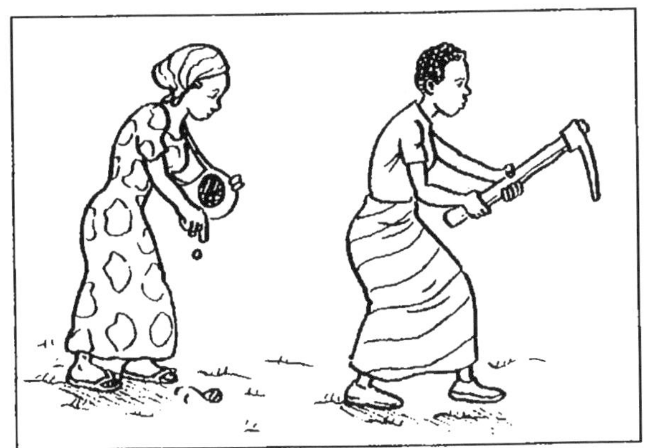

Line drawing

Generally most appropriate
Line drawings are simple, clearly express an idea, and have sufficient detail. These are easier for people to copy to make their own materials to take home.

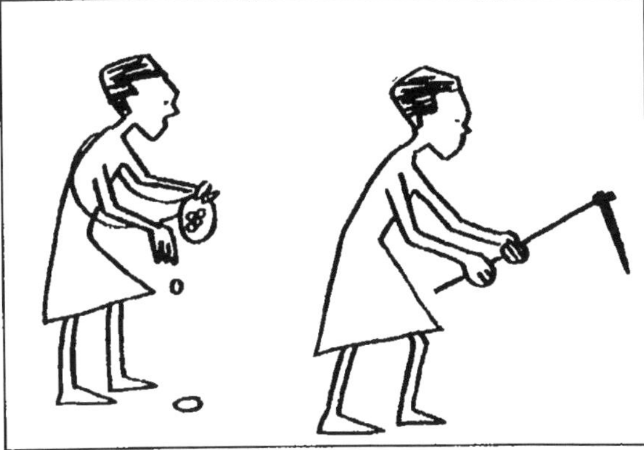

Stylized drawing

Stylized drawings are usually less appropriate. They are too simple and the expressions of the people can't be seen. People may not see themselves in one of these drawings. Not as good in stimulating discussion.

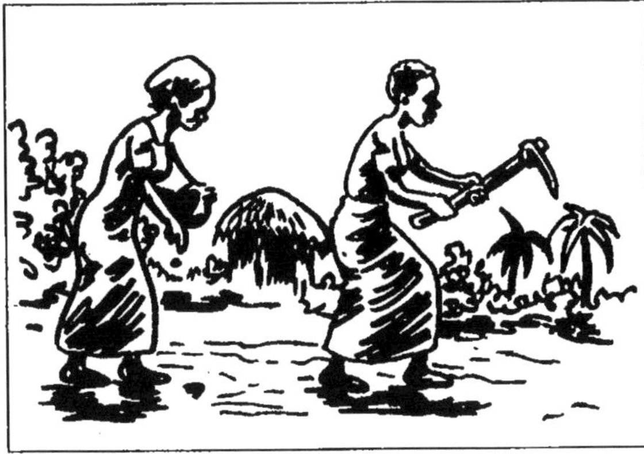

Shaded drawing

Shaded drawings are usually less appropriate. The shadows can be confusing. The background can distract from the drawing, and people may concentrate more on the background. They cannot easily be copied.

In this book and in all of our training pictures we use line drawings. We often will use simple pastels for colors to make the pictures brighter and more interesting. All of the drawings in this book can be copied for training.

Communicating respect and concern

By the way we draw, we communicate what we think and feel about the people in the drawings.

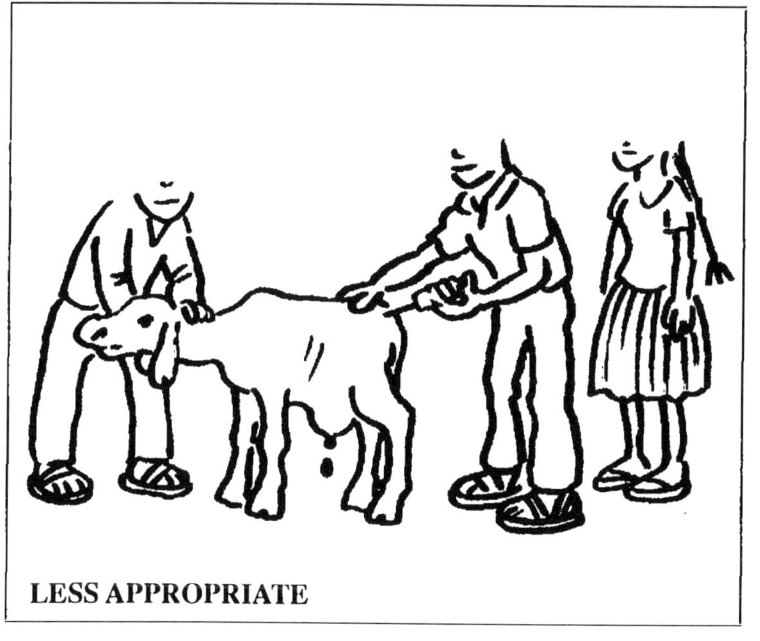

LESS APPROPRIATE

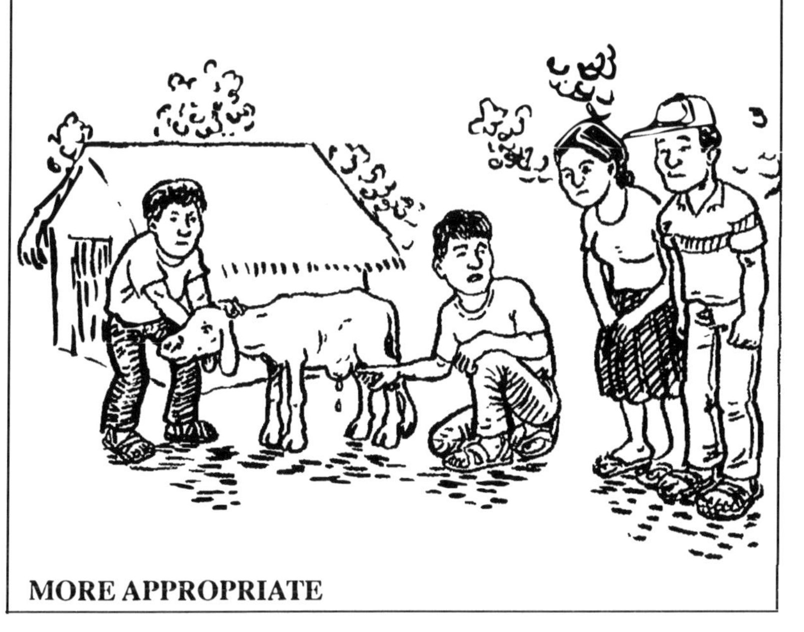

MORE APPROPRIATE

Make your drawings look human, friendly and real.

Who is in the picture?

Often, because men usually train men in agricultural training sessions, the pictures they draw have men doing all of the tasks.

What does this communicate to the women?

- If it is a new task, it suggests that the women cannot do the new task.
- If it is a task traditionally done by women it makes their role in agricultural production invisible.
- If women are shown only in menial tasks, this reinforces the idea that they can only do menial tasks.

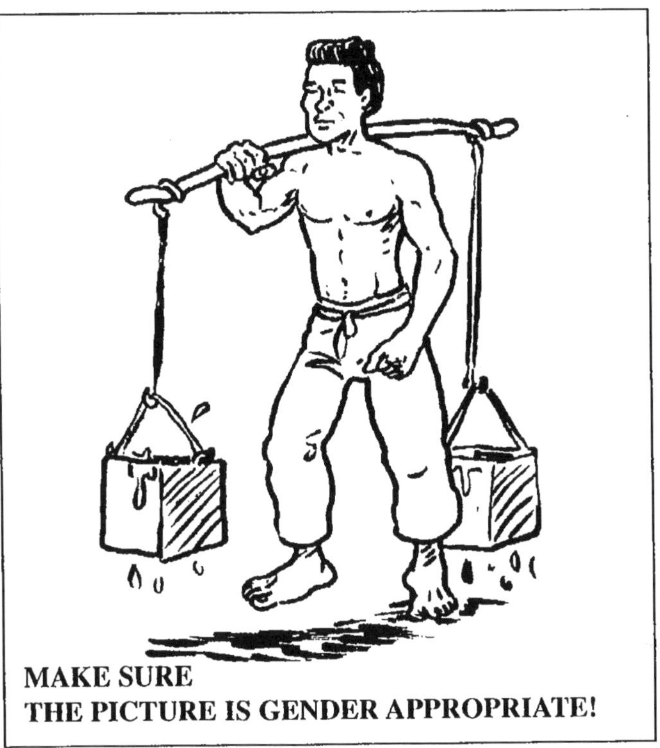

MAKE SURE
THE PICTURE IS GENDER APPROPRIATE!

Don't make a picture of a man performing a task which a woman performs in real life.

As you are developing training materials – be they posters, leaflets, or manuals – make sure women are present in the drawings doing highly respected tasks.

Gender is not the only area where drawings should be appropriate.

When you make a drawing be sure the people are:

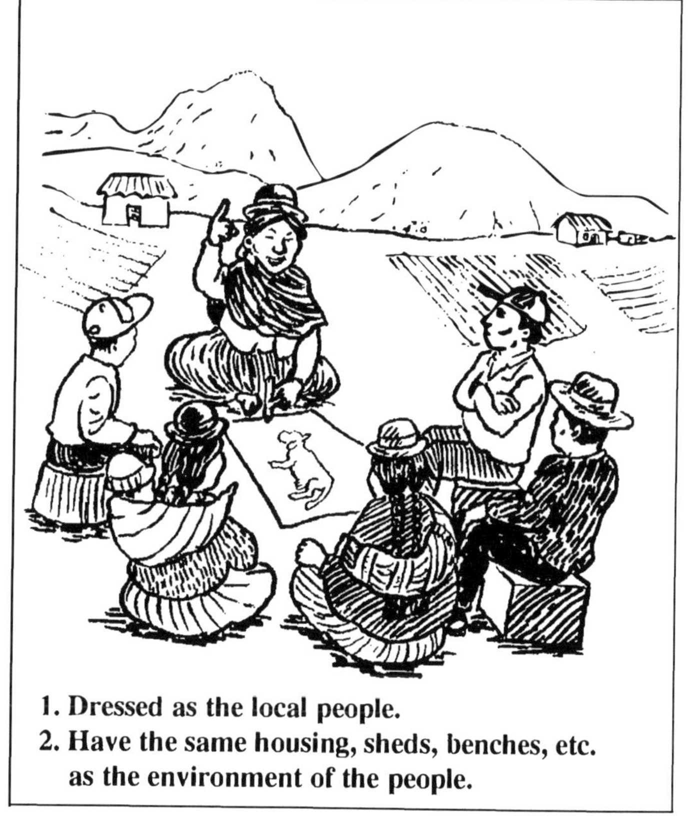

1. Dressed as the local people.
2. Have the same housing, sheds, benches, etc. as the environment of the people.

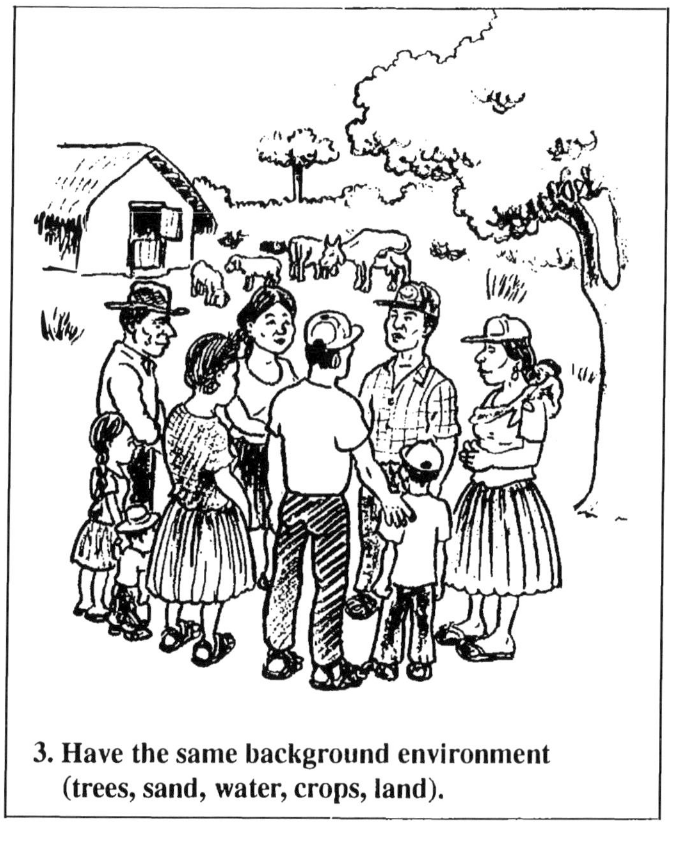

3. Have the same background environment (trees, sand, water, crops, land).

People's expressions communicate what they are feeling

By showing expressions on people's faces, your illustration communicates much more. The expressions tell the message more clearly than words.

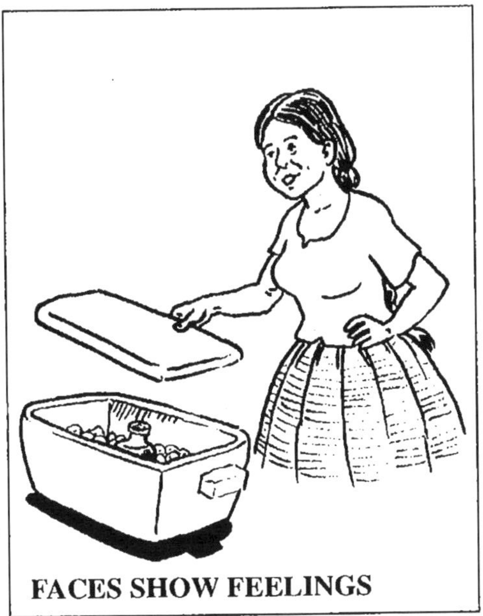

FACES SHOW FEELINGS

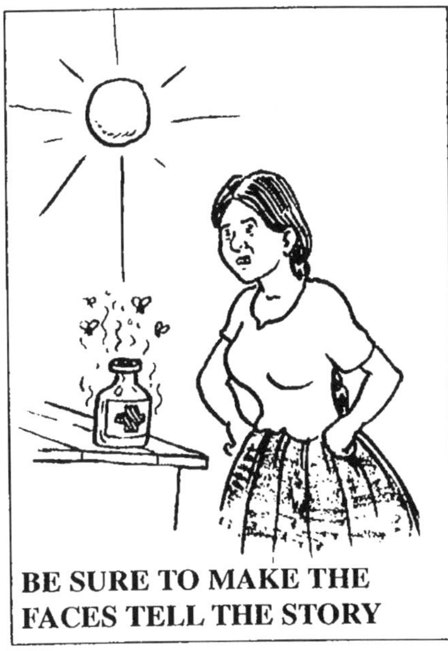

BE SURE TO MAKE THE FACES TELL THE STORY

Make sure your drawings include the expressions on people's faces.
Do not draw their backs only or faces without expressions.

When to use cartoons

There is a great tendency in leaflets and training manuals to draw all the people as cartoon figures. Generally speaking, cartoon figures are appropriate only where criticism or social comment is being made. Cartoon figures change the shape and relative size of people's faces and bodies. This makes fun of them and causes laughter. It shows disrespect for the local people if real situations are expressed as cartoons.

If you want to express something from the people's reality, or need to express fine detail in a technical subject, cartoon characters are not appropriate.

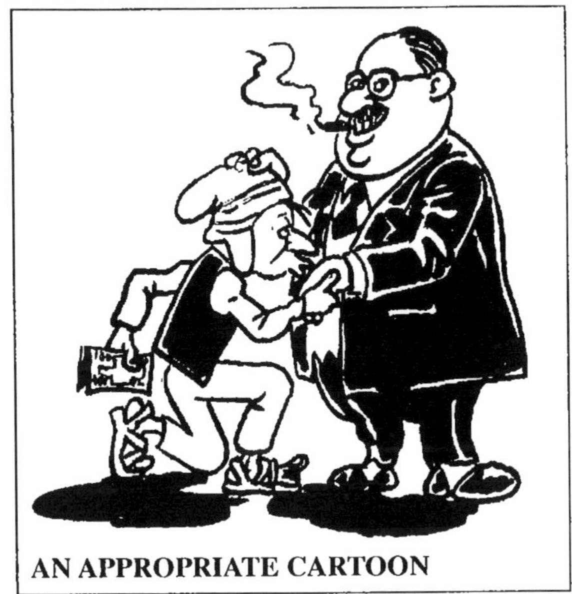

AN APPROPRIATE CARTOON

A sketch with less detail is appropriate when the detail is not necessary.

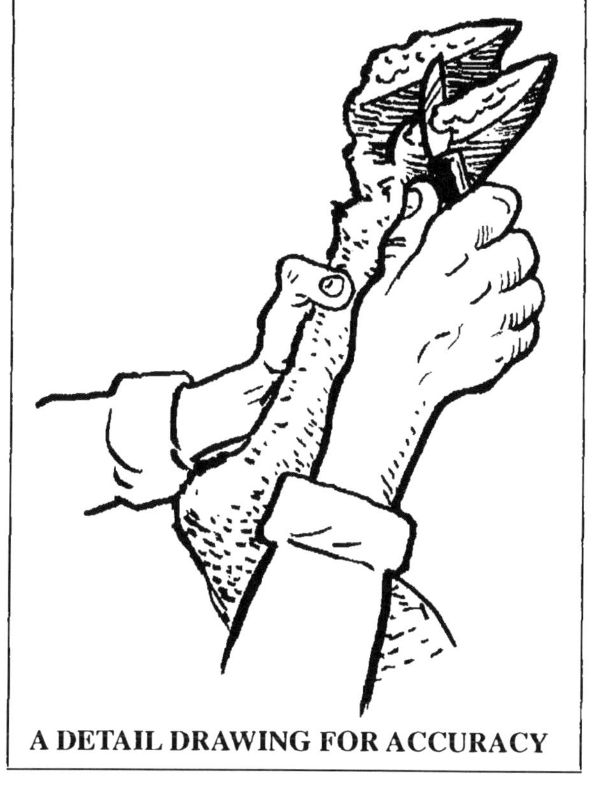

A DETAIL DRAWING FOR ACCURACY

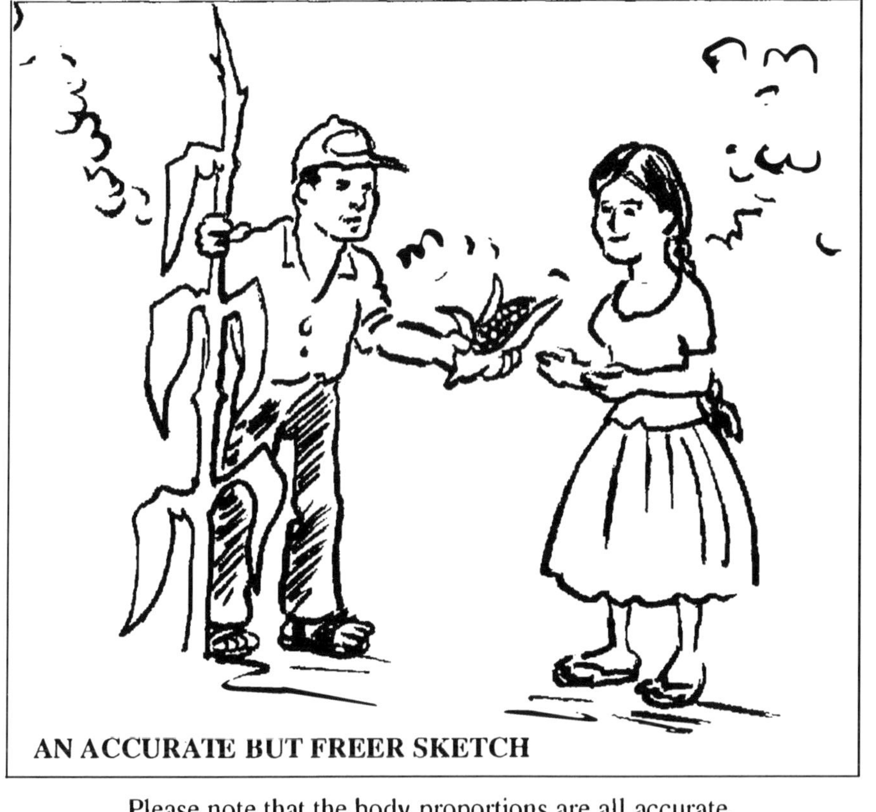

AN ACCURATE BUT FREER SKETCH

Please note that the body proportions are all accurate.
This is what makes the drawing real to the participants.

Show people actively doing things

A picture which shows people actively involved in doing an activity will generate discussion.

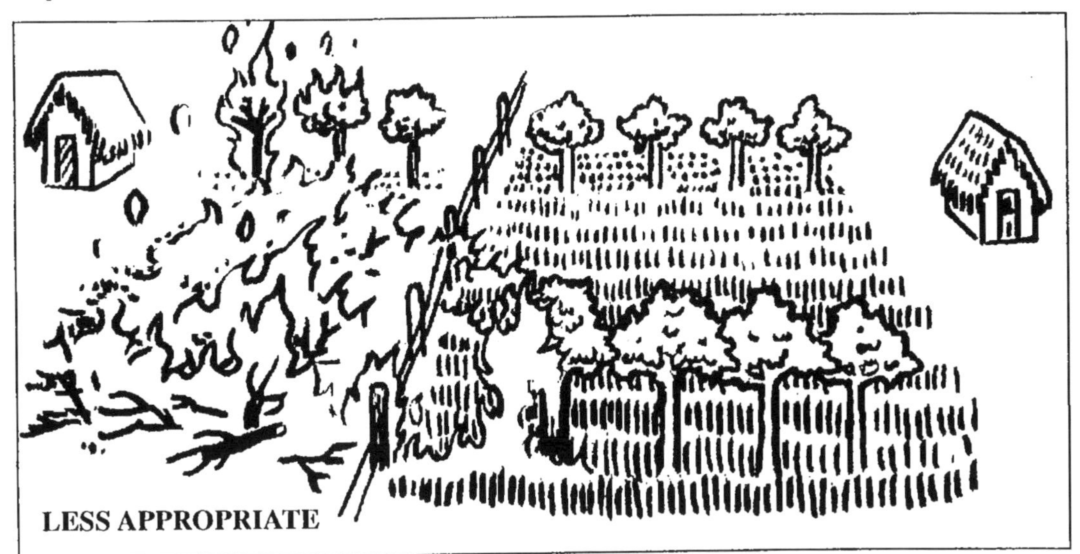

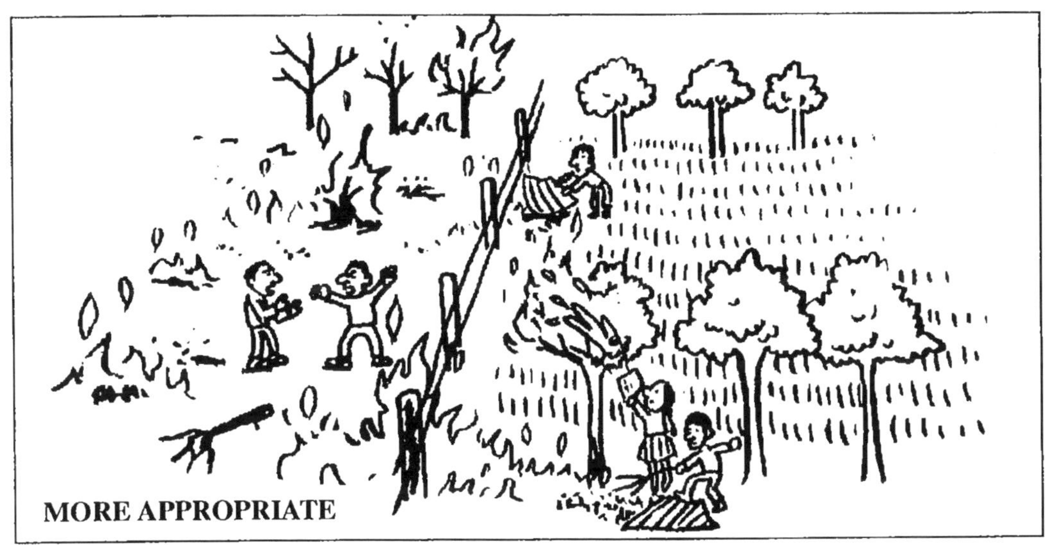

When people are active in the drawing, it helps participants to see themselves in the same situation and generates a lively discussion.

Show how the animal gets the disease

Pictures of symptoms of disease do not generate the same discussion as a picture of the process of the animal contracting the disease which includes the human factor.

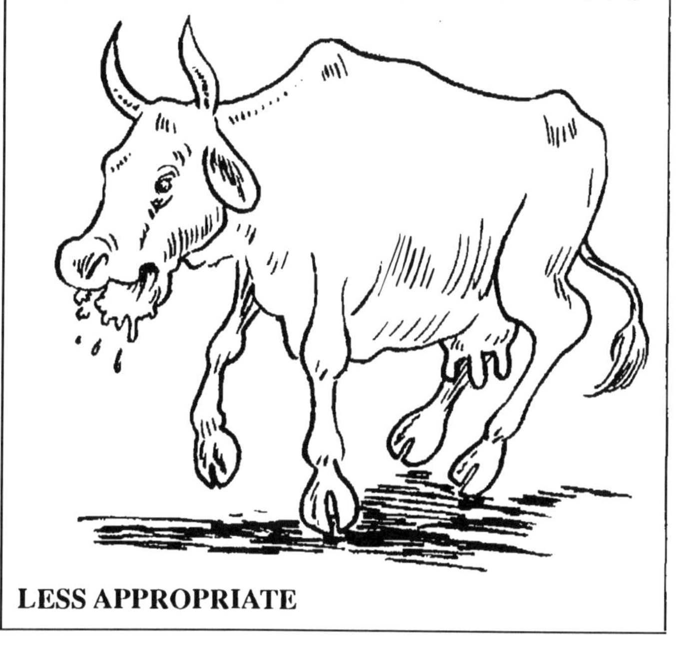

LESS APPROPRIATE

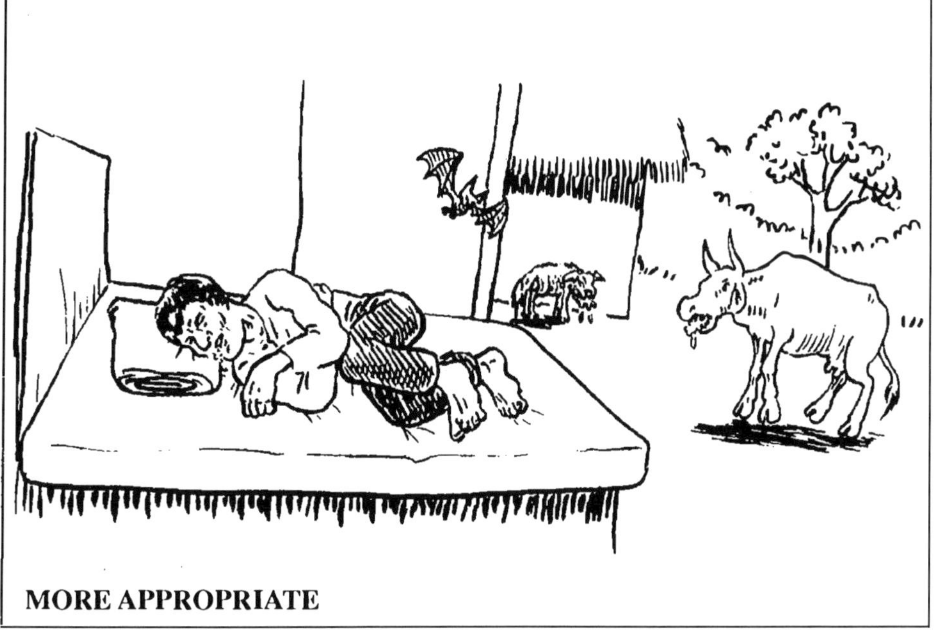

MORE APPROPRIATE

Communicating what you want people to see

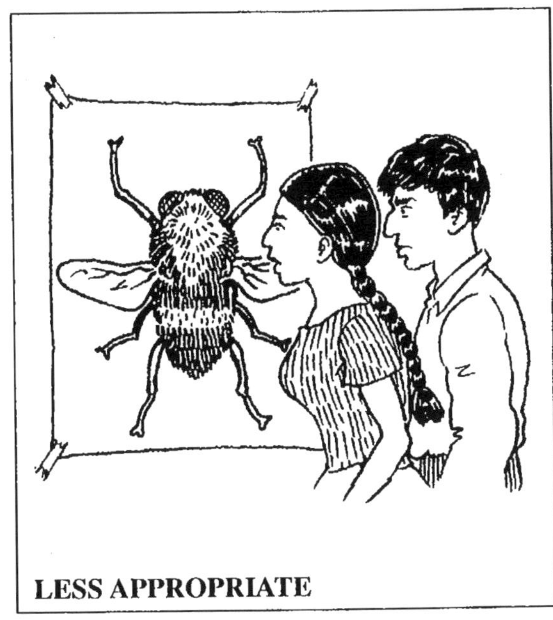

LESS APPROPRIATE

Sometimes we change size and shape or minimize external body parts to help illustrate a technical point. These types of drawing should always be field tested before they are used. If you have to explain them to people for them to be understood, they are most likely not appropriate.

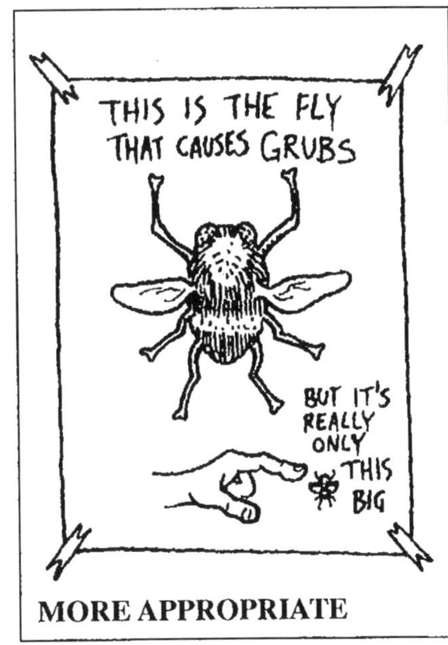

MORE APPROPRIATE

People will not recognize these insects because of their large size on the poster. It is better to have a poster with a large and a small drawing together.

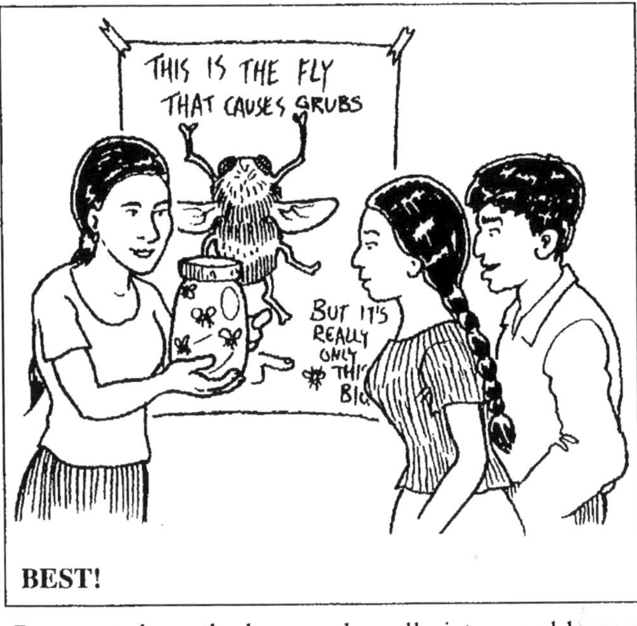

BEST!

Better yet, have the large and small picture and have a real bot fly in a jar so people can see which fly it is. It is better if the fly is alive.

Make sure there is enough of the body of the animal or the part of the plant or tree for the participants to recognize the plant, animal or area.

LESS APPROPRIATE

Here we have to read the caption to know what the picture is about.

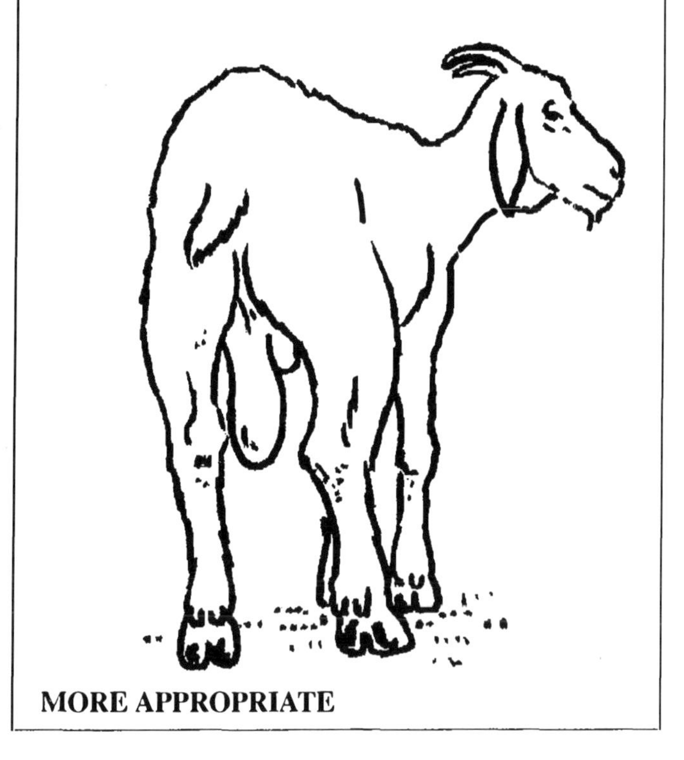

MORE APPROPRIATE

Here the picture is self explanatory.

When you use pictures to illustrate skills, be sure to include enough of the outside landmarks of the body to make the picture clearly recognizable:

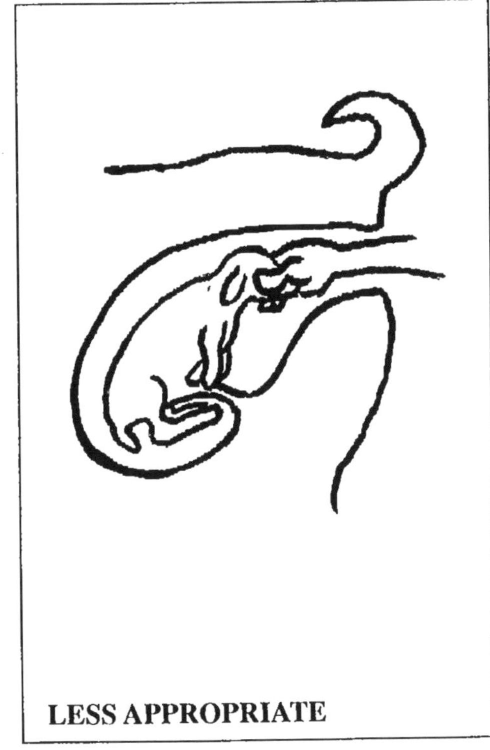

LESS APPROPRIATE

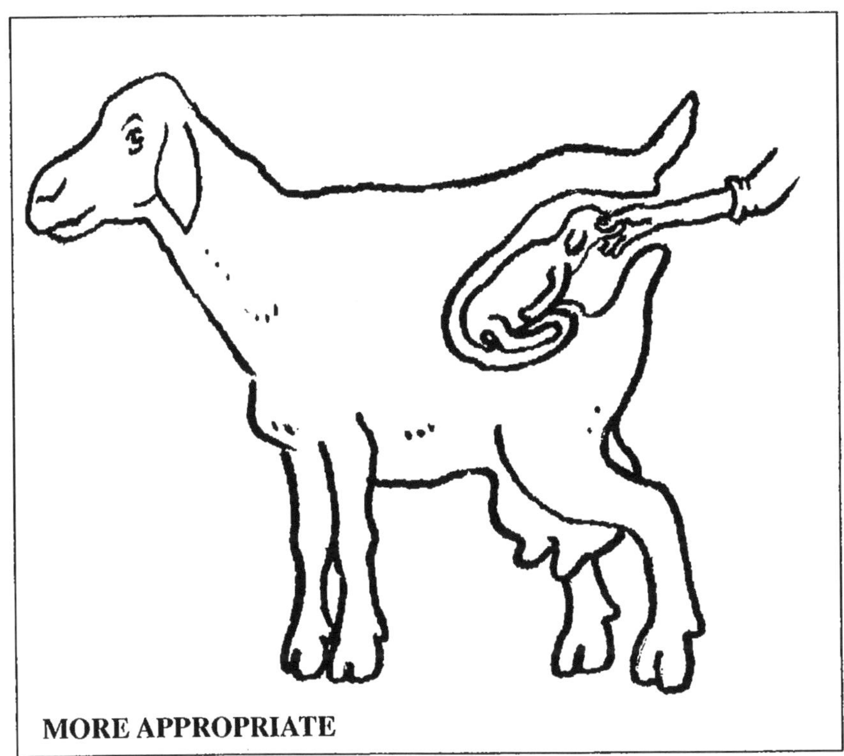

MORE APPROPRIATE

Using symbols in drawing

Sometimes symbols can be confusing in a drawing. This is especially true if the symbol means one thing to the artist and another thing to the viewer. But sometimes symbols can be very powerful in expressing a thought or idea.

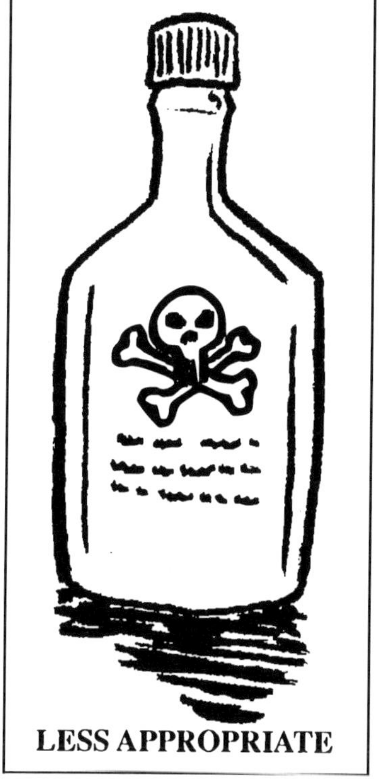

LESS APPROPRIATE

This is less appropriate because different people may not see the same meaning from this symbol.

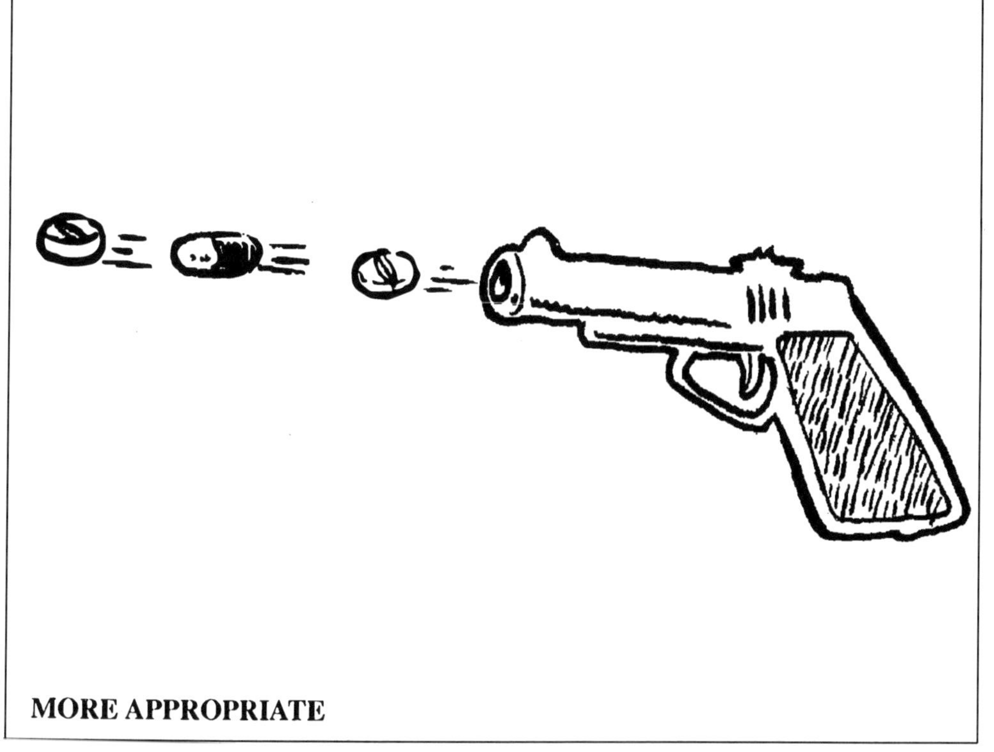

MORE APPROPRIATE

Here the symbol can express a very strong concept which people will remember. Use symbols carefully and generally in such situations as workshops where people can discuss their meaning. Unless the symbol is very clear it may be less appropriate for a manual, leaflet, or poster.

Learning to draw

Almost any person can learn to draw. It is a skill which is very useful for any trainer or livestock worker. Learning to draw takes practice and care and good observation skills.

Most artists spend some of their time learning to draw by copying the work of other artists. Tracing and copying is a very good way to begin to learn to draw. By tracing you start to see how sizes and perspective fit into a drawing.

When you make posters and leaflets do not hesitate to copy from other materials and manuals. Most manuals are there to be copied and put to their greatest use. Many times it is much easier to copy from another picture or photograph than to draw something from real life.

When you copy from other pictures you may need to trace, copy, enlarge, and otherwise make the drawing more appropriate.

Tracing

One of the easiest ways to trace another drawing, especially a large one, is on a window during the day. A glass window works best if it is available, but a screen can also work if the tracer does not press too hard with the pencil.

Stand inside the building in the day, with the sunlight on the back of your drawing. Tape the drawing to the window and tape a fresh piece of paper over it. At night you can stand outside if there is enough light inside.

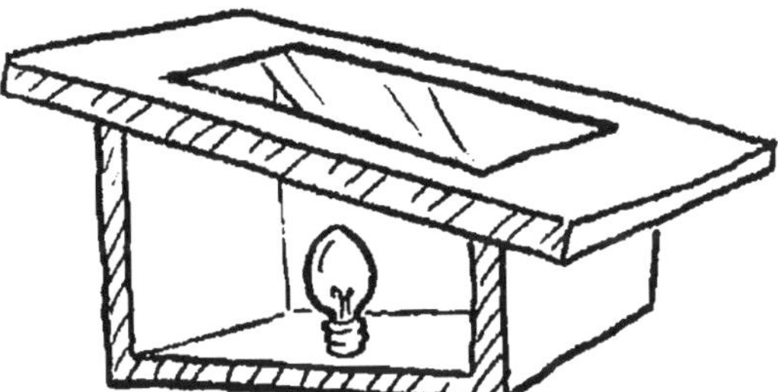

If there are no windows available, you can use a piece of plate glass propped against a wall. If you know you will be tracing often, you can set up a frame with a glass pane on the top and an electric light bulb inside, if electricity is available.

Copying and enlarging

When copying it is important to make sure all of the proportions are correct.
Heads and hands need to be their proper size.

The square method for copying

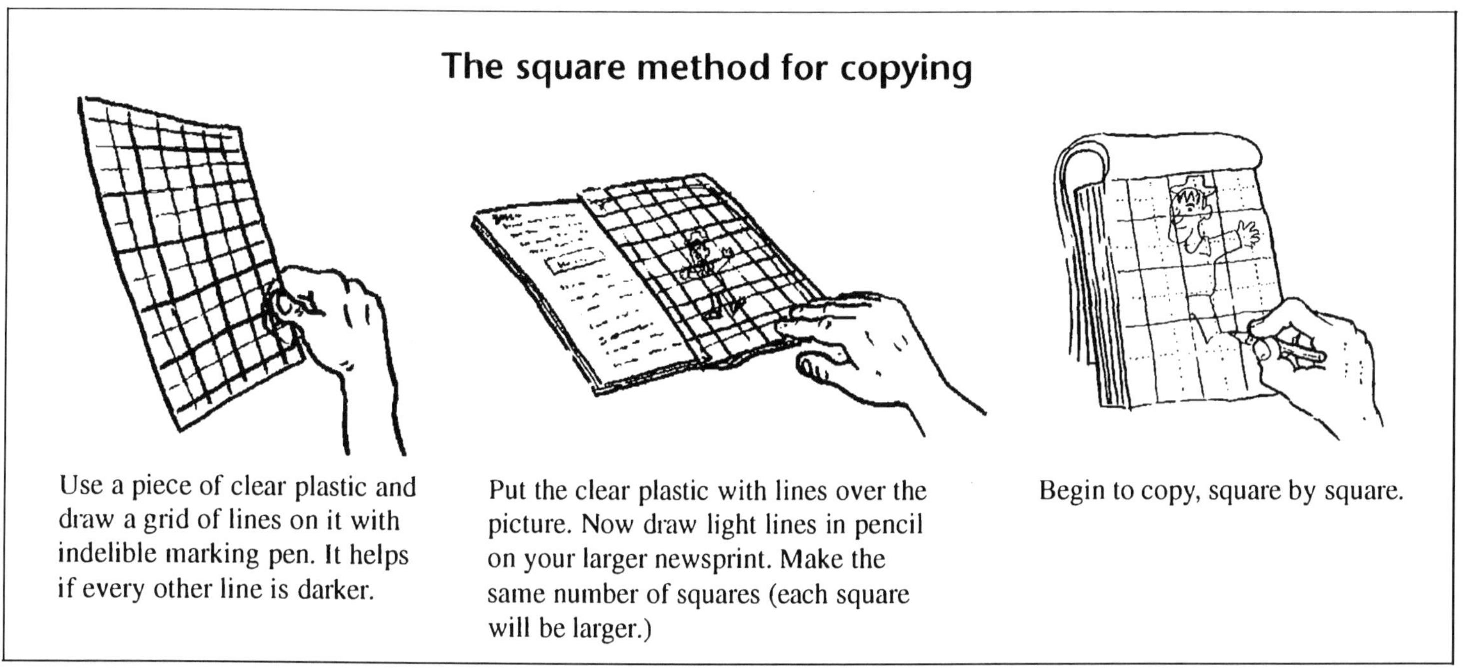

Use a piece of clear plastic and draw a grid of lines on it with indelible marking pen. It helps if every other line is darker.

Put the clear plastic with lines over the picture. Now draw light lines in pencil on your larger newsprint. Make the same number of squares (each square will be larger.)

Begin to copy, square by square.

There are good pictures available in manuals, magazines, posters, copy books and many other places. But sometimes when you want to use them, they are hard to find. It is helpful to **keep a file or notebook of good pictures** so that they are available when you need them. We have pictures filed by body parts, activities, people, plants and animals. You can also buy sheets of line drawings to use for this purpose. See references for suggestions of places to get pictures.

Materials for drawing

It is always best to look for materials which are readily available locally, to use for your drawings and posters. This is so that local Livestock Workers will feel free to use these items in their own communities. Drawings should be on paper. They should be temporary and appropriate for each workshop.

Newsprint

Newsprint is the paper most widely available, inexpensive paper in most parts of the world. In areas where paper is made locally, use the local paper wherever possible to support the local industry. Try not to use expensive art tablets. If large paper is very difficult to find, try to use some other relatively inexpensive form for your drawings. Newsprint can also usually be obtained very inexpensively from the end rolls at newspapers. Visit your daily newspaper and ask what they charge for the end rolls.

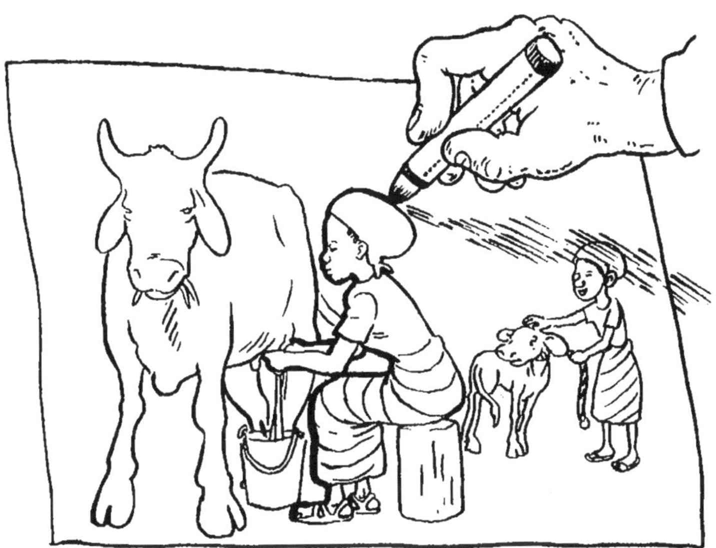

Marking pens

We use marking pens to make the drawings clearer. It is very helpful to draw the major outline of a line drawing with a thicker line than the rest of the drawing. This makes the central characters stand out and makes tracing much easier.

Black, dark blue, or dark green pens are the best for posters. Other colors tend to be difficult to see and distinguish in a group.

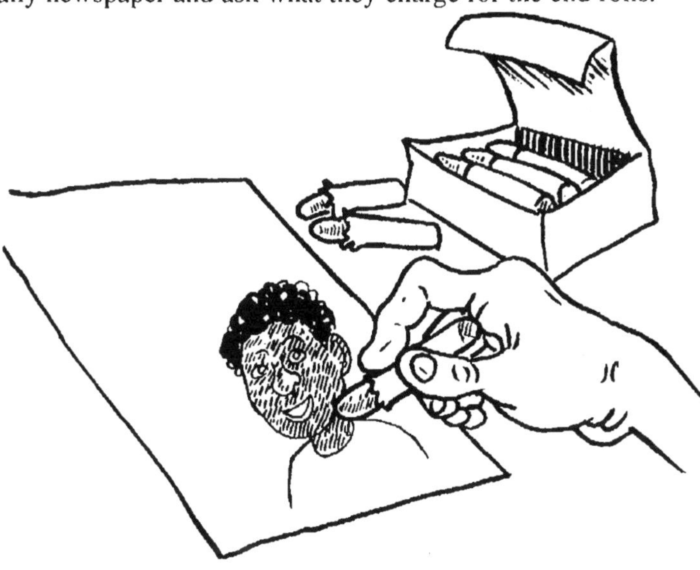

Pastels

Pastel pens are very useful for bringing life to drawings, posters, flipcharts, and puzzles. Pastels may be inexpensive and they are ideal because their colors can be blended for skin tone and more interesting pictures.

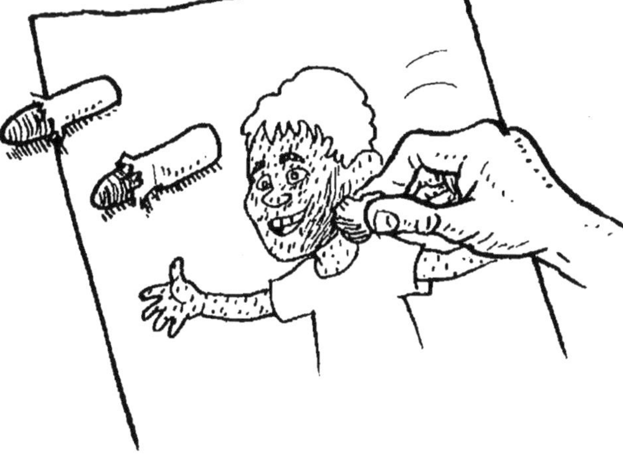

To obtain a bright and vibrant picture:

Begin with your line drawing with the outlines drawn in black marking pen. Outline the drawing with the darker colors desired – for example, a dark brown for the skin of people and for tree trunks and animals, a dark green for tree outlines, etc. Fill in the lighter colors as appropriate. Use the side of the pastel to fill in larger areas and cover the area consistently. Any area of highlighting can be done with darker colors.

Now, using small pieces of torn paper, rub the drawing to blend the colors and discourage smudging. Change the small papers as you change objects and colors on the paper.

Make sure you do not rub outside the drawn lines, since the scrap of paper will color as well as a pastel.

Once the entire drawing has been rubbed, the pastels will not smudge and the drawing can be stacked and rolled with others for carrying.

Protecting Pictures

In some special cases, a drawing or poster may be used many times. In these cases people have been very innovative in devising ways to protect these drawings.

In Nepal, trainers draw their permanent pictures on clear plastic with colored markers. When they arrive at the community for the training they use a big piece of newsprint behind the clear plastic drawing during the training. With their drawings on plastic, they can carry them in the rain and over rough terrain.

Other programs have made their drawings on cloth to enable easier transporting of them.

Be careful! The big disadvantage of permanent drawings is that trainers tend to depend on stock drawings which may or may not be appropriate. Or they develop their training based on the materials they have made permanent, rather than on the expressed needs of the participants.

Plastic water pipes

Because the trainers in Bolivia make their pictures on newsprint and there is much rain, they use **pieces of plastic tubing (PVC pipe) for water systems as a carrying case.** They can then lash the drawings onto their bicycle or back and not worry about arriving with ruined drawings.

Methods to hang and present charts and posters

Hanging flipcharts and posters

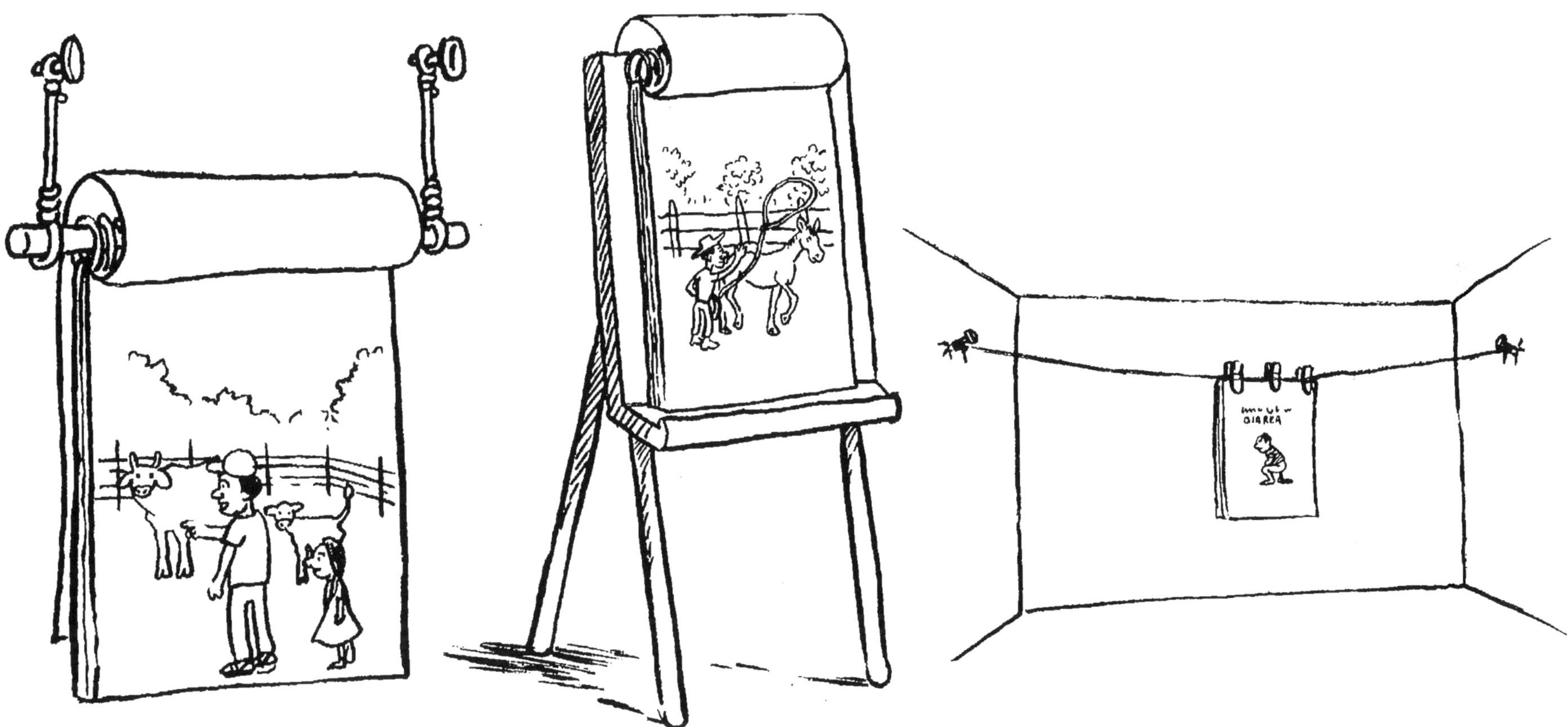

You can hang a flipchart in this way:
Put the top of the flipchart between two sticks or pieces of bamboo. Nail the two sticks together securely. Attach two pieces of rope or string to nails on the wall. Slip the ends of the sticks through loops in the rope. This way you can flip over each page of a flipchart.

Many people use an easel where it is available to hang a flipchart.

You can also hang a flipchart from a suspended piece of rope. Use strong clothes pins to hang the flipchart.

If there is writing on the bottom of the flipchart and you would like the participants to analyze the picture alone, use clothes pins to pin up the bottom of page and cover the writing.

Models for training

Practice is important to the participatory approach to training because it allows participants to discover for themselves how to do a skill. It also allows them to understand potential problems and pitfalls.

The best model to practice with is the real thing! It is always best to use real animals and plants wherever possible. But sometimes the animal and plant population does not oblige with the appropriately sick animal to use to discuss a disease, or a birthing animal to use to discuss difficult birth. Or there may be one sick animal, but not enough for everyone to practice on.

In these cases, models can often be developed to give an opportunity for practice.

Models should be:
As simple as possible.
Made from simple and locally available materials where possible.
Easy to transport.

Here are some sample models which have been developed by different programs.

For teaching about wound management:

The participants were divided into small groups. Each small group was given a different type of wound to treat. They discussed the treatment among themselves, made a decision, and treated the wound. Then each small group taught the whole group about their wound and how they managed it.

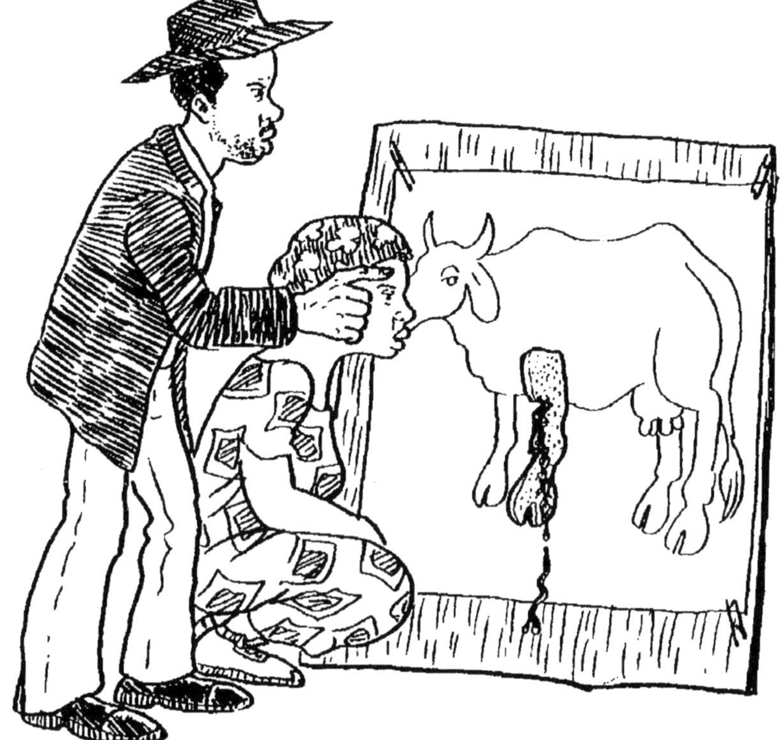

- One was a fresh wound with dirt and pebbles in it.
- One was an old wound which dribbled pus (we used condensed milk)
- One wound actually had a small plastic tube connected to a syringe, and a person behind the picture was putting red liquid through the tube. This was so the group could discuss controlling bleeding.
- One was a simple, fresh, but large wound.

These same models were used to teach about treating an abscess. Buried in the foam rubber was a balloon full of condensed milk. The small groups had the opportunity to treat each abscess and discuss potential problems.

Mastitis recognition and treatment

In an area where mastitis is a severe problem in cattle and sheep, the training program felt it was very important to give hands-on practice with different types of mastitis. Each time there was a possibly affected animal, the participants would do an examination and treatment of the animal. But the trainers felt all participants had not had an adequate opportunity for practice. So they developed a simple model of an udder.

Udder model

The first models were used during a training workshop about sheep. They were made from children's cloth-lined baseball caps, very inexpensive and widely available in the market.

The lining was split, and two holes were poked in the cap. Two fingers from rubber gloves were attached through the holes and glued in place. Each gloved finger had a small hole in the end.

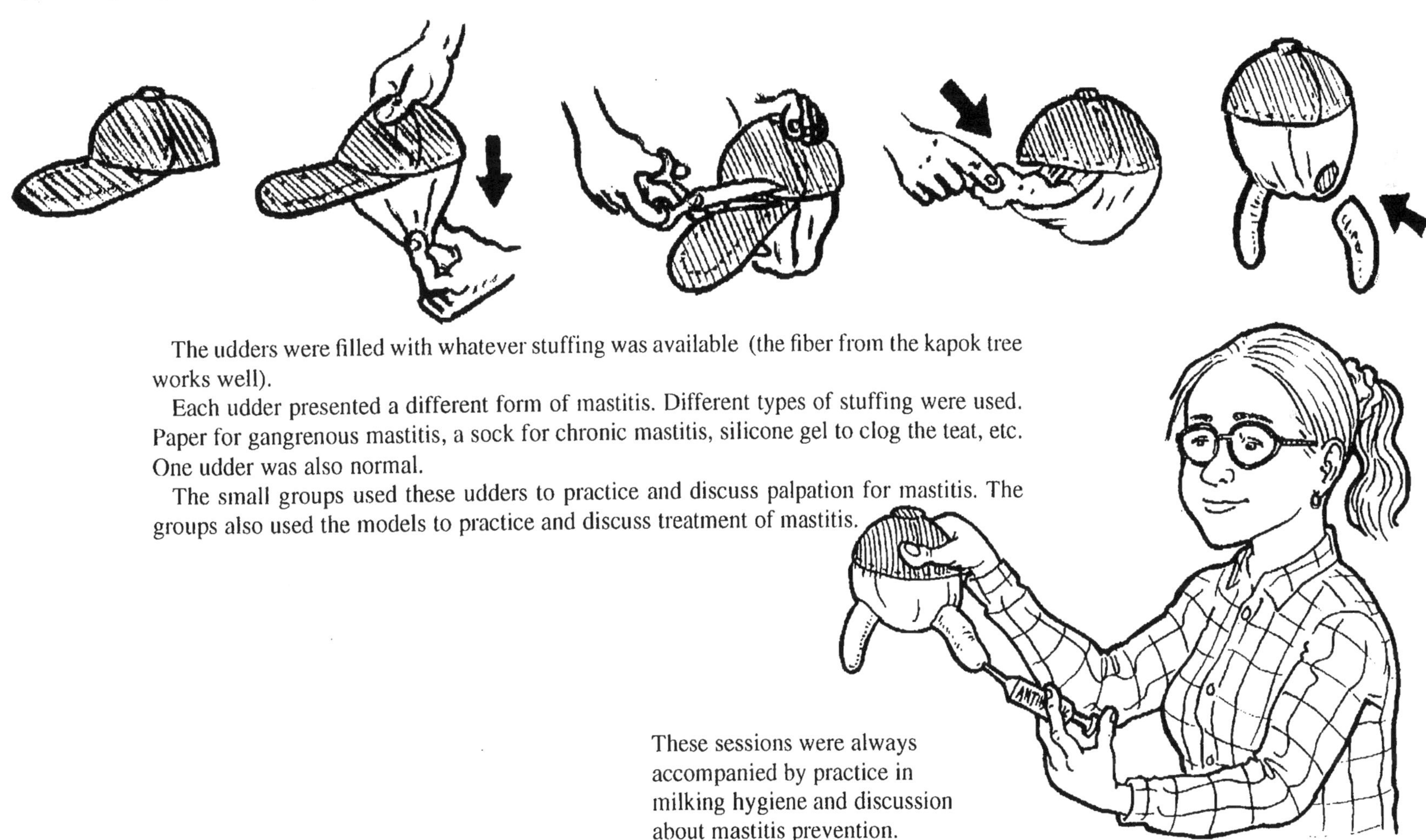

The udders were filled with whatever stuffing was available (the fiber from the kapok tree works well).

Each udder presented a different form of mastitis. Different types of stuffing were used. Paper for gangrenous mastitis, a sock for chronic mastitis, silicone gel to clog the teat, etc. One udder was also normal.

The small groups used these udders to practice and discuss palpation for mastitis. The groups also used the models to practice and discuss treatment of mastitis.

These sessions were always accompanied by practice in milking hygiene and discussion about mastitis prevention.

Two models for a uterus

Problems of difficult birth, retained placenta, and prolapsed vagina require a model for participants to practice treatment skills. No model is as good as really helping animals with difficult birth, but here are two which have been used:

1. Welded uterus with stuffed animal

The metal frame is covered with a blanket or wrap, and a stuffed animal of appropriate size is placed in different positions for delivery practice. The stuffed lamb was made with sticks in the joints which would only bend in the proper directions.
Source: RDC Nepal

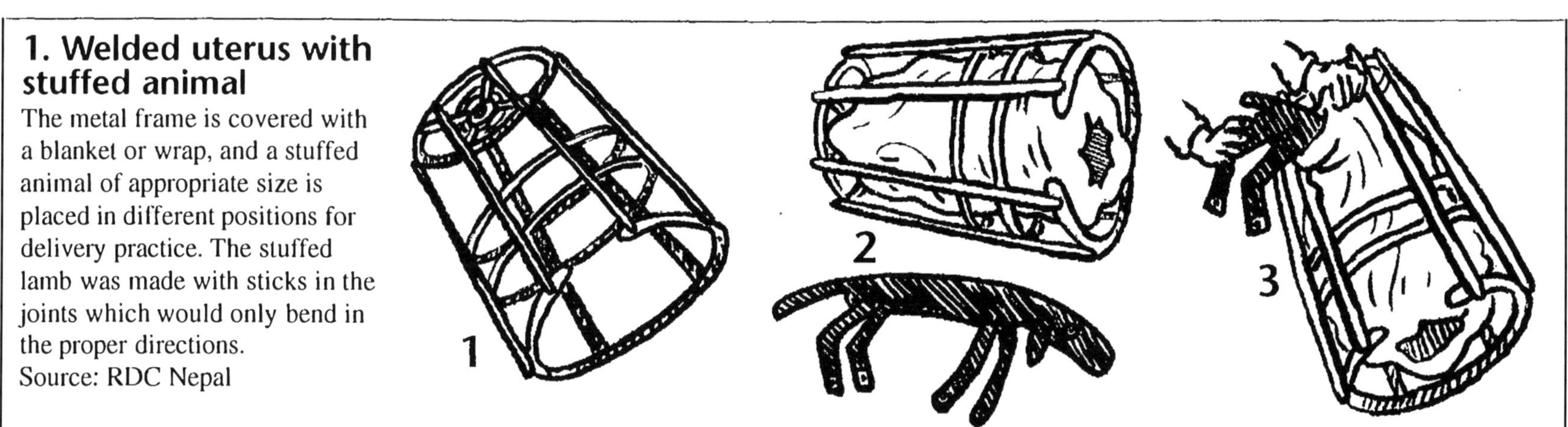

2. Inner tube uterus

Old inner tubes were heat-patched one inside of another (by a man who fixes flat tires), with the valve for air on the outside. With a bicycle pump, air is pumped into the space between the two tubes. This gives a sense of pressure against the calf or lamb.

The uterus is elevated on a stand or tied to a chair and covered with a blanket. A stuffed animal with mobile legs is used in different positions.

The same models can be used with plastic bags, rags, or inflated balloons to practice diagnosis and treatment of retained placenta and prolapsed vagina.

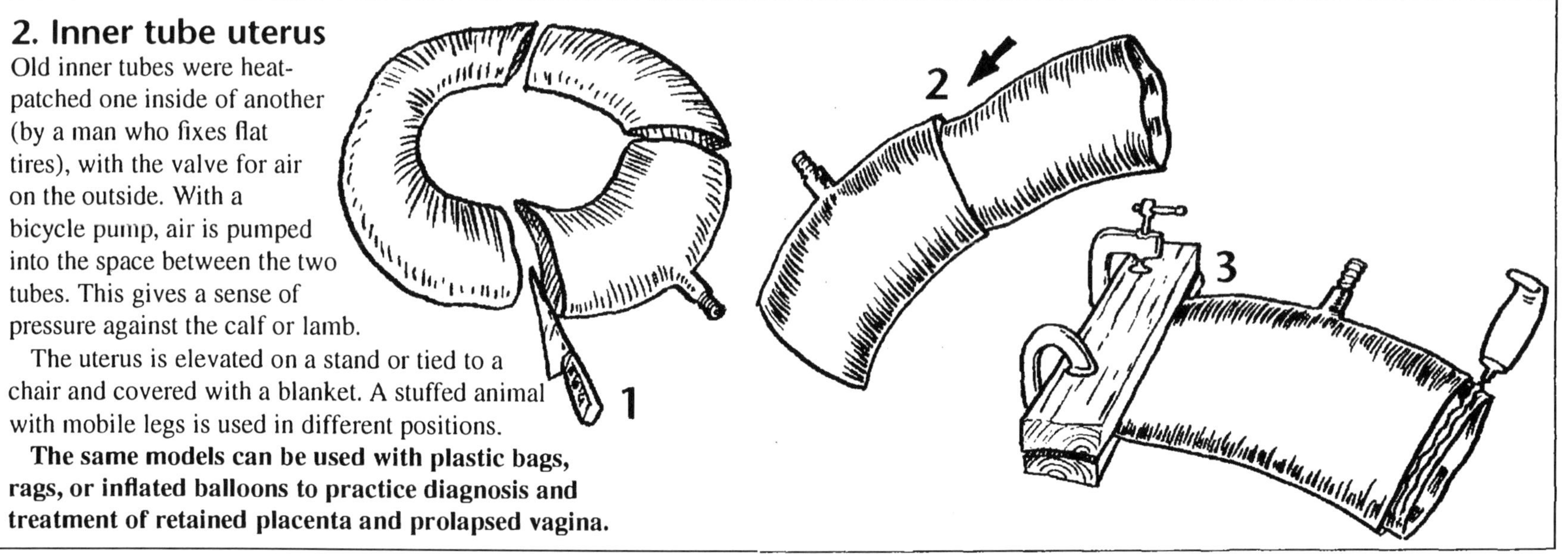

To discuss anatomy:

1. Draw the anatomy on the side of the animal.

This works very well with cattle and hair sheep. You can use a water-soluble marker, or a livestock paint stick.

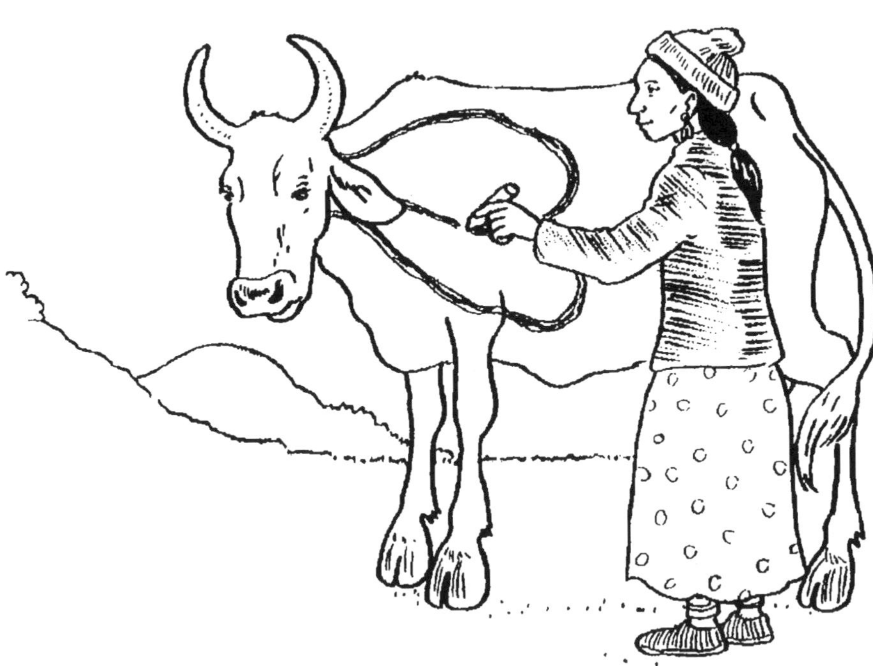

When you discuss pneumonia or other lung problems, draw the lungs on the cow and discuss how they are effected.
Be sure to use a tame animal, one which will cooperate and will not be overly stressed by this process.

2. Wherever possible necropsy an animal to discuss anatomy.

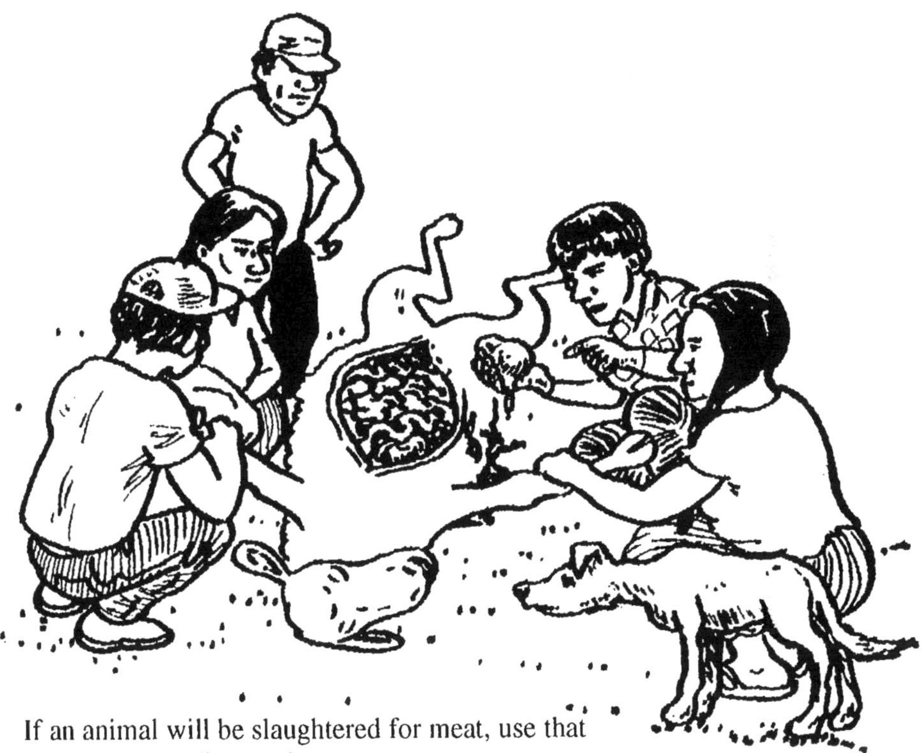

If an animal will be slaughtered for meat, use that opportunity to discuss the organs.
Make sure everyone uses the same names for the organs.

A model for soil erosion

Many times the land itself can be used to discuss erosion.
The group can go out to look at a planted hillside and see for themselves that the plants grow better at the bottom.
They can discuss and decide why this is, and what could be done to prevent the erosion.

Sometimes a model will help to talk about erosion.

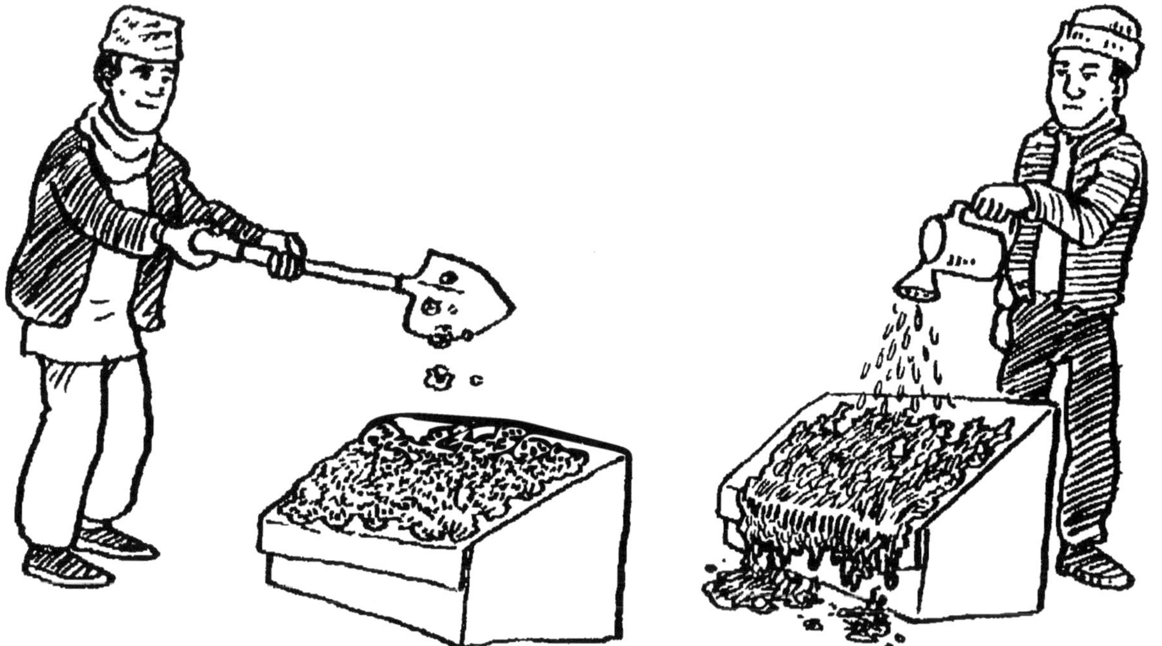

A simple model of a hillside can be made from a cardboard box. The box is shaped with an incline on it.

Dirt is placed on the incline.

The area is then sprinkled with a watering can to represent rain.

The participants discuss if this is what happens, and what evidence they have seen of it.

Then a stone barrier can be made and more water sprinkled to see the effect of terracing.

Source: Irene Christiansen, Nepal

Making our own puppets

Puppets can be made out of almost anything!

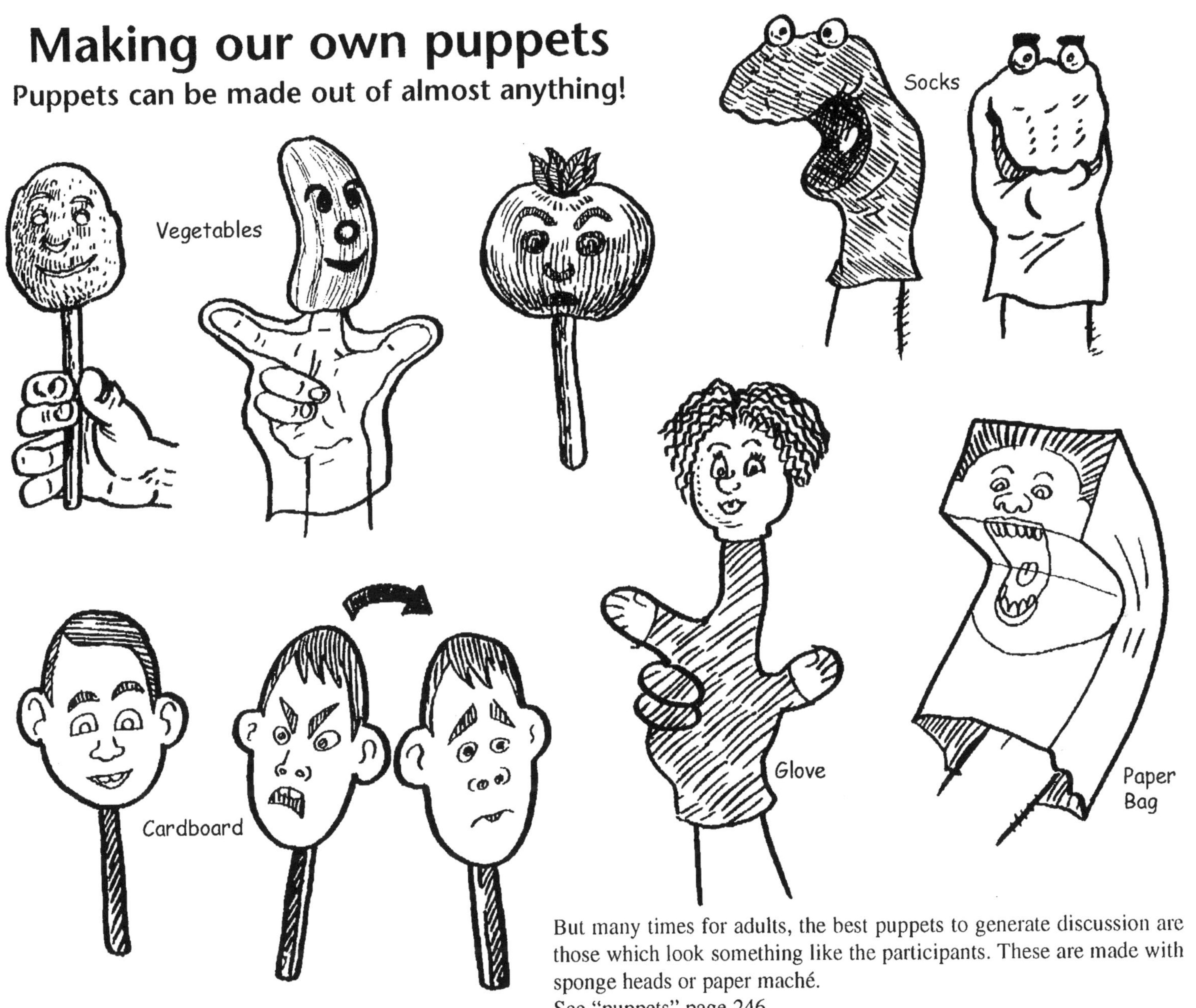

But many times for adults, the best puppets to generate discussion are those which look something like the participants. These are made with sponge heads or paper maché.

See "puppets" page 246.

Paper maché puppets

A good puppet head which has appropriate features, skin coloring, and hair is one made from paper maché. The basic head is made this way:

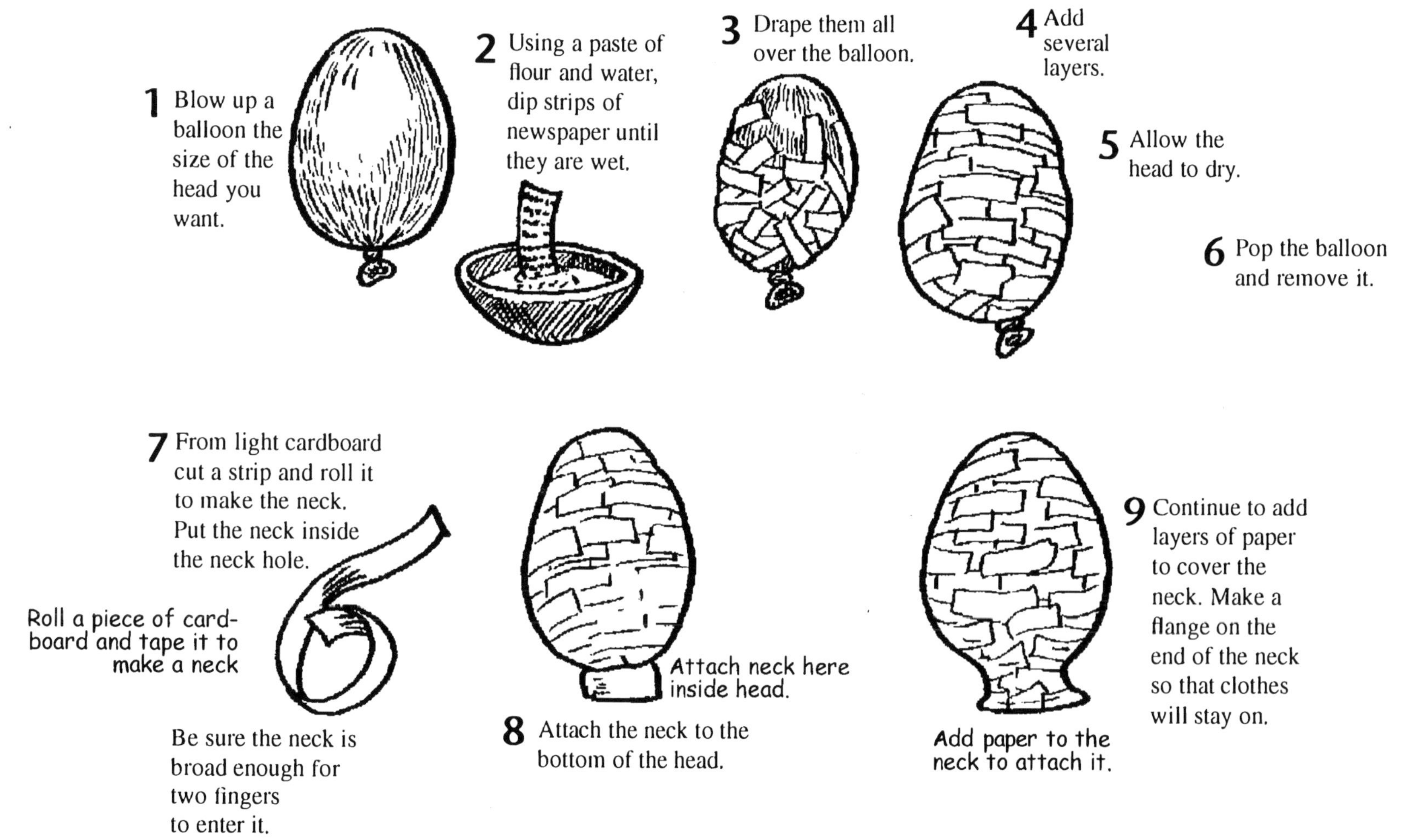

To add realistic features (Make this a day ahead):

Rip the newspaper into tiny pieces. Soak in water overnight and work the paper until it dissolves. Squeeze all of the water from the paper mix. Mix the dissolved paper with a cooked flour-and-water paste. Knead it like bread until the paper is no longer recognizable as paper. The result will be a soft dough.

10 Rip newspaper, soak in water overnight, work it to dissolve it in water.

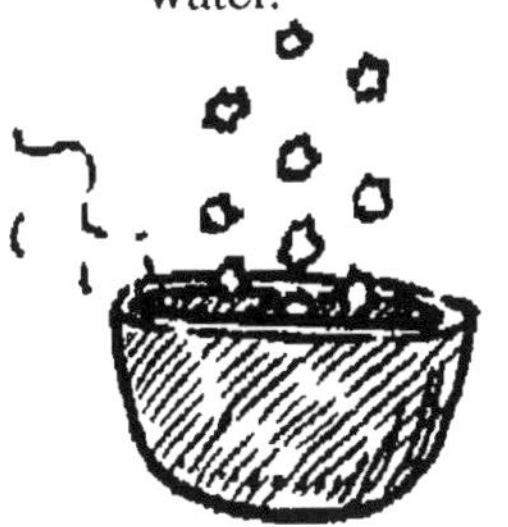

11 Mix dissolved paper with flour and water paste to form a dough.

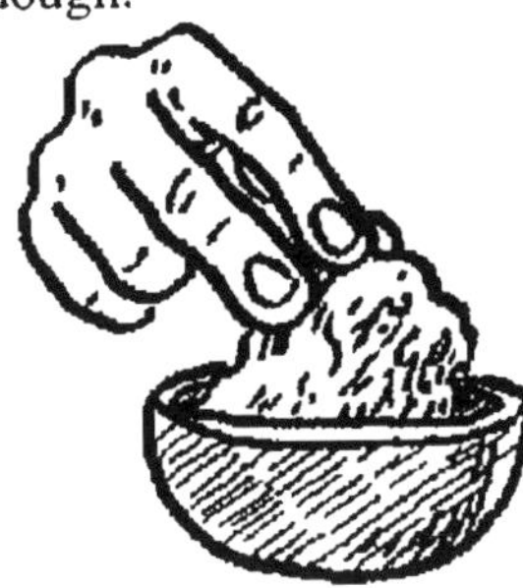

12 Form the dough into the features you desire for the puppet.

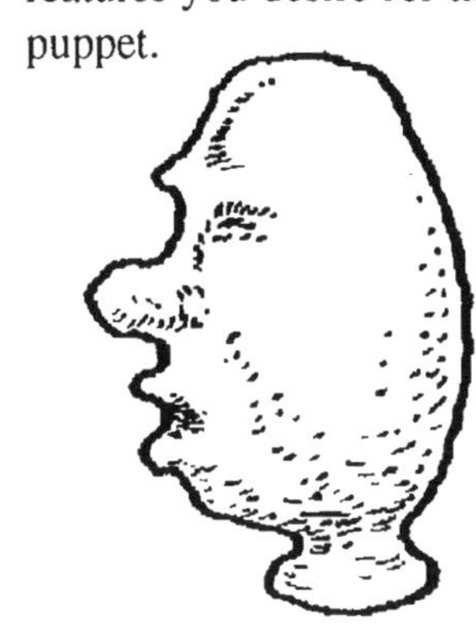

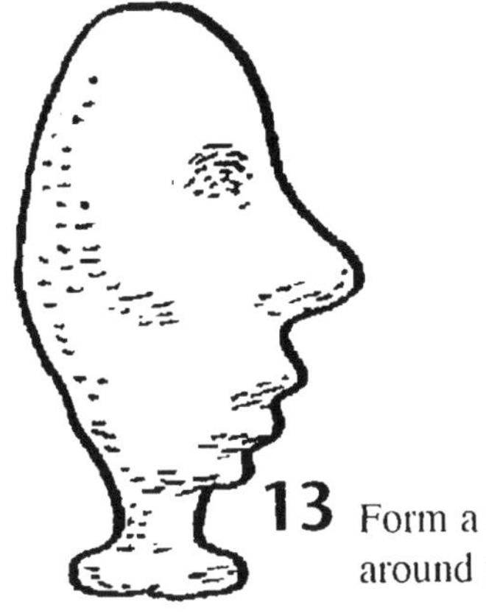

13 Form a flange around the neck.

14 Allow the puppet to dry. Paint the face of the puppet with acrylic paints. Be sure the face is the same color as the faces of the people.

15 Make a template for the clothing from lightweight cardboard.

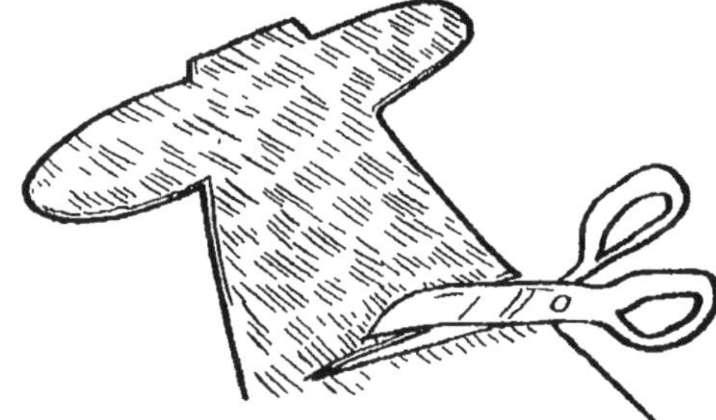

Use scraps of cloth and make clothing for the puppets which looks like local clothing. The heads and the clothing are interchangeable.

16 Use yarn to make hair in braids or straight.

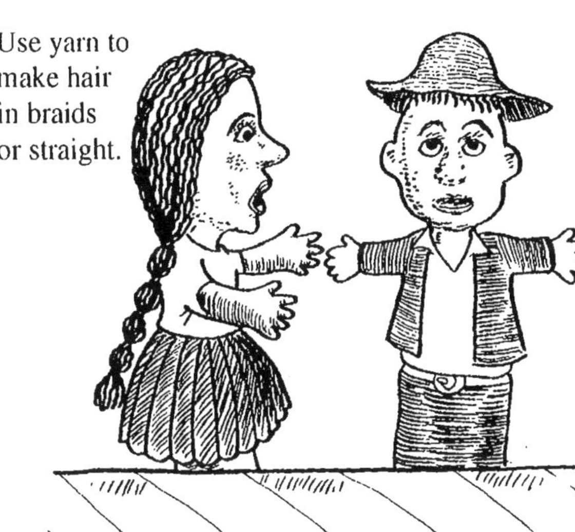

Homemade low cost equipment

Helping your role plays come alive

Props for role plays are often helpful to illustrate what is happening, or to give people practice.
See "role plays" page 244.

Animals and plants

Because animal and plant health care are so important to production problems, many role plays will include animals or plants. **There may be real animals and plants available for use in the role play. This is often best.**

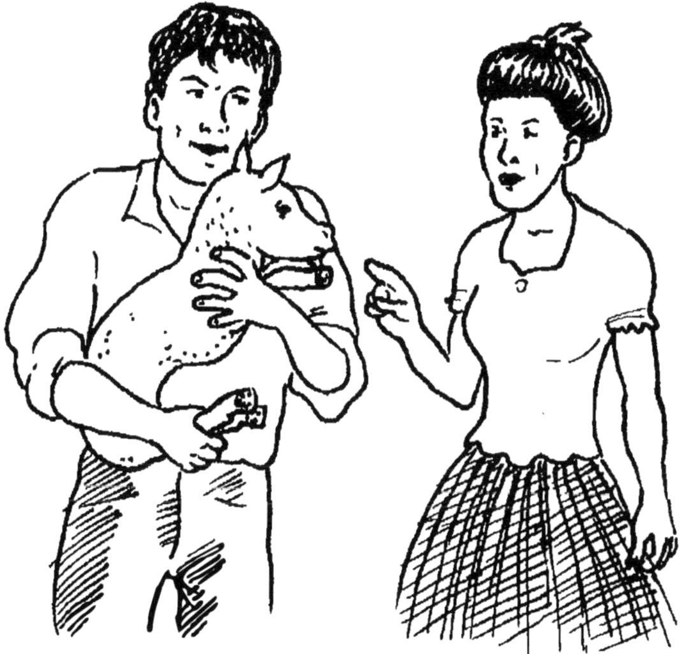

But sometimes it is more distracting to use a real animal, or one which is tame enough to use is not available. Sometimes the specific plant or tree needed cannot be brought to the classroom.

For these cases, you can do these things:

Use cardboard or stuffed animals and plants

The participants can make the animals. They can be thin, normal, or fat according to the need of the role play.

Colored spots, or sores can be added with tape and removed later.

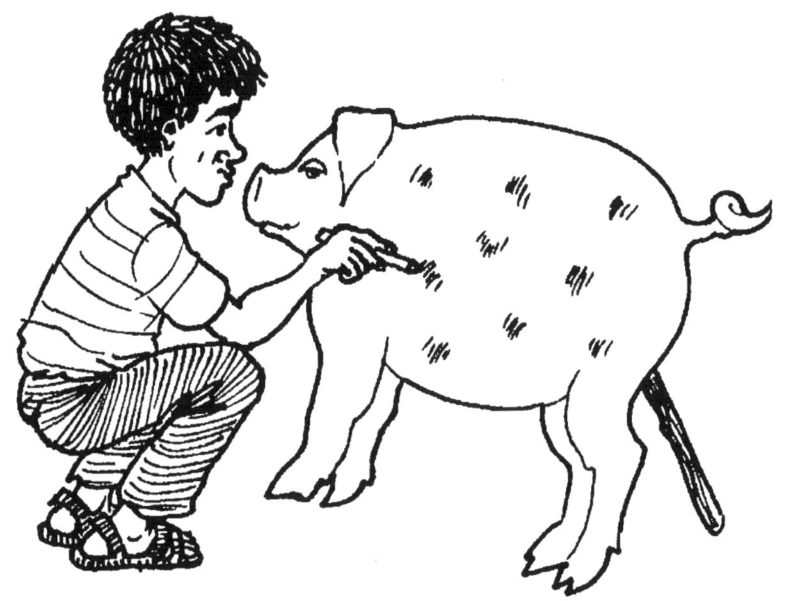

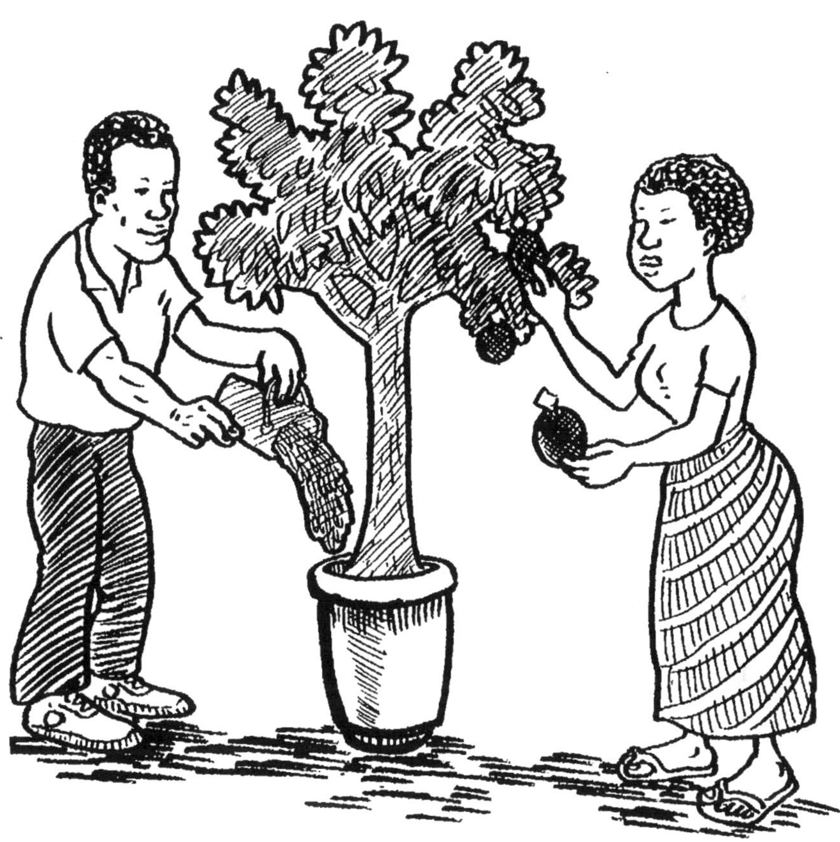

Cardboard plants can show all the steps in a plant's development, or can represent a plant with and without fruit for a role play.

Stuffed animals

These are the eggs I will choose to raise and these are the ones we will eat.

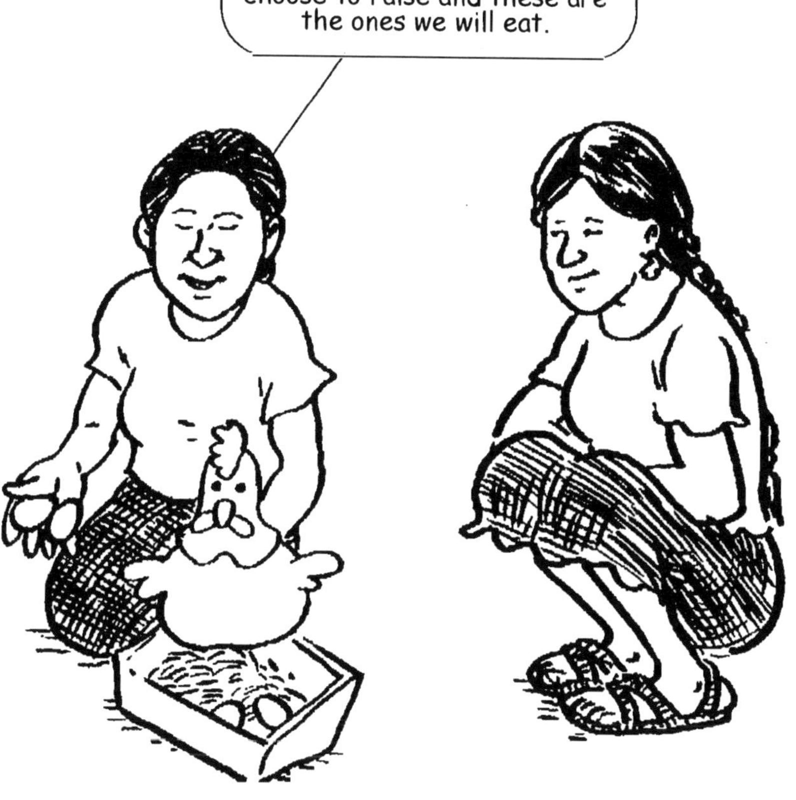

Stuffed animals can also be used, especially if you can find realistic ones or if someone likes to sew. Stuffed chickens were used throughout a workshop about birds. In one small group activity, the small group defined their reasons for choosing eggs.

Stuffed lambs and calves are good for practicing help with difficult birthing.

The more lifelike the cardboard and stuffed animals are, the better.

Use people for the animals in role plays

People acting like sick or injured animals can also be effective in a role play. This can often draw laughter from the group. Be sure the group is not too distracted by the antics of the human animal in the role play.

Masks for animal actors

Animal masks can be made by cutting and shaping cardboard boxes. Once they are shaped they can be glued, taped or stapled in place. Then features like ears can be added with cardboard, or eyes with marker pen, or fur, hair or whiskers with yarn or feathers or plant fibers.

Simple costumes can also be used. And as with cardboard animals, spots, wounds, bites and scabs can be added by taping them on the person's clothing.

Example thermometers

A simple thermometer, larger than reality, can be made from cardboard.

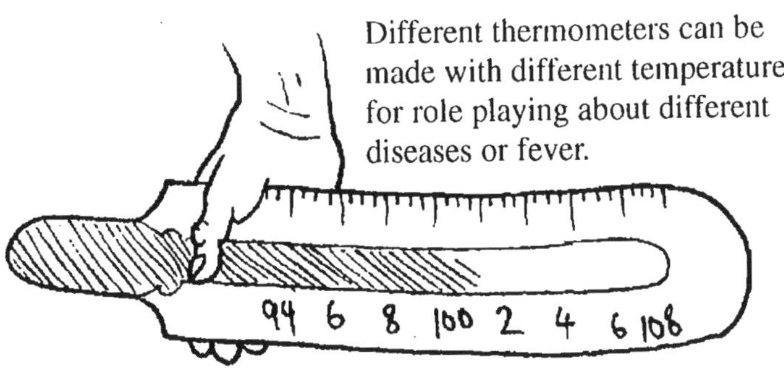

Different thermometers can be made with different temperatures for role playing about different diseases or fever.

This adjustable thermometer was made from two colors of heavy paper in Nepal:

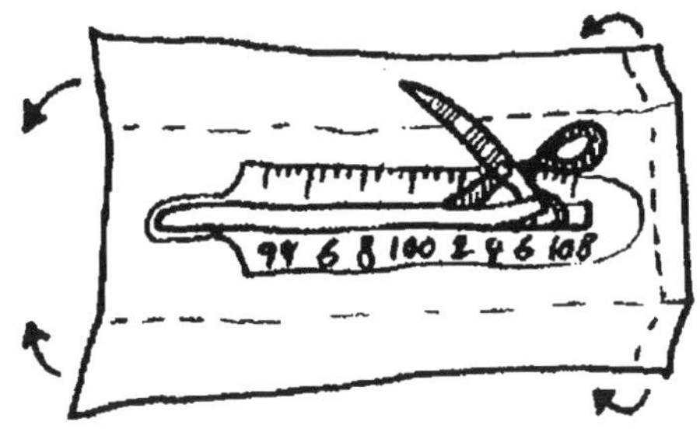

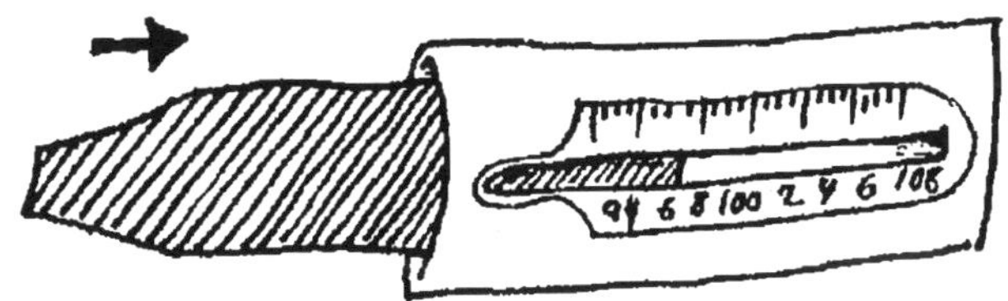

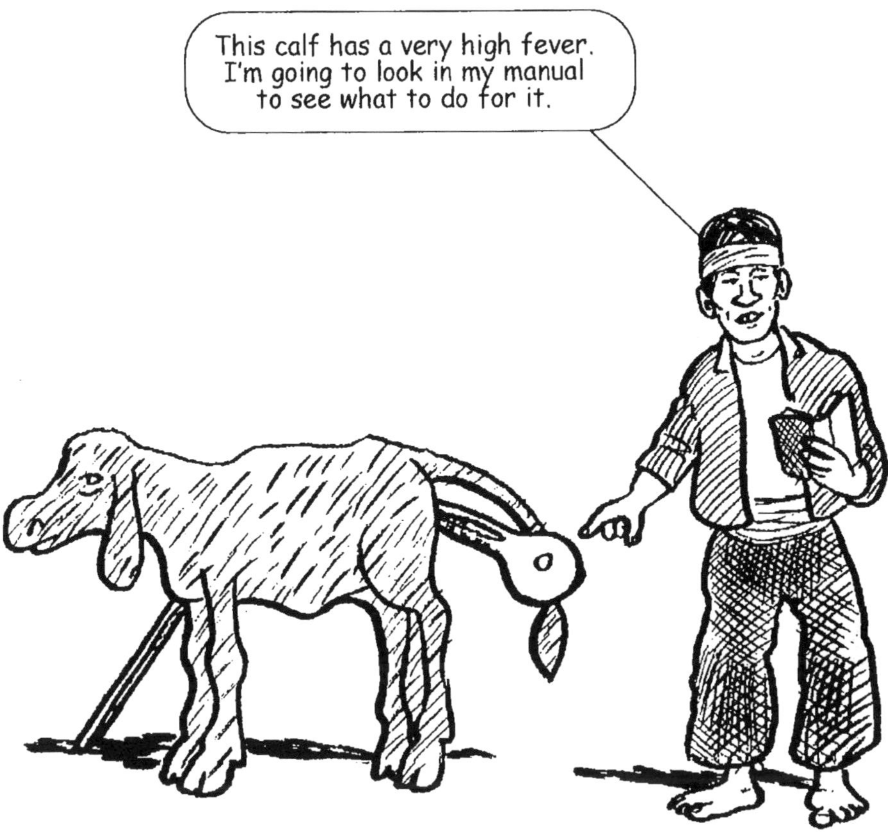

Role playing with thermometers at different temperatures can provide practice about how to deal with fever or other emergencies.

Simple aids for game playing

Cardboard spinner

Many games can use a 'roulette wheel' to help people chose a question or tell them where to move on a game board.

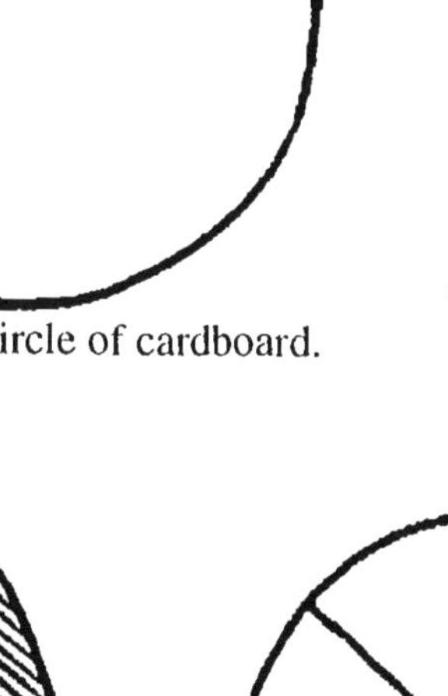

Cut a circle of cardboard.

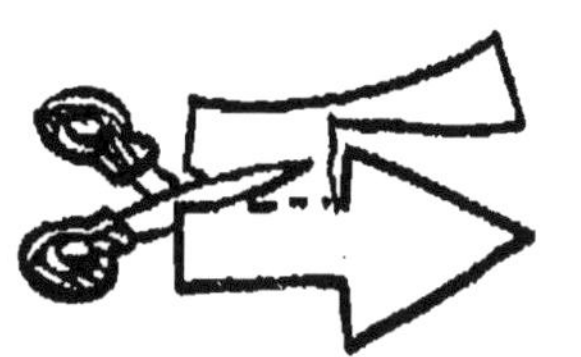

Cut a cardboard arrow which is shorter than the distance from the center of the circle to the edge.

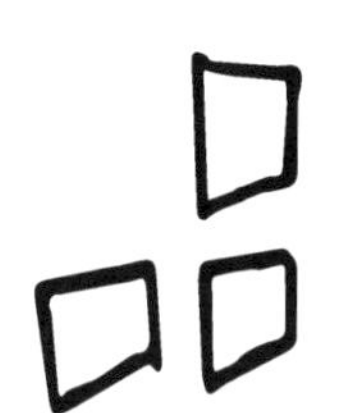

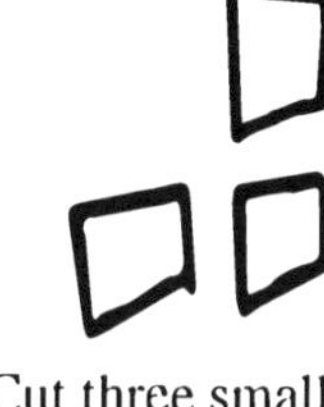

Cut three small squares of cardboard.

Divide the spinner into eight sections and color the sections.
Use four colors and space them evenly around the spinner.

Glue the three small squares to the center of the back of the circle.
Attach the arrow with a small nail or thumbtack.

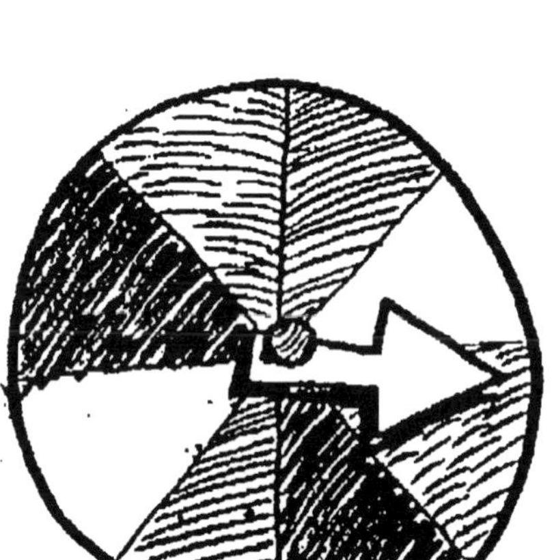

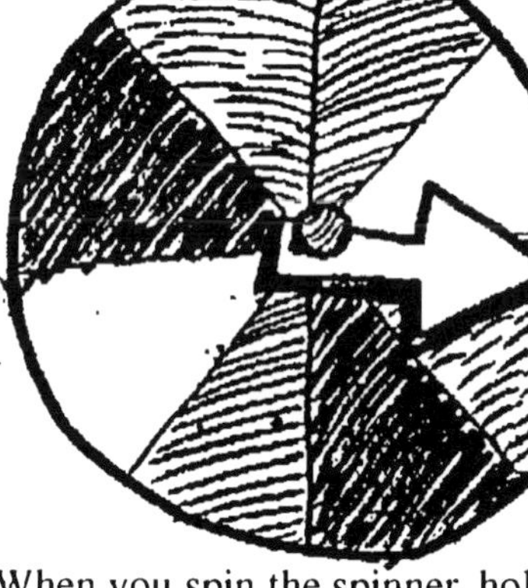

When you spin the spinner, hold the roulette wheel down on the table.

Cardboard Dice

Use this pattern to make a cardboard dice:

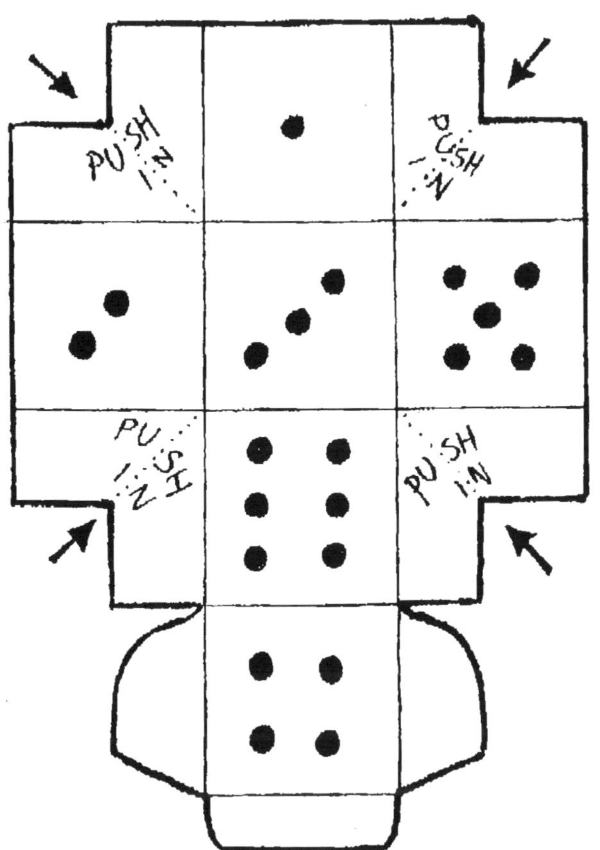

Draw the pattern on thin cardboard. Add dots with a marker pen. Cut out the pattern and assemble it with tape.

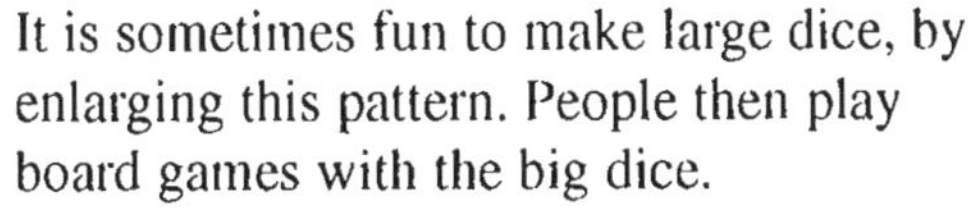

It is sometimes fun to make large dice, by enlarging this pattern. People then play board games with the big dice.

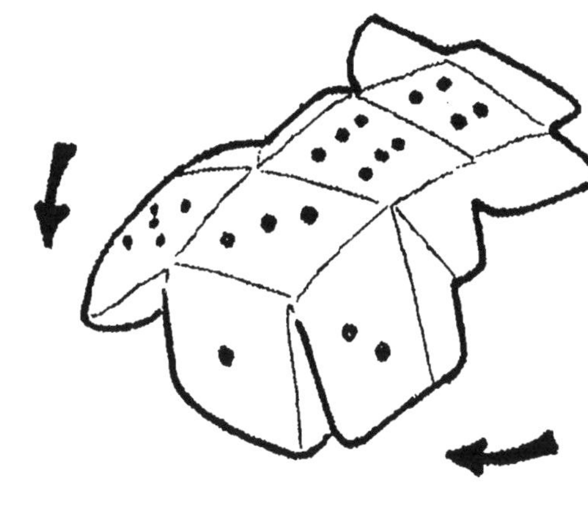

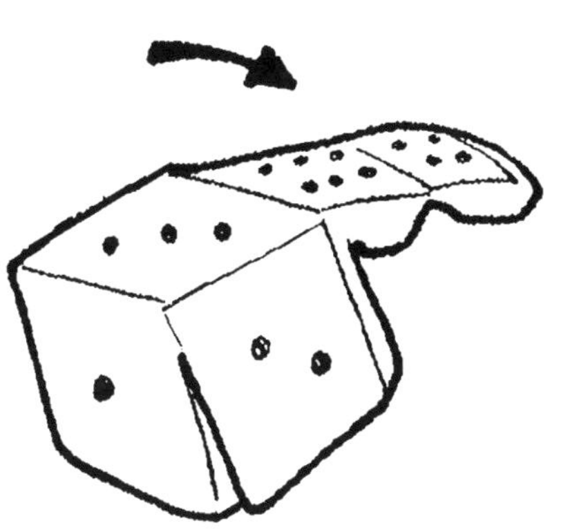

Other equipment

Lap tables

Sometimes, for work in small groups, playing board games, or writing, there may be a need for tables in a workshop. Often in a rural community it is difficult to find enough tables.

CIDE in Chile has invented this useful tool: They use a simple piece of lightweight plywood cut in a circle. The small group puts the plywood circle on their knees, and a table is formed!

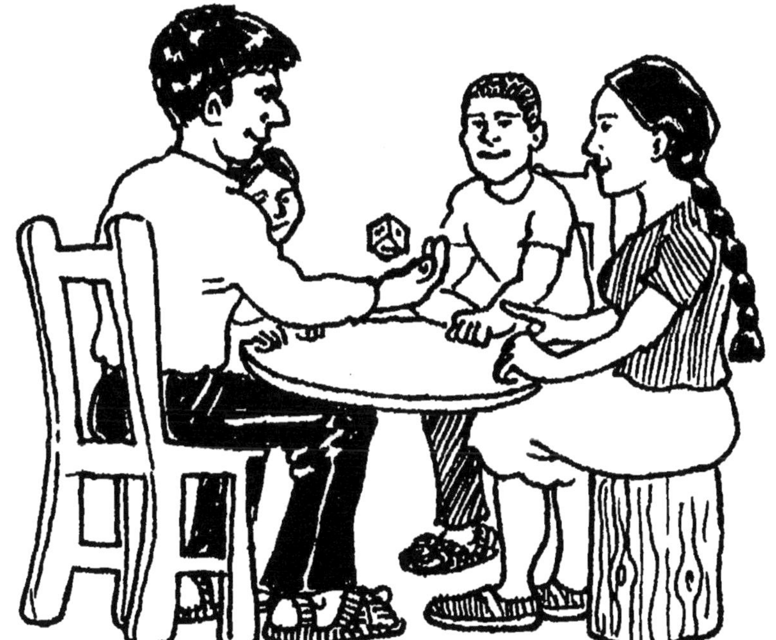

A rectangular piece of plywood can also be converted into a table using anything available to support it.

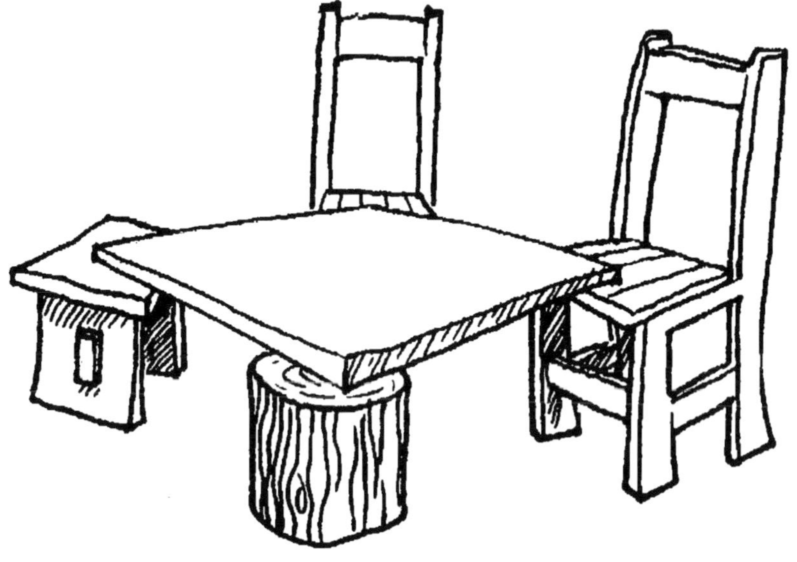

Weights & Measures

Having an easy-to-use, inexpensive tool for estimating the weight of an animal is essential.

- It allows owners and CLWs to know the correct weight **for doses of medicines** such as dewormers and antibiotics.
- Owners can know the real weight gain of their animals to **compare differences in feeds and management.**
- When an owner sells an animal for slaughter, he or she **will not be cheated** by the intermediary who says the animal weighs less.

Weight tapes

A weight tape uses the measurement of the chest size of the animal to estimate the total weight of the animal. They are not the same as a scale, but give a fairly close estimate of the weight.

Commercial weight tapes have the scale printed on the tape. They compare the girth size in inches or centimeters to the weight. In cattle, the breed of the animal will affect the scale, and there are different scales for different breeds. In sheep, the depth of the wool can affect the measurement.

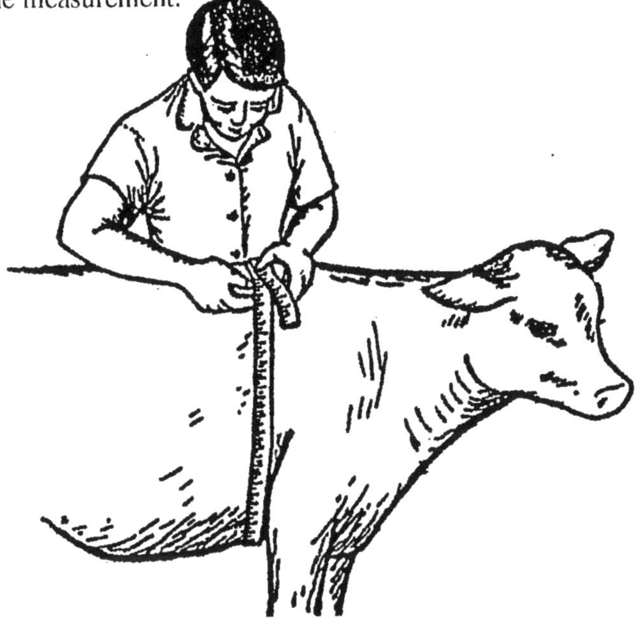

A simple way to make the weight tape available to community people is to use the scale from a commercial weight tape and transfer it to a piece of paper. Then any tape measure for building or for sewing can be used to measure the animal. On the next pages are the scales for cattle, sheep and goats, and pigs with a picture of the place to measure them.

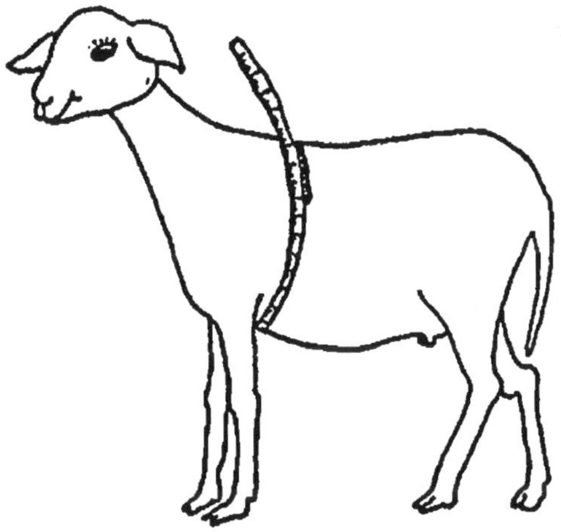

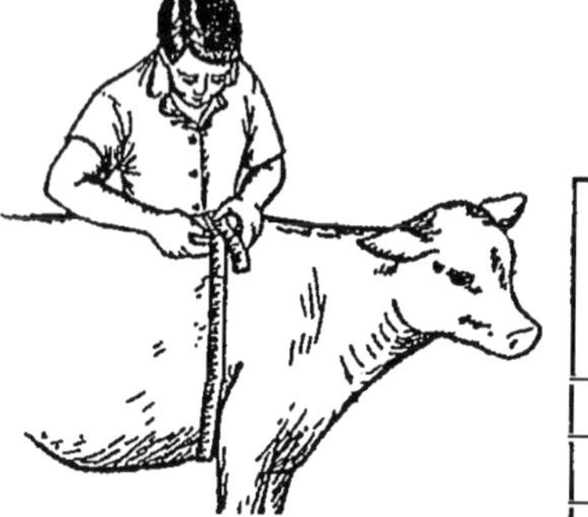

THE ESTIMATED WEIGHT OF CATTLE OF MILK BREEDS FROM MEASURING THE CHEST

Measurement of the chest in centimeters	HOLSTEIN		JERSEY OR MIX	
	Pounds	Kilos	Pounds	Kilos
69	71	38	65	30
71	78	41	72	33
74	86	44	80	37
76	95	46	88	40
79	104	49	97	44
81	113	54	106	47
84	123	58	115	52
86	134	63	125	57
89	145	67	136	62
91	156	72	147	67
94	169	77	159	72
96	181	82	172	78
99	195	87	185	84
102	209	95	199	91
104	224	102	213	97
107	237	109	228	103
109	255	117	244	110
112	272	125	260	118
114	289	134	277	125
117	307	143	295	134
119	326	152	314	143
122	345	161	333	152
124	365	170	353	160
127	386	179	373	170
130	408	189	395	179
132	430	197	417	189

Measurement of the chest in centimeters	HOLSTEIN		JERSEY OR MIX	
	Pounds	Kilos	Pounds	Kilos
135	453	207	440	200
137	477	217	464	210
140	502	227	489	222
142	527	239	515	234
145	553	251	541	246
147	580	263	568	258
150	608	276	597	271
152	637	289	626	284
155	667	303	655	298
157	697	318	686	312
160	728	332	718	327
163	761	348	751	341
165	794	363	784	357
168	828	379	819	372
170	863	395	855	389
173	899	412	891	405
175	935	430	929	421
178	973	448	967	440
180	1012	466	1007	457
183	1052	485	1048	476
185	1092	504	1089	496
188	1134	523	1132	515
191	1177	543	1176	535
193	1220	563	1221	555
196	1265	583	1267	576

THE ESTIMATED WEIGHT OF SHEEP FROM MEASURING THE CHEST

Measurement of the chest in centimeters	Pounds	Kilos
25	4	2
28	5	2.5
30	6	3
33	8	4
36	10	5
38	12	6
41	15	7
43	19	9
46	23	10
48	27	12
51	31	14
53	35	16
56	39	18
58	45	20
61	50	23
63	57	26
66	63	28
68	69	31
71	75	34
73	81	37
76	87	39
79	93	42
81	101	46
84	110	50
86	120	55
89	130	59
91	140	64
94	150	68
96	160	73
99	170	77
102	180	82
104	190	86
107	200	91

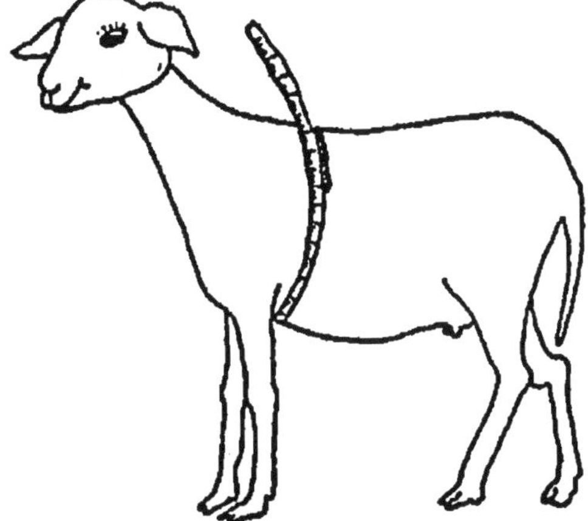

BE CAREFUL! This table does not give a good estimate of the weight of thin animals. In thin animals the weight will be too heavy.

BE CAREFUL! In sheep with heavy wool this table will not give an accurate weight! The table can give a weight which is too high. When measuring the animal put the tape measure directly on the skin by parting the wool.

THE ESTIMATED WEIGHT OF A PIG FROM MEASURING THE LENGTH AND DIAMETER

Use the length and diameter measurements in **centimeters** with this table

Length	80	90	100	110	120	130	140	150	160	170
Diameter 80	36	42	50	58	69	80	93	107	121	137
Diameter 90	40	47	54	65	74	86	98	111	126	143
Diameter 100	48	55	63	72	82	94	106	120	135	151
Diameter 110	60	67	75	84	94	105	118	132	146	162
Diameter 120	75	82	90	99	109	120	133	147	161	177
Diameter 130	94	101	108	117	120	139	161	165	180	196
Diameter 140	118	123	130	139	150	161	173	187	202	218
Diameter 150	141	148	156	165	175	186	189	212	227	243
Diameter 160	170	177	184	193	203	215	227	241	256	272

Estimated weight in kilos

Use a tape measure to measure the length of the pig like this:

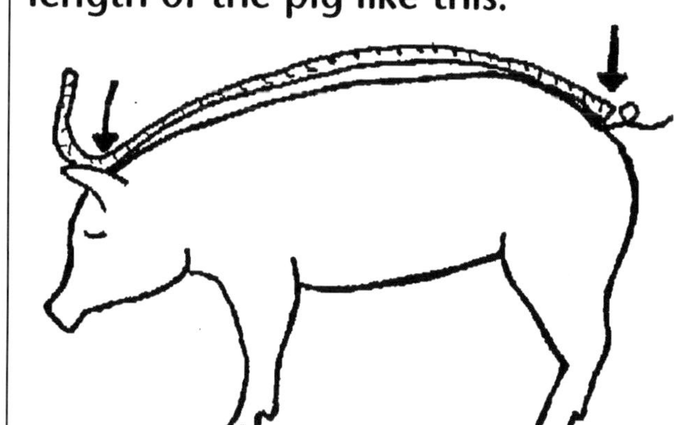

Measure the diameter of the pig like this:

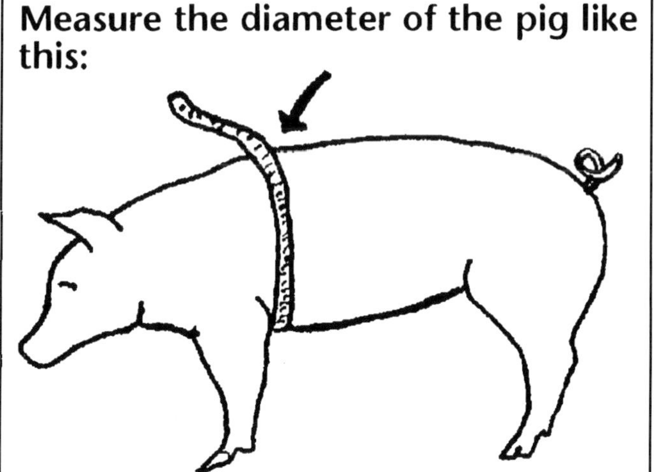

Other measuring tools

For measuring quantities of feed:

When teaching about animals raised in zero-grazing housing, people need to know how much to feed their animals. Look for the way people measure things locally, and measure or weigh out feeds together. Adapt the feed measuring to the local system.

Three ways to measure a meter

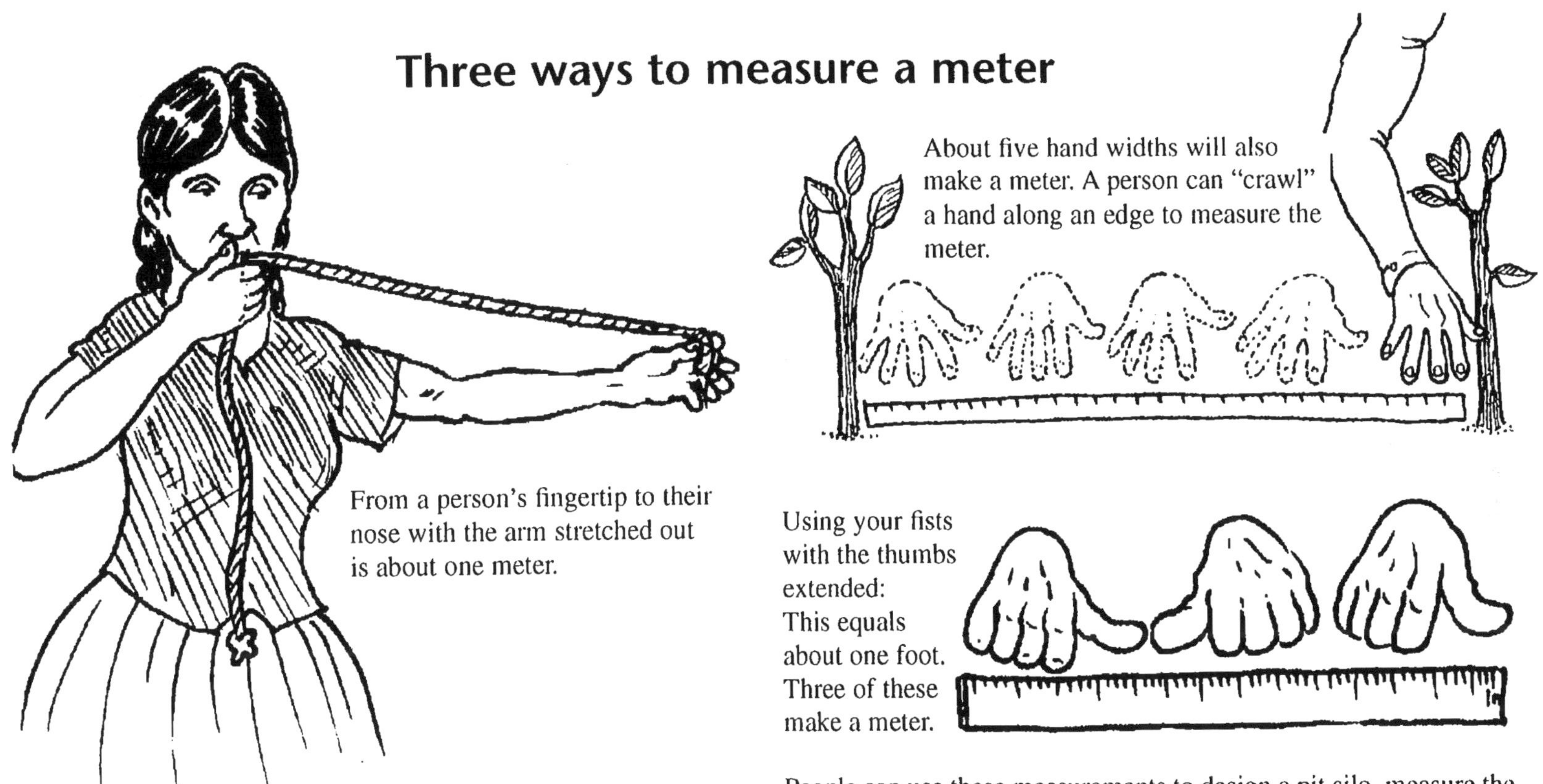

From a person's fingertip to their nose with the arm stretched out is about one meter.

About five hand widths will also make a meter. A person can "crawl" a hand along an edge to measure the meter.

Using your fists with the thumbs extended: This equals about one foot. Three of these make a meter.

People can use these measurements to design a pit silo, measure the quantity of feed, or measure the size of a zero-grazing stall for building.

Animal crate and head gate

In some areas, and for some treatments, having a head gate to control the animals is necessary.

Here is a simple animal crate built in Nepal during every CLW training workshop. The CLWs build the crate early in the workshop. They use it every day to examine and treat animals which are brought from the surrounding areas.

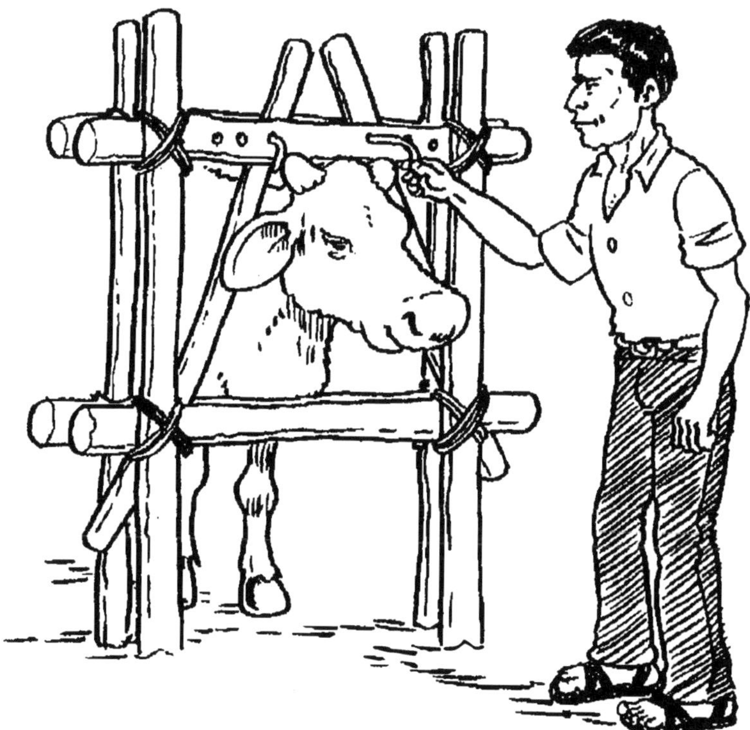

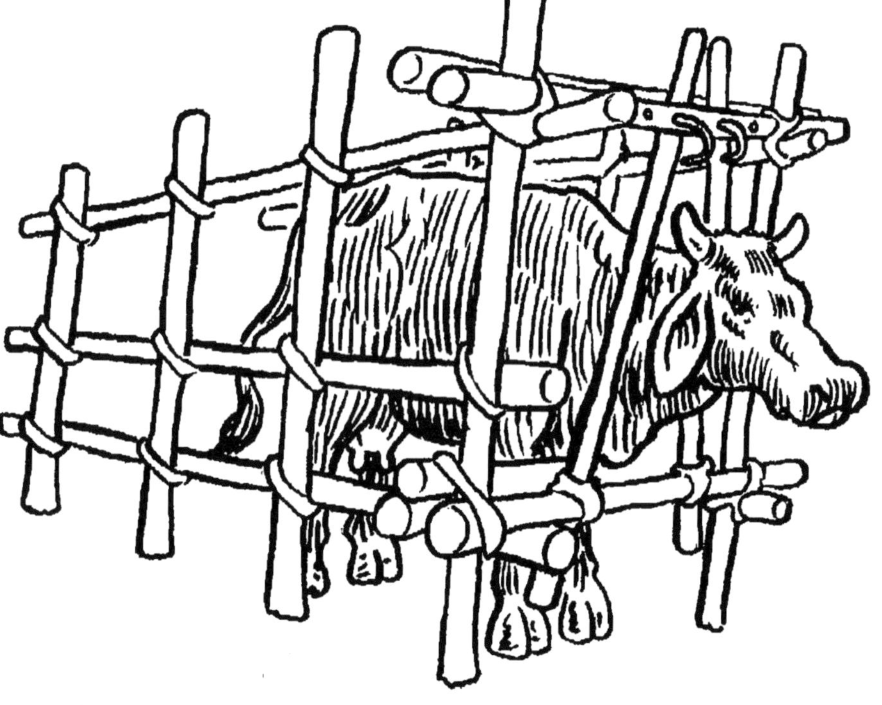

This crate is made from bamboo and requires a half day to make. They dig into the ground to hold it. The bamboo is tied with strings.

The only thing brought to the workshop are two metal stakes used to hold and adjust the head gate. These can easily be made in the community of each CLW.
Source: RDC Nepal

For dosing medicines

A practical medicine doser can be made from mature bamboo to give pills or liquids to animals.

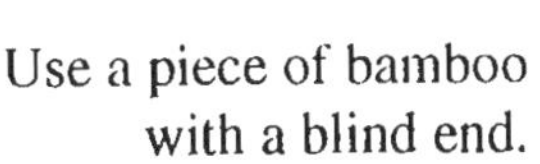

Use a piece of bamboo
with a blind end.

To give pills:

- Grind the pills first and mix with water.
- Put the liquid mix into the bamboo.
- Put the bamboo into the mouth of the animal and lift the head so the liquid flows into the mouth.

The tube of bamboo can be rinsed with more water so all of the medicine goes into the mouth.

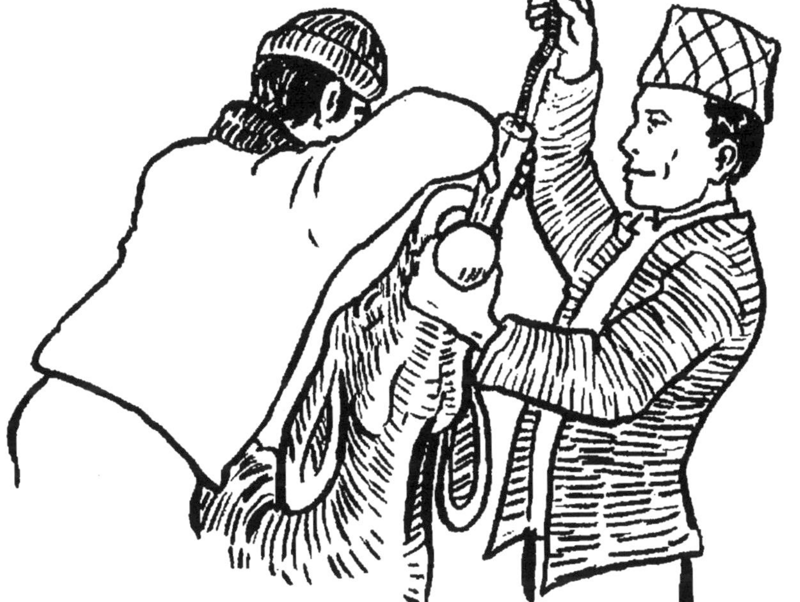

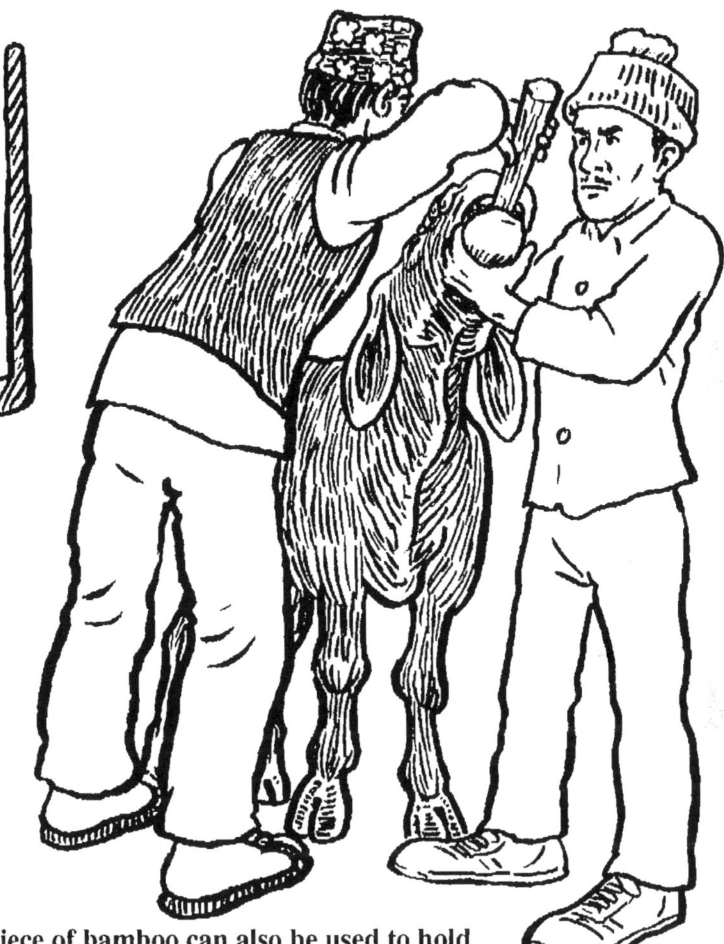

A piece of bamboo can also be used to hold the mouth of a goat or sheep open to pass a tube. The tube can then be passed through the bamboo. This is used for treatment of bloat.
Source: RDC Nepal

Chapter 14
Resources

This chapter is a listing of helpful resources

This is a listing of extremely helpful resources for facilitators of participatory adult learning in agricultural situations. All of these and other resources were consulted in the development of this Sourcebook.

Books and Manuals on Participatory Methods

For Training of Facilitators:

Case, D'Arcy Davis. *The Community's Toolbox The Idea, Methods and Tools for Participatory Assessment, Monitoring and Evaluation in Community Forestry.* Community forestry field manual 2. FAO, 1990. Director Publications Division, Food and Agriculture Organization of the United Nations, Via delle Terme di Caracalla, 00100 Rome, Italy. Spanish title: *Herramientas para la Comunidad.*

CEDPA. *Training Trainers for Development: Conducting a Workshop on Participatory Training Techniques.* 1994. Available from PACT 777 UN Plaza, New York, NY 10017 USA tel: 212-697-6222.

Haaland, Ave. *Pretesting Communication Materials: With a Special Emphasis on Child Health and Nutrition Education.* The PSC Section, UNICEF. P.O. Box 1435. Rangoon, Myanmar (no cost). 1984.

Haciendo Camino al Andar: Guia Metodologica para la Accion Comunitaria. OEF Intl. 1815 H St. NW. 11th Floor, Washington, DC 20016 USA. 1991.

Hope, A., S. Timmel. *Training for Transformation A Handbook for Community Workers* Vols 1,2,&3. Mambo Press PO Box 779 Gweru, Zimbabwe, 1984. Available from PACT 777 UN Plaza New York, NY 10017 Tel: 212-697-6222. Revised 1996. Revised edition available from Women Inc in the US and Intermediate Technology Publications in the UK.

Narayan, Deepa & Lira Srinivasan. Participatory *Development Tool Kit: Training Materials for Agencies and Communities.* World Bank.1994. Available from UNIPUB 4611-F Assembly Drive, Landham, MD 20706-4391 World Bank order # WB2687

Pretty, Jules N. et al. *Participatory Learning and Action. A Trainer's Guide.* Sustainable Agriculture Programme International Institute for Environment and Development (IIED) 3 Endsleigh St, London WC1H ODD, UK 1995.

Srinivasan, Lyra. *Tools for Community Participation: A Manual for Training Trainers in Participatory Techniques.* New York: Prowess/UNDP.1990. Available from PACT 777 UN Plaza, New York, NY 10017. Tel: 212-697-6222

Training Manual for Change Agent Training. Published by Uganda Change Agents Association P.O. Box 2922, Kampala, Uganda. 1994.

Van Veldhuizen, Laurens, Ann Waters-Bayer, & Henk deZeeuw. *Developing Technology With Farmers: A Trainer's Guide for Participatory Learning.* ZED Books, 7 Cynthia St, London N19JF, UK. In Press 1997.

Vella, Jane. *Learning to Teach. Training of Trainers for Community Development.* OEF International, 1815 H St.,NW 11th Floor, Washington, DC 20006 USA and Save the Children Federation, P.O. Box 950, Westport, CT 06881. 1989.

Vella, Jane. *Training Through Dialogue: Promoting Effective Learning and Change With Adults.* Jossey-Bass Publishers, 350 Sansome St. San Francisco, CA 94104. 1995.

Werner, David and Bill Bower *Helping Health Workers Learn.* Hesparian Foundation P.O. Box 1692 Palo Alto, CA 94302 USA, 1982.

Participatory Method

Arnold, Rick et al. *Educating for a Change.* Co-Published: Between the Lines 394 Euclid Ave, Toronto, Ontario M6G 2S9 and Dorsi Marshall Institute for Education and Action. 818 College St, No 3, Toronto, Ontario M6G 1C8. 1991.

Bergdall, Terry D. *Methods for Active Participation, Experiences in Rural Development from East and Central Africa.* Oxford University Press, 1993.

Crone, C.D. and C Hunter. *From the Field: Tested Participatory Activities for Trainers.* World Education 210 Lincoln St Boston, MA 02111 Tel: 617-482-9485 Fax: 617-482-0617 US$ 15.50. 1980.

Freire, Paulo. *Pedagogy of the Oppressed.* The Continuum Publishing Company. 370 Lexington Ave, New York, NY 10017 USA. 1973.

Lansdale, Bruce M. *Master Farmer.* 1986. Direct order inquiries to: American Farm School, Box 23, GR55102 Kalamaria, Greece or 1133 Broadway New York, NY 10010 USA.

Srinivasan, Lyra. *Options for Educators.* PACT/CDS, Inc. 777 UN Plaza, New York, NY 10017 USA Tel 212/697-6222 Fax 212/692-9748. 1992.

Livestock Related

Pena-Olvera, Benjamin. *Investigación Accion Participativa con Grupos de Mujeres Campesinas: Manual Para Capacitación y Operación.* Colegio de Postgrados, CILCA, CEICADAR. Apdo postal 1247 Puebla, Puebla, Mexico. 1988.
This is a succinct manual for a program which works with women's groups in business projects including livestock rearing. It clearly describes techniques and tools used in the program.

Ruwa, Rachael and Margaret Belewa *Extension for Livestock Groups A Guide to the Participatory Method.* Ministry of Agriculture, Livestock Development and Marketing, Kenya and Heifer Project Intl. P.O. Box 808 Little Rock, AR 72202 tel 501/376-6836 fax 501/ 376-8906. 1994.

Participatory Investigation and Planning

Aaker, Jerry and Jennifer Shumaker. *The Cornerstones Model: Values Based Planning and Management.* Heifer Project International. P.O. Box 808 Little Rock, AR 72203 USA Tel: 1-800-422-0474. 1996.

Haverkort, Bertus (Ed) *Joining Farmer's Experiments. Experiences in Participatory Technology Development.* Intermediate Technology. 1031105 Southampton Row, London WC1B 4HH, UK. 1991.

PLA Notes. *Notes on Participatory Learning and Action.* International Institute for Environment and Development. 3 Endsleigh St, London WC1H ODD UK Tel +44 171/388 2117. Fax +44 171/388 2826. email: iiedagri@gn.apc.org
These are an excellent series of papers on different uses and tools in PRA. The April 1994 issue was a special issue on livestock. These include case studies, discussions of theory, and presentations of methods used to share ideas. Back issues can be requested. Free to people in the south.

Waters-Bayer, Ann and Wolfgang Bayer. *Planning with Pastoralists: PRA and more.* A review of Methods Focused on Africa. GTZ GmbH Division 422, Postfach 5180, D-65726 Eschborn, Germany. 1994.
This working paper has a very complete annotated Bibliography of resource materials in PRA in English, German and French. The comments are very helpful when choosing additional resources. It also has a good overview of PRA and good descriptions of many of the tools.

Valarezo, Galo Ramon. *Manual de Planeamiento Andino Comunitario El PAC en le Región Andina.* COMUNIDEC Apartado 554 Suc. 12 de Octubre, Quito, Ecuador. 1993. A descriptive manual of Andean Community Planning.

Evaluation

Aaker, Jerry and Jennifer Shumaker. *Looking Back and Looking Forward: A Participatory Approach to Evaluation.* Little Rock, AR: Heifer Project Intl. 1994. A very useful, practical step-by-step manual.

de Voogd, Stanley and Jodi-Beth McCain. *Técnicas de la Evaluación Participativa.* Habitat for Humanity Bolivia, mimeographed 1994.

Feuerstein, Marie-Therese. *Partners in Evaluation: Evaluating Development and Community Programs with Participants.* MacMillan Education Ltd, London available from T.A.L.C. Box 49 St Albans, Herts. AL1 4AX, UK. 1990.

Marsden, David and Peter Oakley. *Evaluating Social Development Projects.* Oxfam 274 Banbury Rd, Oxford OX2 7DZ UK. 1990.

Patton, Michael Quinn. *How to Use Qualitative Methods in Evaluation.* Sage Publications 2455 Teller Rd, Newbury Park, Calif, USA 91320. 1987.

Pfohl, Jake. *Participatory Evaluation: A User's Guide.* New York: PACT Publications 777 United Nations Plaza New York, NY 10017 USA. 1989.

Rugh, J. *Self-Evaluation: Ideas for Participatory Evaluation of Rural Community Development Projects.* Oklahoma City: World Neighbors, 1986.

Weaver, Jane. *How Much Did I Change the World Today? Evaluating Development Education – a Handbook.* Password Publishing Services 38-40 Exchange Street, Norwich NR2 1AX UK. Tel: (0603)761507 fax: (0603) 761645. 1993.

Woodhill, Jim and Lisa Robbins. *Participatory Evaluation for Landcare and Catchment Groups. A Guide for Facilitators.* Greening Australia Limited. PO Box 74. Yaralumla ACT 2600 Tel: 0262818585 Fax: 0262818590 E-mail: general@greeningaustralia.com.au. 1998.

Working With Organizations

Gonzales, Rafael Solorzano and Rafael Morales Vela. *Organización y Participación Comunitaria en el Marco de la Educación No Formal.* Altertec. Avenida 5-27, Zona 1, Ciudad de Guatemala, Guatemala. Mimeograph. 1993.

Kindervatter, Suzanne. Women Working Together for Personal, Economic, and Community Development. OEF Intl, 1991. Available from Women Inc. 777 UN Plaza, New York, NY 10017 USA.

Magnani, Nanette Bray. *Building Organizational Effectiveness Through Participation and Teamwork.* World Education. PACT 777 UN Plaza, New York, NY 10017 tel: 212/697-6222.

Mutua, Elvina *SAIDIKA Tototo Trainer's Manual for Trainers of Women's Groups.* Tototo Home Industries. P.O. Box 1636, Mombasa, Kenya. Tel 220490.

Dynamics and Games

Book of Starters for the Training of Community Health Workers. Kampala, Uganda: Uganda Community Based Health Care Assn & the Government of Uganda, UNICEF, World Neighbors, 1992.

Brown, Guillermo. *Que tal si Jugamos.* CESAP, Apartado 4240 Caracas 1010- A, Venezuela. Tel 81-38-85.

Eitington, Julius E. *The Winning Trainer.* Gulf Publishing Co, Book Division. P.O. Box 2608. Huston, TX 77252-2608 USA. 2nd Ed 1989.

Junes, Ken. *Imaginative Events for Training: A Trainer's Sourcebook of Games, Simulations, and Role-Play Exercises.* McGraw Hill, 1993. Available from Women Inc. 777 UN Plaza, 3rd Floor New York, NY 10017.

Nilson, Carolyn. *Team Games for Trainers.* McGraw-Hill, 1993. Available from Women Inc. 777 UN Plaza, 3rd floor. New York, NY 10017.

Vargas Vargas, Laura and Graciela Bustillos de Nunez. *Técnicas Participativas para la Educación Popular.* Vols. 1 and 2. ALFORJA, Tarea, Asociación de Publicaciónes Educativas. Horacio Urteaga 970, Lima 11, Peru Tel 230935.

Resources for Pictures

The Copy Book Copyright-free Illustrations for Development. Intermediate Technology Publications Ltd. 103-105 Southampton Row, London WCIB 4HH, UK, reprinted in 1991.

Woman: The Password is Action. Clip Art for Women. International Women's Tribune Center. 777 United Nations Plaza, New York, NY 10017 USA, 1988.

Fussel, Diana & Ane Haaland. *Communicating With Pictures in Nepal.* UNICEF, Lazimpath. P.O. Box 1187. Kathmandu, Nepal, 1976.

Rohr-Rouendaal, Petra. *Where There is no Artist - Development Drawings and How to Use Them.* Intermediate Technology Publications. 103-105 Southampton Row, London WC1B 4HH, UK Tel:44 171 436 9761 email: itpubs@itpubs.org.uk, 1996.

Rural Women in Action. A Clip Art Book. International Women's Tribune Center 777 United Nations Plaza, New York, N.Y. 10017 USA, 1991.

Small Enterprise Development

Buzzard, Shirley y Elaine Edgcomb Eds. *A Step by Step Guide to Monitoring and Evaluation of Small Business Projects for Development Organizations.* SEEP. PACT, 777 United Nations Plaza, New York, NY 10017, USA, 1987.

Commonwealth Secretariat. *Entrepreneurial Skills for Young Women: A Manual for Trainers.* London: Women & Development Programme, Human Resource Development Group. Commonwealth Secretariat, Marlborough House, Pall Mall, London SW1Y 5HX, UK, 1992.

Edgcomb, Elaine and James Cawley Eds. *An Institutional Guide for Enterprise Development Organizations.* Includes a comprehensive Tools Section. SEEP Network. PACT Publications 777 United Nations Plaza, New York, NY 10017 USA, 1993.

Kobak, Sue Ellen and Nina McCormack. *Workshop on Developing Feasibility Studies for Community Based Business Ventures.* The Highlander Center Rt 3, Box 370, New Market, Tennessee 37820 USA. 615/933-3443, 1988.

Luttrell, Wendy. *Claiming What is Ours: An Economics Experience Workbook.* Highlander Center. 1959 Highlander way, New Market, TN 37820.

Svendsen, D.S. & Wijetetilleke. *Navamaga: Training Activities for Group Building, Health, and Income Generation.* OEF Intl, 1983. Available from Women Inc. 777 United Nations Plaza, 3rd floor, New York, NY 10017 USA. English, Spanish, & French.

Gender Analysis

Antwi-Saiah, C. *Registry of Gender Training Materials.* Available from Office of Women International Development, Univ of Illinois, 320 International Studies Bld, 910 S Fifth St, Champaign, IL, 61810 USA, 1991.

Balarezo,Susana. *Gúia Metodologica para Incorporar la Dimensión de Género en el Cíclo de Proyectos Forestales Participativos.* FTPP - FAO. 10 de Agosto 5470 y Villalengua POB 17-21-0190. Quito, Ecuador. Fax 593-2 441 348, 1994.

CEDPA. *Volume 3: Gender and Development.* Volume three of the CEDPA Training Manual Series. CEDPA, 1996. Available from Women Ink.

CIDA. *A Handbook for Social Gender Analysis.* Ottawa, Canada Coady Intl Inst: Antigonish and Social and Human Resources Devel Div of CIDA, 1989.

Feldstein, H.S. & S.V. Poats (Eds). *Working Together: Gender Analysis in Agriculture. Vol I Case Studies. Vol II Teaching Notes.* West Hartford & Kumarian Press, 1990.

Parker, A Rani. *Another Point of View: A Manual on Gender Analysis Training for Grassroots Workers.* UNIFEM, 1989. 304 East 45th St., New York, NY 10017 USA.

Parker, A Rani, Itziar Lozano, Lyn A. Messner. *Gender Relations Analysis: A Guide for Trainers.* Save the Children. 54 Wilton Rd, Westport, CT 06880 USA Tel: 203-221-4000,1995. Available from Women Ink.

Rao, A., M.B. Anderson, & C.A. Overholt (Eds). *Gender Analysis in Development Planning.* West Hartford & Kumarian Press, 1991. Also Teaching Notes. Available from Women Ink.

Williams, Suzanne with Janet Seed and Adelina Mwau. *The Oxfam Gender Training Manual.* Oxfam, 1994. Available from Women Ink.

Traditional Knowledge

Blunt, Peter, and D. Michael Warren. *Indigenous Organizations and Development.* Intermediate Technology Publications, 1996.

Gamser, Matthew S. ED with Helen Appleton and Nicola Carter. *Tinker, Tiller, Technical Change.* Intermediate Technology Publications, 1990.

McCorkle, Constance, Evelyn Mathias-Mundy, Tw Schillhorn van Veen (Eds). *Ethnoveterinary Research and Development.* Intermediate Technology Publications 103-105 Southampton Row, London WC1B 4HH, UK, 1996. Also available from Women Inc.

McCorkle, Constance (Ed). *Plants, Animals, and People. Agropastoral Systems Research.* Westview Press. 5500 Central Ave. Boulder, CO 80310-2847, 1992.

Warren, D. Michael, L. Jan Slikkerveer and David Brokensha. *The Cultural Dimension of Development - Indigenous Knowledge Systems.* Intermediate Technology Publications, 1995.

Reijntjes, Coen, Bertus Haverkort, and Ann Waters-Bayer. *Farming for the Future An Introduction to Low-External-Input and Sustainable Agriculture.* Macmillan, 1992. Available from ILEIA PO Box 64, NL-3830 AB Leusden, Netherlands. Also available in Spanish.

Sources of Training and Technical Materials

Christian Veterinary Mission
Series on Raising Animals
Email: vetbooks@cvm.org
Website: www.cvm.org

Dinah-Might Activities, Inc
P.O. Box 39657
San Antonio, TX 78218 Tel: 210/ 657-5951

Educational Resources Information Clearing House
Document Reproduction Service
EDR/CBIS Federal, 7420 Fullerton Rd Suite 110
Springfield, VA 22153-2852 USA

Heifer Project International
Participatory Training Resources for the Fieldworker. A Listing of Manuals, Books, & Training Tools for Agriculture and Rural Development
P.O. Box 808
Little Rock, AR 72203

Highlander Research and Education Center
1959 Highlander Way
New Market, TN 37820

Intermediate Technology Publications
103-105 Southampton Row
London WCIB 4HH, UK
Tel: 44 1714369761 Fax: 44 1714352013
Email: itpubs@itpubs.org.uk
Website: http://www.oneworld.org/itdg/publications.html

International Institute for Environment and Development (IIED)
Email: resource.centre@iied.org
Website: www.oneworld.org/iied/resource

International Institute for Rural Reconstruction
475 Riverside Drive, Room 1270
New York, NY 10115 USA

PACT Publications
777 United Nations Plaza
New York, NY 10017 Tel: 212/ 697-6222
Email: books@pactpub.org
Website: www.pactpub.com

Peace Corps
A Catalogue of Manuals, Reprints and Training Materials 1995
Information Collection and Exchange
1990 K St NW
Washington, DC 20526 USA

Teaching Aids at Low Cost (TALC)
PO Box 49
St. Albans,
Hertfordshire ALI 4AX, UK

Women Inc.
777 United Nations Plaza, 3rd Floor
New York, NY 10017
Email: wink@igc.apc.org

Institute of Development Studies
University of Sussex, Brighton BNI 9RE
Tel: +44 1273 606261 Fax: +44 1273 621202
Email: ids.books@sussex.ac.uk
Website: http//: www.ids.ac.uk/ids

References Cited

Ariyaratne, A.T. *Transformation of Vision Into Reality - Planning for Development (Awakening).* Manilla, Phillippines: Asian Institute of Management, 1990.

Bergdall, Terry D. *Methods for Active Participation Experiences in Rural Development from East and Central Africa.* Oxford Univ. Press, 1993.

Covey, Stephen R. *The Seven Habits of Highly Effective People.* New York: Fireside, 1989.

DeVries, James. *Development or Transformation? Reflections on a Wholistic Approach to People-Centered Change.* Heifer Project International Paper, 1992.

Freire, Paulo. *Pedagogy of the Oppressed.* The Continuum Publishing Co., 1973.

Kiamba, Suzanne & Gilbert Namwonja. *Notes on Participatory Development Workshop for CARE Uganda.* PREMESE April 1994.

Nyerere, Julius K. *Freedom and Development.* Oxford University Press, 1973.

Orito, Charles. *ITDG's Decentralized Animal Health Care, an overview.* From Proceedings from 5th Annual Vet's Workshop, Intermediate Technology Kenya, October 1995.

Uganda Change Agents Association and Quaker Service Norway. *Training Manual for Change Agent Training.* 1994

Vella, Jane. *Training Through Dialogue.* Jossey-Bass Inc.,1995.

Werner, David & Bill Bower. *Helping Health Workers Learn.* Hesperian Foundation, 1982.

Young, John. *Kamujne Farmer's Center, Wasaidizi Wa Mifugo Instruction Plan.* Intermediate Technology Development Group.

Young, John (Ed). *A Report on a Village Animal Health Care Workshop.* Kenya: Rugby, Intermediate Technology Development Group, 1992.

Young, John, Karen Stoufer, Narayan Ojha, & Henk Peter Dijkema. *Animal Health Care Training. Nepal's Animal Health Improvement Training Programme.* Intermediate Technology Publications, 1994.

INDEX

If you are thinking a year ahead, sow seed.

If you are thinking ten years ahead, plant a tree.

If you are thinking one hundred years ahead, educate the people.

By sowing seed once, you will harvest once.

By planting a tree, you will harvest tenfold.

By educating the people, you will harvest one hundredfold.

–Anon Chinese poet

Made in the USA
Middletown, DE
30 September 2021